Enzyme Inhibitors from Marine Resources

Enzyme Inhibitors from Marine Resources

Guest Editors

Francesc Xavier Avilés
Isel Pascual Alonso

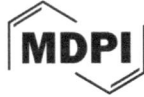 Basel • Beijing • Wuhan • Barcelona • Belgrade • Novi Sad • Cluj • Manchester

Guest Editors

Francesc Xavier Avilés
Universitat Autònoma de
Barcelona
Cerdanyola del Vallès,
Barcelona
Spain

Isel Pascual Alonso
University of Havana
La Habana
Cuba

Editorial Office
MDPI AG
Grosspeteranlage 5
4052 Basel, Switzerland

This is a reprint of the Special Issue, published open access by the journal *Marine Drugs* (ISSN 1660-3397), freely accessible at: https://www.mdpi.com/journal/marinedrugs/special_issues/Marine_Enzyme_Inhibitors.

For citation purposes, cite each article independently as indicated on the article page online and as indicated below:

Lastname, A.A.; Lastname, B.B. Article Title. *Journal Name* **Year**, *Volume Number*, Page Range.

ISBN 978-3-7258-2445-8 (Hbk)
ISBN 978-3-7258-2446-5 (PDF)
https://doi.org/10.3390/books978-3-7258-2446-5

Cover image courtesy of C. Jose Antonio Espinosa
Instituto de Ciencias del Mar (ICIMAR), Ministerio de Ciencia, Tecnología y Medio Ambiente (CITMA), Cuba

Contents

About the Editors . . . . **vii**

Preface . . . . **ix**

Isel Pascual Alonso, Fabiola Almeida García, Mario Ernesto Valdés Tresanco, Yarini Arrebola Sánchez, Daniel Ojeda del Sol, Belinda Sánchez Ramírez, et al.
Marine Invertebrates: A Promissory Still Unexplored Source of Inhibitors of Biomedically Relevant Metallo Aminopeptidases Belonging to the M1 and M17 Families
Reprinted from: *Mar. Drugs* **2023**, *21*, 279, https://doi.org/10.3390/md21050279 . . . . **1**

Maria Hayes, Rotimi E. Aluko, Elena Aurino and Leticia Mora
Generation of Bioactive Peptides from *Porphyridium* sp. and Assessment of Their Potential for Use in the Prevention of Hypertension, Inflammation and Pain
Reprinted from: *Mar. Drugs* **2023**, *21*, 422, https://doi.org/10.3390/md21080422 . . . . **38**

Andrea Córdova-Isaza, Sofía Jiménez-Mármol, Yasel Guerra and Emir Salas-Sarduy
Enzyme Inhibitors from Gorgonians and Soft Corals
Reprinted from: *Mar. Drugs* **2023**, *21*, 104, https://doi.org/10.3390/md21020104 . . . . **53**

Irina Bakunina, Tatiana Imbs, Galina Likhatskaya, Valeria Grigorchuk, Anastasya Zueva, Olesya Malyarenko and Svetlana Ermakova
Effect of Phlorotannins from Brown Algae *Costaria costata* on α-N-Acetylgalactosaminidase Produced by Duodenal Adenocarcinoma and Melanoma Cells
Reprinted from: *Mar. Drugs* **2023**, *21*, 33, https://doi.org/10.3390/md21010033 . . . . **83**

Jed F. Fisher and Shahriar Mobashery
β-Lactams from the Ocean
Reprinted from: *Mar. Drugs* **2023**, *21*, 86, https://doi.org/10.3390/md21020086 . . . . **101**

Xiaoshan Long, Xiao Hu, Shaobo Zhou, Huan Xiang, Shengjun Chen, Laihao Li, et al.
Optimized Degradation and Inhibition of α-glucosidase Activity by *Gracilaria lemaneiformis* Polysaccharide and Its Production In Vitro
Reprinted from: *Mar. Drugs* **2022**, *20*, 13, https://doi.org/10.3390/md20010013 . . . . **116**

Federico Gago
Computational Approaches to Enzyme Inhibition by Marine Natural Products in the Search for New Drugs
Reprinted from: *Mar. Drugs* **2023**, *21*, 100, https://doi.org/10.3390/md21020100 . . . . **138**

Aymara Cabrera-Muñoz, Yusvel Sierra-Gómez, Giovanni Covaleda-Cortés, Mey L. Reytor, Yamile González-González, José M. Bautista, et al.
Isolation and Characterization of NpCI, a New Metallocarboxypeptidase Inhibitor from the Marine Snail *Nerita peloronta* with Anti-*Plasmodium falciparum* Activity
Reprinted from: *Mar. Drugs* **2023**, *21*, 94, https://doi.org/10.3390/md21020094 . . . . **166**

Seong-Yeong Heo, Nalae Kang, Eun-A Kim, Junseong Kim, Seung-Hong Lee, Ginnae Ahn, et al.
Purification and Molecular Docking Study on the Angiotensin I-Converting Enzyme (ACE)-Inhibitory Peptide Isolated from Hydrolysates of the Deep-Sea Mussel *Gigantidas vrijenhoeki*
Reprinted from: *Mar. Drugs* **2023**, *21*, 458, https://doi.org/10.3390/md21080458 . . . . **183**

Jianlin Xu, Zhifeng Liu, Zhanguang Feng, Yuhong Ren, Haili Liu and Yong Wang
Rapid Mining of Novel α-Glucosidase and Lipase Inhibitors from *Streptomyces* sp. HO1518
Using UPLC-QTOF-MS/MS
Reprinted from: *Mar. Drugs* **2022**, *20*, 189, https://doi.org/10.3390/md20030189 . . . . **194**

About the Editors

Francesc Xavier Avilés

Francesc Xavier Avilés (ORCID: 0000-0002-1399-6789) is a Senior Researcher interested in the molecular and structural biology of proteins and proteomics, particularly proteases and protease inhibitors and their basic and applicative (biotech/biomed/pharma) properties. He has published 281 peer-reviewed papers and supervised 43 PhD theses. He was formerly a full professor (until 2018), director of the Department of Biochemistry and Molecular Biology (2008–2014) and director of the Institute for Biotechnology and Biomedicine (IBB, 1991–2002) at the Universitat Autonoma de Barcelona. He is now an active Emeritus Professor there.

Isel Pascual Alonso

Isel Pascual Alonso (ORCID: 0000-0002-6316-9327) is a titular Professor and Senior Researcher at the Center for Protein Studies, Faculty of Biology, University of Havana, Cuba. She is specialized in the biochemistry of proteins and enzymes, particularly aminopeptidases and aminopeptidase inhibitors and their fundamental and applicative (biotech/biomed/pharma) properties. She has published 50 peer-reviewed papers and supervised 3 PhD, 8 MSc and 34 basic sciences theses. She has also organized and/or lectured at more than 60 national and international congresses/workshops, and is the President of the Scientific Council of the University of Havana, Cuba (2022–now).

Preface

Marine living organisms and their main and secondary compounds and metabolites are among the richest in biological diversity. Many of their fundamental qualities and applications are still fully or partially unexplored. Given that enzymes are essential in the plethora of biological functions of these organisms, it is increasingly evident that enzyme inhibitors are also involved in the control of these functions, as well as in many diseases and attack–defense processes. Research on the natural inhibitors found in marine organisms is, therefore, of great interest at present in a myriad of research perspectives.

It is known that the diversity of species is much greater in marine than in terrestrial habitats, regarding phyla and classes, doubling the numbers of the former compared to the latter. This provides marine species with a large variety of biomolecules and metabolites, particularly at the secondary level, a point of great fundamental and applicative interest. Consequently, the number and array of specific enzymes required for the synthesis and modification of such compounds are very rich, as well as for their control, as happens with enzyme inhibitors, many of them of great specificity. The challenge to characterizing them is therefore formidable and, at the same time, very interesting and rewarding. We hope that such interest is reflected in the series of articles assembled in this Special Issue.

Dedication of this Special Issue to the Memory of Profs. Maria de los Ángeles Chavez (UH) and Josep Vendrell (UAB). This Special Issue is dedicated to the memory of these two respected and beloved colleagues and friends lost in the last few years and who, in parallel, had a strong impact on the research and teaching of the fields addressed herein by different research groups, institutions, and countries. More specifically, such impact took place in the fields of proteolytic enzymes (proteases) and their inhibitors and, generically, of the biochemistry and biotechnology of proteins and enzymes, from both colleagues at the Center for Protein Studies (CEP), University of Havana—UH, Cuba, and at the Department of Biochemistry and Molecular Biology, Universitat Autonoma de Barcelona—UAB, Spain, respectively. Both were recognised as leading specialists and innovative contributors in such fields, with more emphasis on the former on protease inhibitors and the latter on proteases, i.e., on the characterization, structure–function and biochemistry, and biotech–biomed applications of inhibitors of different mechanistic classes from Cuban marine biodiversity, and on metallo-carboxypeptidases from European mammals and insects, from each side. In addition, they played an essential role as founders of the bachelor's degrees and teaching of Biochemistry in Cuba (from UH—Havana, CEP and Faculty of Biology), and of Biochemistry and of Biotechnology in Spain (from UAB—Barcelona, Faculty of Biosciences). Our greatest respect and gratitude is devoted to them.

Francesc Xavier Avilés and Isel Pascual Alonso
Guest Editors

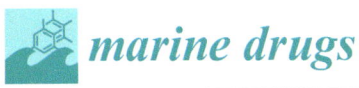

Review

Marine Invertebrates: A Promissory Still Unexplored Source of Inhibitors of Biomedically Relevant Metallo Aminopeptidases Belonging to the M1 and M17 Families

Isel Pascual Alonso [1,*], Fabiola Almeida García [1], Mario Ernesto Valdés Tresanco [1,2], Yarini Arrebola Sánchez [1], Daniel Ojeda del Sol [1], Belinda Sánchez Ramírez [3], Isabelle Florent [4], Marjorie Schmitt [5] and Francesc Xavier Avilés [6,*]

[1] Center for Protein Studies, Faculty of Biology, University of Havana, Havana 10400, Cuba; almeidafabiola0406@gmail.com (F.A.G.); marioe911116@gmail.com (M.E.V.T.); yarini1985@gmail.com (Y.A.S.); dojeda9711@gmail.com (D.O.d.S.)
[2] Department of Biological Sciences, University of Calgary, Calgary, AB T2N 1N4, Canada
[3] Centro de Inmunología Molecular, Habana 11600, Cuba; belinda@cim.sld.cu
[4] Unité Molécules de Communication et Adaptation des Microorganismes (MCAM, UMR7245), Muséum National d'Histoire Naturelle, CNRS, CP52, 57 Rue Cuvier, 75005 Paris, France; isabelle.florent@mnhn.fr
[5] Université de Haute-Alsace, Université de Strasbourg, CNRS, LIMA UMR 7042, 68000 Mulhouse, France; marjorie.schmitt@uha.fr
[6] Institute for Biotechnology and Biomedicine and Department of Biochemistry, Universitat Autònoma de Barcelona, 08193 Bellaterra, Spain
* Correspondence: iselpascual@yahoo.es (I.P.A.); francescxavier.aviles@uab.cat (F.X.A.)

Citation: Pascual Alonso, I.; Almeida García, F.; Valdés Tresanco, M.E.; Arrebola Sánchez, Y.; Ojeda del Sol, D.; Sánchez Ramírez, B.; Florent, I.; Schmitt, M.; Avilés, F.X. Marine Invertebrates: A Promissory Still Unexplored Source of Inhibitors of Biomedically Relevant Metallo Aminopeptidases Belonging to the M1 and M17 Families. *Mar. Drugs* **2023**, *21*, 279. https://doi.org/10.3390/md21050279

Academic Editor: Claudiu T. Supuran

Received: 27 March 2023
Revised: 25 April 2023
Accepted: 26 April 2023
Published: 28 April 2023

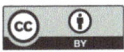

Abstract: Proteolytic enzymes, also known as peptidases, are critical in all living organisms. Peptidases control the cleavage, activation, turnover, and synthesis of proteins and regulate many biochemical and physiological processes. They are also involved in several pathophysiological processes. Among peptidases, aminopeptidases catalyze the cleavage of the N-terminal amino acids of proteins or peptide substrates. They are distributed in many phyla and play critical roles in physiology and pathophysiology. Many of them are metallopeptidases belonging to the M1 and M17 families, among others. Some, such as M1 aminopeptidases N and A, thyrotropin-releasing hormone-degrading ectoenzyme, and M17 leucyl aminopeptidase, are targets for the development of therapeutic agents for human diseases, including cancer, hypertension, central nervous system disorders, inflammation, immune system disorders, skin pathologies, and infectious diseases, such as malaria. The relevance of aminopeptidases has driven the search and identification of potent and selective inhibitors as major tools to control proteolysis with an impact in biochemistry, biotechnology, and biomedicine. The present contribution focuses on marine invertebrate biodiversity as an important and promising source of inhibitors of metalloaminopeptidases from M1 and M17 families, with foreseen biomedical applications in human diseases. The results reviewed in the present contribution support and encourage further studies with inhibitors isolated from marine invertebrates in different biomedical models associated with the activity of these families of exopeptidases.

Keywords: aminopeptidase; aminopeptidase N; aminopeptidase A; TRH-degrading ectoenzyme; leucyl aminopeptidase; enzyme inhibitors; drug-oriented inhibitors; marine invertebrates

1. Introduction

Proteolytic enzymes, known as peptidases or proteases, are critical in all living organisms [1]. Proteases can act as exo- and/or endopeptidases. They are segregated in classes that strongly depend on the chemical nature of the groups involved in catalysis. The recognized mechanistic classes are aspartic, cysteine, glutamic, metallo, asparagine, mixed, serine, threonine, and a group dedicated to unknown catalytic type [1].

Peptidases are one of the most abundant groups of enzymes in living organisms. Thus, in mammals, more than six hundred genes have been assigned to them. They control the activation, synthesis, and turnover of proteins and regulate most biochemical and physiological processes, such as digestion, fertilization, growth, differentiation, cell signaling/migration, immunological defense, wound healing, and apoptosis [1–3]. They are consequently major regulators of homeostasis, ageing, and different human diseases such as cancer, hypertension, diabetes, inflammation, neurodegeneration, and Alzheimer's disease, among others [4–6]. Proteases are also essential for the propagation of infectious agents, being major contributors of pathogenesis in several infectious diseases, including the current coronavirus emergent pandemic SARS COVID-19 [1,7–14].

Among peptidases, aminopeptidases catalyze the cleavage of the N-terminal amino acids of proteins or peptide substrates. They are distributed in many phyla and play critical roles in physiology and pathophysiology [1,8,9,15]. In mammals, they have a widespread cellular distribution in various organs and are found within cells in many subcellular organelles, in the cytoplasm, as integral membrane proteins, or are exposed or secreted extracellularly [8,16–18]. They are mainly metallopeptidases belonging to different families such as M1 and M17, although cysteine and serine peptidases are also included in this group [1]. Among the best representatives of aminopeptidases that are currently in the focus of biomedical investigation, we can pinpoint the M1 family neutral aminopeptidase (APN, EC 3.4.11.2), glutamyl aminopeptidase (APA EC 3.4.11.7) and thyrotropin-releasing hormone-degrading ectoenzyme (TRH-DE; EC 3.4.19.6), and M17 neutral aminopeptidase, also known as leucyl aminopeptidase (LAP, EC 3.4.11.21) (Figure 1). These enzymes are involved in multiple physiological processes as well as in cancer, hypertension, central nervous system disorders, inflammation, immune system disorders, skin pathologies, and infectious diseases, such as malaria, and are current targets for the development of new therapeutic drugs [8,9,19].

A   **B**   **C**

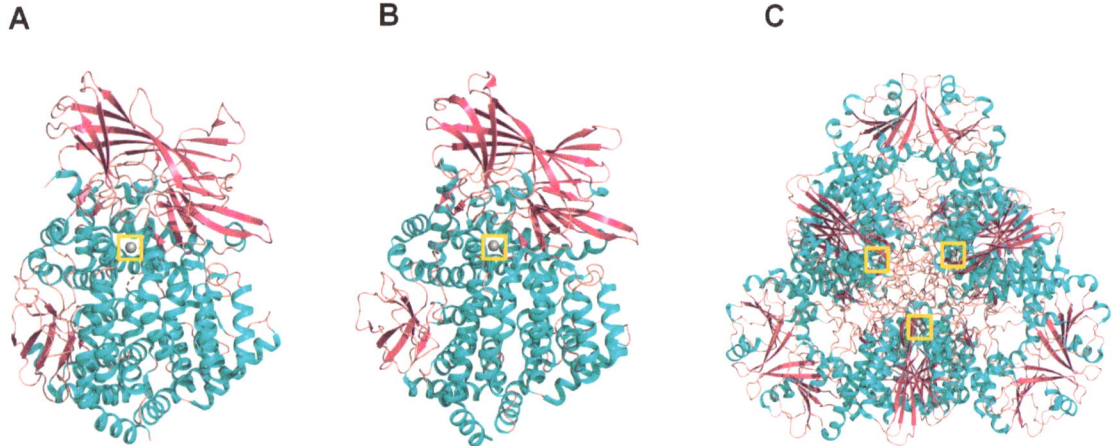

Figure 1. Cartoon representation of the 3D structure of the three aminopeptidases focused on by the present contribution: (**A**) human aminopeptidase N (PDB ID: 4fyq), (**B**) human aminopeptidase A (PDB ID: 4kx7), and (**C**) *Plasmodium* falciparum M17 aminopeptidase PfA-M17 (PDB ID: 4r76). Colors: alpha-helices (cyan), beta sheets (warm pink), and loops (salmon). The zinc atoms are shown as gray spheres highlighted in a yellow box.

Marine habitats are an extraordinary source of structurally complex bioactive metabolites, characterized by unique functions with marked biological activities and polished through evolution. These features can be attributed to varied environmental conditions, such as access to/lack of light, high pressure, aqueous environment, ionic concentration, pH and temperature changes, scarcity of nutrients, and restricted living spaces. Marine organisms are an abundant source of bioactive molecules (including saccharides, polysaccharides, peptides, proteins, polyketides, polyphenolic compounds, sterol-like products, alkaloids, quinones, and quinolones, among others), such as toxins [20,21], antimicrobial peptides [22,23], antiviral compounds [24], enzymes and enzyme inhibitors [25–28], and particularly peptidases [29,30] and peptidase inhibitors of almost all mechanistic classes [31–42]. These bioactive molecules have a great diversity of chemical structures, high potency, and diverse specificities, especially the inhibitors of metalloenzymes (Figures 2–4) [37,43–54]. These inhibitory biomolecules are frequently involved in nutrition, homeostasis, reproduction, and communication of marine organisms [27]. Additionally, the high concentration of coexisting organisms in a limited area also makes them very competitive and complex, resulting in the development of adaptations and behaviors aimed at safeguarding the species. Since most invertebrates (e.g., sponges, bryozoans, tunicates, cnidarians, and mollusca snails, among others) lack morphological defense structures, peptidase inhibitors are also part of mechanisms related with protection against predators, infection, and competition [55]. In the present contribution, we review and summarize the status of metalloaminopeptidase inhibitors isolated from marine organisms with a focus on the M1 and M17 families of enzymes targeted in biomedical studies.

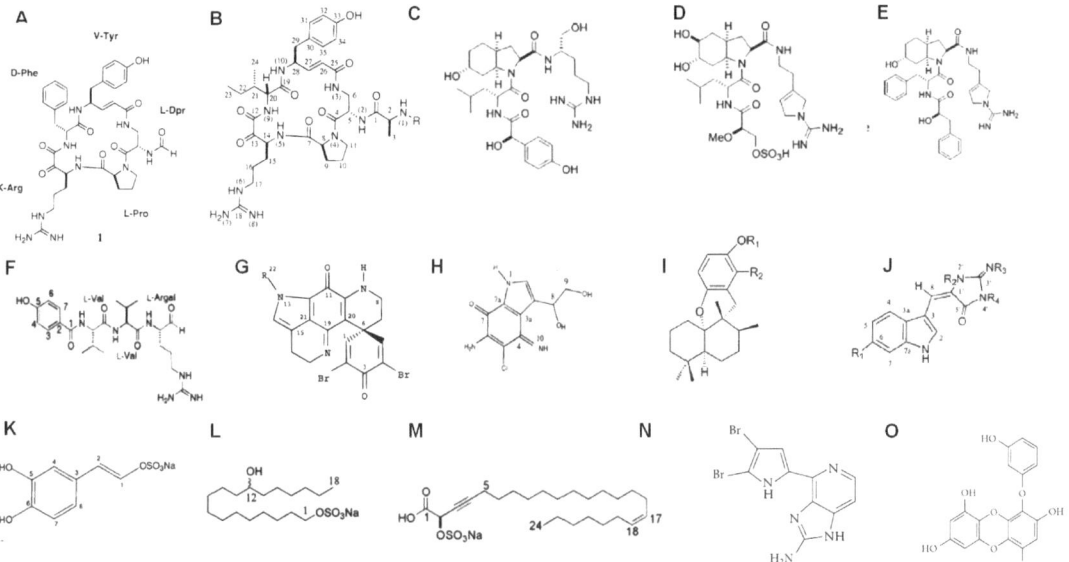

Figure 2. Structures of low molecular weight non-peptidic protease inhibitors of different mechanistic classes isolated from marine organisms. Serine peptidase inhibitors: (**A**) cicloteonamide A [56], (**B**) general structure of cicloteonamide E [56], (**C**) aeruginosine 298-A, (**D**) dinosine, (**E**) oscilarina [57]; cystein peptidase inhibitors: (**F**) tokaramida A [45], (**G**) discorhabdina P [58], (**H**) secobatzellina A [59]; aspartic peptidases inhibitors: (**I**) N,N-dimetiltiocarbamate, (**J**) 6 Br-aplisinopsine [60]; metalloendopeptidase inhibitors: (**K**) jaspisin [43], (**L**) 1-12-hidroxioctadecanil sodium sulphate [61], (**M**) calisponginol sulphate [46], (**N**) Ageladine A [47], (**O**) Eckol [62].

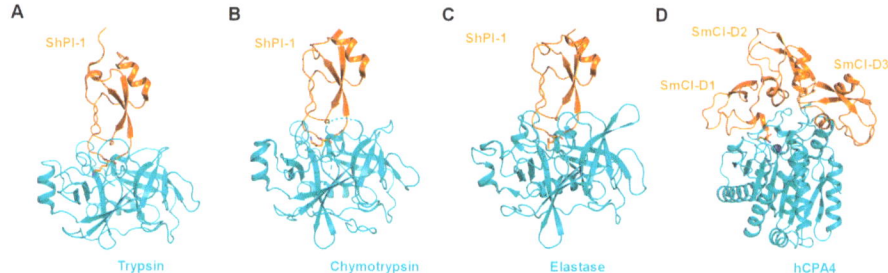

Figure 3. Structures of inhibitors isolated from marine invertebrates in complex with target proteases. (**A**) ShPI-1 isolated from the sea anemone *Stichodactyla helianthus* in complex with bovine trypsin (PDB ID: 3m7q), (**B**) ShPI-1 in complex with bovine chymotrypsin (PDB ID: 3t62), (**C**) ShPI-1 in complex with pancreatic elastase, and (PDB ID: 3m7Q), (**D**) SmCI isolated from marine annelide Sabellastarte magnifica in complex with human carboxypeptidase A4 (hCPA4) [51]. Residues interacting with the S1 subsite have been highlighted as sticks. Proteases and inhibitors are colored cyan and orange, respectively. The zinc atom in hCPA4 is shown as a gray sphere.

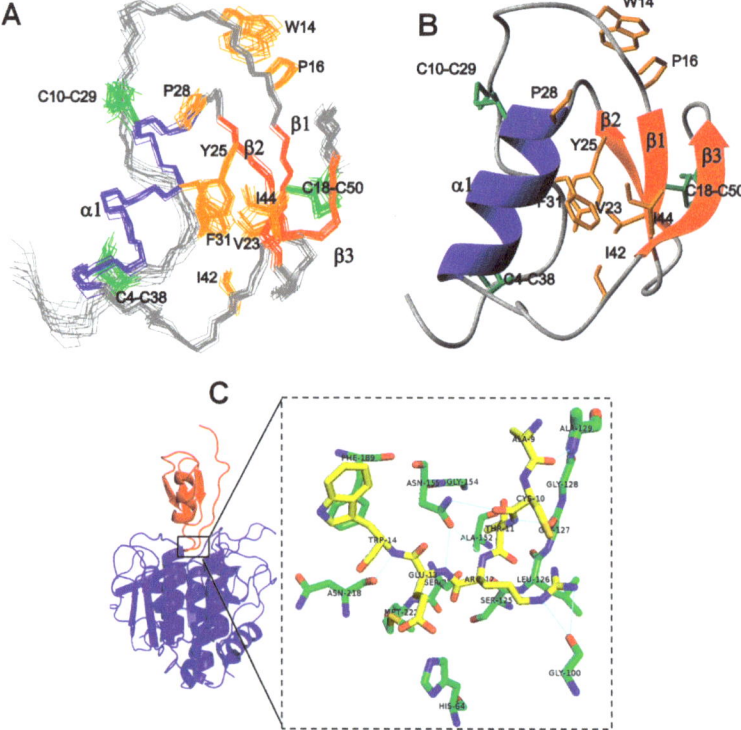

Figure 4. Structure of CmPI-II (a serine protease inhibitor isolated from the marine snail *Cenchritis muricatus*). (**A**) Family of the 15 lowest energy structures of CmPI-II obtained by NMR. (**B**) Ribbons-like representation of the lowest energy structure. The β strands (β1–β3) and the α helix are represented in red and blue, respectively. Orange parts represent the hydrophobic nucleus of the protein and green shows disulfide bridges. (**C**) Prediction of the 3D structure of the CmPI-II/subtilisin A complex. CmPI-II is shown in red and subtilisin A in blue [53]. Courtesy of Prof. Aymara Cabrera Muñoz.

2. M1 and M17 Metalloexopeptidase Inhibitors Isolated from Marine Invertebrates

2.1. Metallopeptidases: General Characteristics and Classification

Metallopeptidases constitute the most diverse catalytic type within proteases, since they include both endopeptidases and exopeptidases, cytosolic enzymes, and others that are secreted to the outside of cells, as well as enzymes associated with the plasma membrane and cell organelles. They are widely distributed in all forms of life such as viruses, bacteria, fungi, and plant and animal cells, indicating the important role they play in biological processes.

Metalloproteases are included among the hydrolases in which the nucleophilic attack on the peptide bond is mediated by a water molecule. This is a feature they share with aspartic-type peptidases, but in metallopeptidases, a divalent metal cation activates the water molecule [63]. This divalent cation is usually zinc (Zn^{2+}) but can sometimes be cobalt (Co^{2+}) or manganese (Mn^{2+}). The metal ion is held in the protein structure by amino acids that act as ligands.

Metallopeptidases can be divided into two large groups based on the number of metal ions required for catalysis. In many metallopeptidases, only one metal ion is required, which frequently is Zn^{2+}; however, there is another group of families in which two cocatalytically acting metal ions are required. Within this group, there are families that have two Zn^{2+} ions and all the families in which Co^{2+} or Mn^{2+} are essential for catalysis. In families where only one metal ion acts, three amino acid residues are required to act as metal ligand coordinators, and in families with cocatalytic ions, only five amino acids are required since one of them acts as a ligand coordinator for both metal ions. All metallopeptidases with cocatalytic ions are exopeptidases, while metallopeptidases with a single metal ion can be both exo- and endopeptidases.

Various attempts have been made to classify proteases. The most accepted today is the one initially proposed by Rawlings and Barrett [64,65] that is continuously updated at (https://www.ebi.ac.uk/merops/, accessed on 9 January 2023) [1]. From the general classification of the nine mechanistic classes, they first group the enzymes of each class into families. A family is defined as a group of (homologous) peptidases in which each member shows significant amino acid sequence identity with the "type enzyme" or at least with another member of the family homologous to the type enzyme, mainly in the region of the peptidase that is related to its catalytic activity. The selection criteria used by these authors were very strict, in such a way that they guarantee a common ancestor for the members of a family, which are, therefore, homologous according to the definition of Reeck et al. [66]. Each family is named with a letter denoting the catalytic type (Example: M for metallopeptidases), followed by an arbitrarily assigned number. At a higher level of hierarchy, we find the clan, which is the term used by these authors to describe a group of families, whose members originate from a common ancestor protein but which have diverged to a point where relationships between them cannot be demonstrated by homology in their primary structures. The main evidence for the clan level is the relationship between families in terms of similarities in the three-dimensional structure of their members, in the arrangement of catalytic residues in the peptide structure, as well as similarities in the amino acid sequence around the catalytic residues [1].

Up to now, 16 clans of metallopeptidases have been described: MA, MC, MD, ME, MF, MG, MH, MJ, MM, MN, MO, MP, MQ, MS, MT, and MU, with six of them comprising exo-peptidases. Overall, they form 76 families, with clans MA and MF being two of the most well characterized with enzymes from all living organisms [1].

2.2. Clan MA: Subclan MA (E)

The clan MA is the largest of the metallopeptidases, with a total of 49 families [1], all consisting of enzymes that contain a single Zn^{2+} in their active sites. This clan is made up of both endopeptidases and exopeptidases, comprising aminopeptidases (families M1, M2, M4, M5, M9, M13, M30, M36, M48, and M61), carboxypeptidases (M2 and M32), peptidyl-dipeptidases (M2), oligopeptidases (M3 and M13), and endopeptidases (families

M4, M10, and M12). In the enzymes of the MA clan, the Zn^{2+} atom is coordinated to the protein through two His residues, which are part of the HEXXH motif. In addition to the His residues, the catalytic Zn^{2+} is coordinated by a water molecule and a third residue, the nature of which determines the clan's subdivision into the MA (E) and MA (M) subclans. In the subclan MA (M), the third ligand can be a residue of His or Asp within the HEXXHXXGXXH/D signature sequence, while in subclan MA (E) the third ligand is a residue of Glu, located at least 14 residues after the carboxyl terminus of the HEXXH motif [1] (Figure 5). The oxygen atom of the water molecule that acts as a metal ligand is the nucleophilic agent that attacks the carbonyl of the peptide bond to be hydrolyzed.

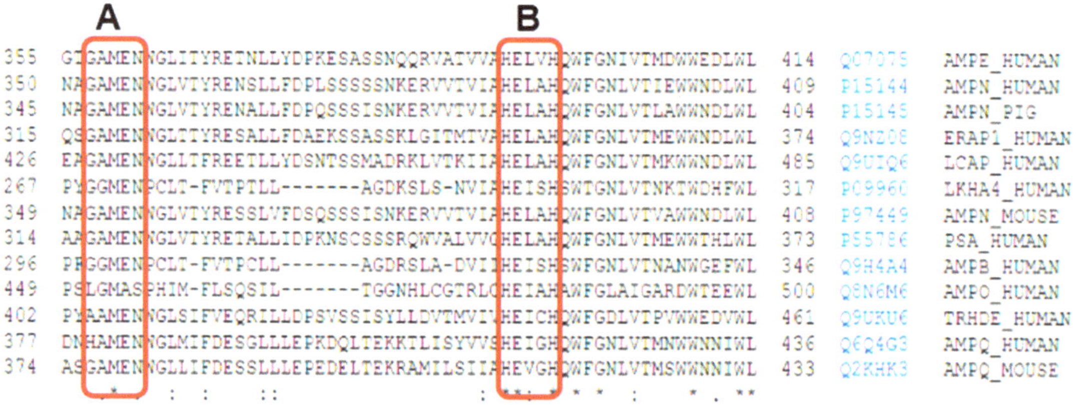

Figure 5. Uniprot alignment of the aminoacidic sequence of the active site of various M1 family aminopeptidases: AMPE_Human: human aminopeptidase E, AMPN_Human: human aminopeptidase N, AMPN_Pig: porcine aminopeptidase N, ERAP1_Human: endoplasmatic reticulum aminopeptidase 1, LCAP_Human: human leucyl-cystinyl aminopeptidase, LKHA4_Human: human leukotriene A4 hydrolase, PSA_Human: human puromycin sensitive aminopeptidase, AMPB_Human: human aminopeptidase B, AMPO_Human: human aminopeptidase O, TRHDE_Human: human thyrotrophin-releasing hormone-degrading enzyme or pyroglutamyl aminopeptidase II, AMPQ_Human: human aminopeptidase Q, AMPQ_Mouse: mouse aminopeptidase Q. On the right of each sequence, the access number and identifiers from Uniprot are included. The short name for each enzyme corresponds to Uniprot abbreviations. The rectangle A encircles the conserved sequence GAMEN related with the aminopeptidase activities of these enzymes from M1 family, and the rectangle B encircles the consensus sequences HEXXH from the active site. Signs below alignment points to other highly conserved amino acid residues inside the M1 family. * indicates residues completely conserved, : indicates position with high degree of conservation of the residues, and . indicates position with mild degree of conservation of the residues.

Thermolysin (EC 3.4.24.27), a secretory endopeptidase, is the model enzyme of the MA clan and its structure, widely characterized, is a point of reference for the study of the enzymes of this clan due to the high structural similarity between them in terms of the organization of the active center [1]. Among the most studied families of the subclan MA (E) is M1, whose members show a wide distribution in the living world (Table 1); furthermore, they are involved in many functions that include cell maintenance, growth, development, and defense [8]. This family includes enzymes of Gram (+) and Gram (−) bacteria, cyanobacteria, archaea, protozoa, fungi, animals, and plants [1,8].

Table 1. Some members of the M1 family of the MA(E) subclan of metallopeptidases. (Compiled from https://www.ebi.ac.uk/merops/cgi-bin/, accessed on 9 January 2023).

Enzyme	IUBMB * Nomenclature	Merops ID	Sources
Aminopeptidase N (APN)	EC 3.4.11.2	M01.001	*Homo sapiens, Sus scrofa*
Lysyl aminopeptidase	-	M01.002	*Escherichia coli*
Aminopeptidase A (APA)	EC 3.4.11.7	M01.003	*Homo sapiens*
Leukotriene A4 hydrolase (LTA4H)	EC 3.3.2.6	M01.004	*Homo sapiens*
Alanyl aminopeptidase (bacterial-type)	EC 3.4.11.2	M01.005	*Escherichia coli, Arabidopsis thaliana*
Ape2 aminopeptidase	-	M01.006	*Saccharomyces cerevisiae*
Aap1' aminopeptidase	-	M01.007	*Saccharomyces cerevisiae*
Thyrotropin-releasing hormone-degrading ectoenzyme or Pyroglutamyl-peptidase II (TRH-DE, PPII)	EC 3.4.19.6	M01.008	*Homo sapiens, Mus musculus, Ratus novergicus*
Aminopeptidase N (actinomycete-type)	-	M01.009	*Streptomyces lividans*
Cytosol alanyl aminopeptidase	-	M01.010	*Homo sapiens, Arabidopsis thaliana, Caenorhabditis elegans*
Insulin-regulated membrane aminopeptidase or cystinyl Aminopeptidase (IRAP)	EC 3.4.11.3	M01.011	*Homo sapiens*
Aminopeptidase G	-	M01.012	*Streptomyces coelicolor*
Aminopeptidase N (insect)	-	M01.013	*Manduca sexta*
Aminopeptidase B (APB)	EC 3.4.11.6	M01.014	*Homo sapiens*
Aminopeptidase H11 (nematode)	-	M01.015	
Aminopeptidase Ey	EC 3.4.11.20	M01.016	*Gallus gallus domesticus*
TMA108 protein	-	M01.017	*Saccharomyces cerevisiae*
Endoplasmic reticulum aminopeptidase 1 ERAP-1	-	M01.018	*Homo sapiens*
Tricorn interacting factor F2	-	M01.020	*Thermoplasma acidophilum*
Tricorn interacting factor F3	-	M01.021	*Thermoplasma acidophilum*
Arginyl aminopeptidase-like 1	-	M01.022	*Homo sapiens*
Endoplasmic reticulum aminopeptidase 2 ERAP-2	-	M01.024	*Homo sapiens*
Aminopeptidase-1 (Caenorhabditis-type)	-	M01.025	*Caenorhabditis elegans*
Aminopeptidase Q	-	M01.026	*Homo sapiens*
Aminopeptidase O (AP-O)	EC 3.4.11.-	M01.028	*Homo sapiens*
M1 aminopeptidase (*Plasmodium* spp.)	EC 3.4.11.2	M01.029	*Plasmodium falciparum*
Aminopeptidase N2 (insect)	-	M01.030	*Manduca sexta*
Cold-active aminopeptidase (*Colwellia psychrerythraea*)-Type peptidase	-	M01.031	*Colwellia psychrerythraea*
Lysyl aminopeptidase 1 (*Streptomyces* sp.)	-	M01.032	*Streptomyces albulus*
Lysyl endopeptidase (*Streptomyces albulus*)	-	M01.033	*Streptomyces albulus*
Leukotriene A4 hydrolase (*Saccharomyces cerevisiae*)	EC 3.3.2.6	M01.034	*Saccharomyces cerevisiae*
LePepA g.p. (*Legionella pneumophila*)	-	M01.035	*Legionella pneumophila*

* IUBMB: International Union of Biochemistry and Molecular Biology.

2.3. M1 Family of Metalloaminopeptidases

The aminopeptidases of the M1 family exist in monomeric or dimeric forms. In eukaryotes, they are generally membrane-associated enzymes such as mammalian APN (i.e., from human or pig), acidic or glutamyl aminopeptidase (APA), adipocyte-derived leucine aminopeptidase, and thyrotropin-releasing hormone-degrading ectoenzyme (TRH-DE), also known as pyroglutamyl peptidase II [16]. Some are cytosolic enzymes, such as leukotriene A4 hydrolase (bifunctional enzyme with aminopeptidase activity) [67] and aminopeptidase B (APB) [68], or associated with the cell wall [9], such as the neutral aminopeptidase (APN, EC 3.4.11.2) of the yeast *Candida albicans* [69]. The structure of the membrane-bound aminopeptidases of the M1 family, in general, comprises a short intracellular tail attached to the transmembrane domain and a large ectodomain formed, in turn, by 2- or 3-folded and conserved domains. Domain I, N-terminal, has a β-sheet nucleus that, although it is widely exposed to the solvent, contains a hydrophobic region that continues in an anchorage region in the membrane. Catalytic domain II, such as that of thermolysin, contains an active site flanked by a mixed structure of β-sheet and α-helix that is highly conserved throughout the family. Domain III, which is composed of an immunoglobulin-like fold, does not appear in some family members (such as leukotriene A4 hydrolase). Domain IV, C-terminal, is the most variable region within the family. It is completely helical, with such an arrangement that it covers the active site; it is also involved in the dimerization of the mammalian isoforms [8]. Disulfide bridges and abundant glycosylations are generally seen in this extracellular region, and some of these enzymes are surface antigens [1,16].

In the M1 family, a well-conserved motif is the Gly-Ala/X-Met-Glu-Asn (GAMEN/GXMEN) sequence. This sequence, also known as the exopeptidase motif, frequently shows variations in the first two residues, and is very useful for the identification of family members [8,16,70] (Figure 5).

Through the technique of crystallography and X-ray diffraction, the three-dimensional structures of several members of this family have been elucidated, such as leukotriene A4 hydrolase in complex with its inhibitor bestatin [71]; tricorn-interacting factor 3 of *Thermoplasma acidophilum* [72]; *Escherichia coli* APN (Pep N) in complex with its inhibitor bestatin [73]; *Plasmodium falciparum* (PfA-M1) alone and in complex with bestatin and low molecular mass analogs [74–76]; human APA [77]; human ERAP-1 [78]; and porcine and human APN in complex with substrates and bestatin [70,79], among others (Table 2) (Figure 6). In all these structures, it can be seen that the catalytic domain of this enzymatic family presents a high structural similarity with thermolysin, despite the fact that in some cases, there is only 7% identity in sequence with the corresponding polypeptide chains [71]. The high availability of M1 aminopeptidase structures, the well-studied active site able to the binding of small molecules, and the well characterized reaction mechanisms, make M1 aminopeptidases ideal candidates for the application of structure-guided inhibitor discovery, including high-throughput screenings in different databases of marine and other natural compounds. These inhibitors have potentialities in different infectious and chronic human diseases [80,81].

2.4. Inhibitors of M1 Family Isolated from Marine Invertebrates

2.4.1. A Specific Inhibitor of Thyrotropin-Releasing Hormone-Degrading Ectoenzyme/Pyroglutamyl Aminopeptidase II Isolated from a Marine Organism

Thyrotropin-releasing hormone (TRH), an N-terminal blocked tripeptide (pGlu-His-ProNH2), is mainly produced by brain neurons. Expressed by neurons of the paraventricular nucleus of the hypothalamus, TRH is a hypophysiotropic factor that increases the synthesis and release of thyroid stimulating hormone (TSH) and prolactin (PRL) from the adenohypophysis. In other central nervous system (CNS) circuits, it functions as a neurotransmitter and/or neuromodulator [82]. This peptide has therapeutic properties in the treatment of brain and spinal damage and various neurodegenerative disorders [83]. However, TRH effects are of short duration, in part because the peptide is hydrolyzed in blood and extracellular space by TRH-DE, the thyrotropin-releasing hormone-degrading ectoenzyme, a M1 family metallopeptidase. TRH-DE is enriched in various brain regions but is also expressed in peripheral tissues including the anterior pituitary and the liver, which secretes a soluble form into blood. Among the M1 metallopeptidases, TRH-DE is the only member with a very narrow specificity, hydrolyzing preferentially the pGlu-His bond of TRH, its best characterized biological substrate, making it a target for the specific manipulation of TRH activity. TRH-DE presents an anatomical location that correlates partially with TRH receptors in various regions and is very strictly regulated by different hormones and hypothalamic factors, as well as by various pharmacological and pathophysiological conditions that alter the transmission of TRH-mediated signals. The regulation of TRH-DE activity may be very important for the adjustment of communication mediated by this peptide [84]. Therefore, TRH-DE inhibitors are important tools for studying the physiological functions of this enzyme and TRH in the CNS, as well as for enhancing the different actions of TRH by protecting the degradation of endogenous TRH or exogenously administered analogues [85]. TRH-DE inhibition may be used to enhance TRH activity in different pathologies (Figure 7). Only a few synthetic PPII inhibitors have been described [86–88].

Table 2. Crystallographic structures reported for members of the M1 family of metallopeptidases (Compiled from https://www.ebi.ac.uk/merops/cgi-bin/, accessed on 10 January 2023).

Enzyme	Source	Crystallographic Codes of the Structures at Protein Data Bank (PDB)
aminopeptidase N	*Plasmodium falciparum*	3EBG, 3EBH, 3EBI, 3Q43, 3Q44, 3T8V, 4J3B, 4K5L, 4K5M, 4K5N, 4K5O,4K5P, 4R5T, 4R5V, 4R5X, 4ZQT, 4ZW3, 4ZW5, 4ZW6, 4ZW7, 4ZW8, 4ZX3, 4ZX4, 4ZX5, 4ZX6, 5XM7, 5Y19, 5Y1H, 5Y1K, 5Y1Q, 5Y1R, 5Y1S, 5Y1T, 5Y1V, 5Y1W, 5Y1X, 6EA1, 6EA2, 6EAA, 6EAB, 6EE3, 6EE4, 6EE6, 6EED, 6SBQ, 6SBR
aminopeptidase N	*Escherichia coli*	2DQ6, 2DQM, 2HPO, 2HPT, 2ZXG, 3B2P, 3B2X, 3B34, 3B37, 3B3B, 3KED, 3PUU, 3QJX,4Q4E, 4Q4I, 4XMU, 4XMV, 4XMW, 4XMX, 4XM2, 4XN1, 4XN2, 4XN4, 4XN5, 4XN7, 4XN8, 4XN9, 4XNA, 4XNB, 4XND, 4X03, 4X04, 4X05, 5MFR, 5MFS, 5MFT, 5Y01, 5YQ1, 5YQ2, 5YQB, 6G8B
aminopeptidase N	*Homo sapiens*	4FYQ, 4FYR, 4FYS, 4FYT, 5LHD, 6AKT
aminopeptidase N	*Sus scrofa*	4FSC, 4FKE, 4FKH, 4FKK, 4HOM, 4NAQ, 4NZ8, 4OU3
ERAP 1	*Homo sapiens*	2XDT, 2YD0, 3MDJ, 3QNF, 3RJO, 6Q4R
ERAP 2	*Homo sapiens*	3SE6, 4E36, 4JBS, 5AB0, 5AB2, 5CU5, 5J6S, 5KIV
aminopeptidase A	*Homo sapiens*	4KX7, 4KX8, 4KX9, 4KXA, 4KXB, 4KXC, 4KXD
leukotriene A4 hydrolase	*Homo sapiens*	1G6W, 1H19, 1HS6, 1SQM, 2R59, 2VJ8, 3B7R, 3B7S, 3B7T, 3B7U, 3CHO, 3CHP, 3CHQ, 3CHR, 3CHS, 3FH5, 3FH7, 3FH8, 3FHE, 3FTS, 3FTU, 3FTV, 3FTW, 3FTX, 3FTY, 3FTZ, 3FU0, 3FU3, 3FU5, 3FU6, 3FUD, 3FUE, 3FUF, 3FUH, 3FUI, 3FUJ, 3FUK, 3FUL, 3FUM, 3FUN, 3U9W, 4DPR, 4L2L, 4MKT, 4Ms6, 4RSY, 4RVB, 5AEN, 5BPP, 5FWQ, 5N3W, 5NI2, 5NI4, 5NI6, 5NIA, 5NID, 5NIE, 6ENB, 6ENC, 6END
leukotriene A4 hydrolase (*Saccharomyces cerevisiae*)	*Saccharomyces cerevisiae* (ATCC 204508/S288c)	2XPY, 2XPZ, 2XQ0
cold-active aminopeptidase (*Colwellia psychrerythraea*)-type peptidase	*Colwellia psychrerythraea* (34H/ATCC BAA-681)	3CIA
tricorn interacting factor F3	*Thermoplasma acidophilum* (ATCC 25905/DSM 1728/JCM 9062/NBRC 15155/AMRC-C165)	1Z1W,1Z5H, 3Q7J
LePepA g.p. (*Legionella pneumophila*)	*Legionella pneumophila*	5ZI5, 5ZI7, 5ZIE
TATA-binding protein-associated factor	*Homo sapiens*	5FUR, 6MZC, 6MZL, 6MZM
IRAP (cystinil aminopeptidase)	*Homo sapiens*	4P8Q, 4PJ6, 4Z7I, 5C97, 5MJ6

A joint project of the Faculty of Biology, University of Havana, Cuba, with the Institute of Biotechnology of UNAM, Mexico, involving a screening in aqueous extracts from 26 Cuban coastline marine organisms (Table 3) resulted in the first natural inhibitor of TRH-DE identified and isolated from the marine annelid *Hermodice carunculata* (Figure 8); it was named HcPI. As a result of this screening, we also detected inhibitory activities of porcine kidney cortex dipeptidyl peptidase IV in the species *Phallusia nigra, Mycale microsigmatosa*, *Condylactis gigantea*, *Stichodactyla helianthus*, and *Palythoa caribbaeroum*. HcPI is a 580 Da compound (molecular mass determined by ESI-TOF mass spectrometry), with a possible polymeric structure and the presence of bromine in its structure, as well as amide-type bonds. HcPI potently inhibits TRH-DE with a Ki value of 70.3 nmol/L in a slow and reversible way, making it one of the most powerful inhibitors described against this enzyme [49] (Figure 9A).

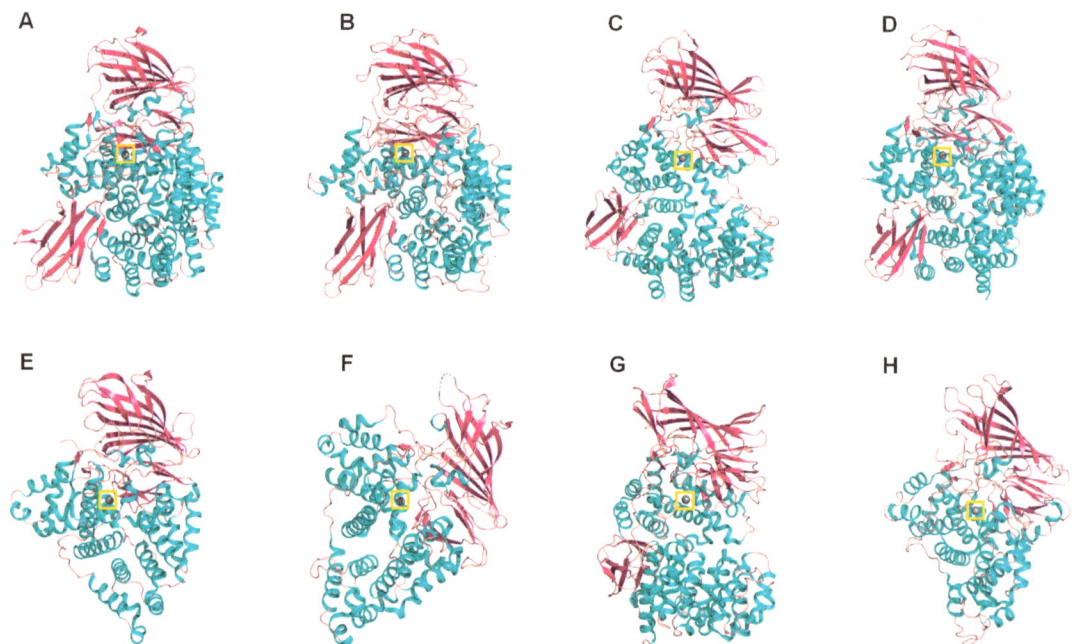

Figure 6. Cartoon representation of different M1 family aminopeptidases: (**A**) pepN from Escherichia coli (PDB ID: 2dq6), (**B**) Plasmodium falciparum aminopeptidase N PfA-M1 (PDB ID: 3ebh), (**C**) human ERAP 1 (PDB ID: 3mdj), (**D**) human ERAP 2 (PDB ID: 3se6), (**E**) human leukotriene A4 hydrolase (PDB ID: 1hs6), (**F**) Saccharomyces cerevisiae leukotriene A4 hydrolase (PDB ID: 2xq0), (**G**) Thermoplasma acidophilum tricorn interacting factor F3 (PDB ID: 1z1w), (**H**) Colwellia psychrerythraea cold-active aminopeptidase (PDB ID: 3cia). Colors: alpha-helices (cyan), beta sheets (warm pink), and loops (salmon). The zinc atoms are shown as gray spheres highlighted in a yellow box.

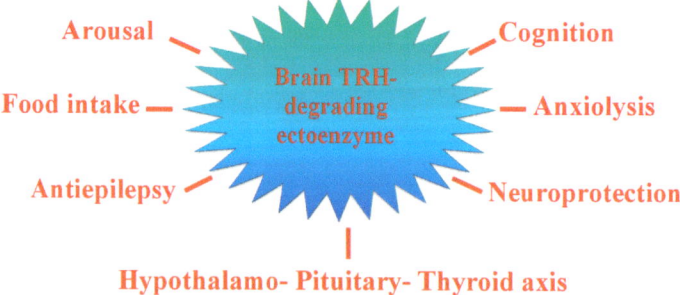

Figure 7. Potential therapeutic applications of targeting central TRH-degrading ectoenzyme activity.

Table 3. Screening of inhibitory activity of TRH-DE and DPP-IV in aqueous extracts from marine invertebrates collected at the Havana coastline, Cuba (adapted from Pascual et al. [49]).

Species	Phylum	[Protein] Crude Extract (mg/mL)	Inhibit Activity of DPP-IV (U/mg)	Inhibit Activity of TRH-DE (U/mg)
Caulerpa racemosa	*Chlorophyta*	5.86	-	-
Dictyosphaeria cavernosa	*Chlorophycota*	8.73	-	-
Halimeda opuntia	*Chlorophycota*	14.72	-	-
Halimeda incrassata	*Chlorophycota*	10.23	-	-
Bidens pilosa	*Magnoliophyta*	22.78	-	-
Ascidia sidneyense	*Chordata*	57.27	-	-
Molgula occidentalis	*Chordata*	31.41	-	-
Pyura vittata	*Chordata*	58.53	-	-
Phallusia nigra	*Chordata*	25.90	93.00	-
Microcosmus gamus	*Chordata*	24.45	-	-
Tectitethya cripta	*Porifera*	0.90	-	-
Mycale microsigmatosa	*Porifera*	43.50	56.59	-
Lima scabra	*Mollusca*	51.55	-	-
Aplisia dactilomela	*Mollusca*	24.00	-	-
Zoanthus pullchelus	*Cnidaria*	15.57	-	-
Plexaura homomalla	Cnidaria	15.25	-	-
Condylactis gigantea	Cnidaria	36.60	79.46	-
Stichodactyla helianthus	Cnidaria	79.50	17.48	-
Cassiopea xamachana	Cnidaria	3.14	-	-
Physalia physalis	*Cnidaria*	13.84	-	-
Palythoa caribaeorum	*Cnidaria*	16.80	133.00	-
Bartholomea annulata	*Cnidaria*	56.50		-
Hermodice carunculata	*Annelida*	62.41	-	24.00
Sabellastarte magnifica	*Annelida*	67.24	-	-
Holothuria floridiana	*Echinodermata*	18.84	-	-
Holothuria mexicana	*Echinodermata*	29.63	-	-

Inhibitory specificity studies carried out against proteases of all mechanistic classes indicate that HcPI is highly specific for TRH-DE. The specificity of the inhibitory activity was assayed using several enzymes from each mechanistic class of proteinases. In a concentration range from 33 to 660 ng/mL and preincubation times at 37 °C of 5, 10, or 30 min, HcPI was not active against serine (trypsin, chymotrypsin, elastase, and DPP-IV), cysteine (papain, bromelain, and PPI), or aspartic (pepsin and PR-HIV) proteases nor against metalloproteinases (collagenase, gelatinase, ACE, aminopeptidase N, and carboxypeptidase A). It was further confirmed that HcPI inhibits, in vitro, thyroliberinase, a soluble version of TRH-DE that inactivates TRH in the bloodstream. The inhibition is dose-dependent, with a Ki value of 51 nmol/L, similar to that previously described for TRH-DE. The specificity results support the idea that HcPI should be useful to study the role of TRH-DE in different experimental models. HcPI is not toxic in vivo and its intraperitoneal injection in BalbC mice decreases TRH-DE activity in the pituitary and in different brain regions such as the hypothalamus, cerebellum, and olfactory bulb [49] (Figure 9C). The inhibition of TRH-DE in vivo in this experimental model causes a transient increase in the serum concentrations of prolactin (PRL) and thyrotropin (TSH), which indicates an in vivo enhancement of the actions of endogenous TRH when degradation by TRH-DE is decreased. Additionally, studies on cells were performed. First, in primary cultures of adenohypophyseal cells, 45 min of incubation with HcPI produces a decrease in the activity of membrane-associated TRH-DE, highly dependent on the dose of inhibitor tested with an IC_{50} of 8.3 μg/mL (Figure 9B). Incubation with 8 μg HcPI/mL decreases enzyme activity by 42% from 5 min, an effect stable for at least one hour. Once enzyme inhibition was demonstrated in cultures, the effect of the enzyme on TRH-mediated communication was evaluated, and it was detected that in the absence of TRH in the system, the presence of HcPI (50 μg/mL) does not change the basal levels of secretion of TSH, or PRL. On the other hand, in the presence of TRH (10 nmol/L), the inhibition of TRH-DE by HcPI caused an increase in the levels of PRL released after 30 min by lactotrophs, specialized cells of the adenohypophysis. These results were confirmed in parallel by inhibition of TRH-DE synthesis with the use of antisense RNA, which demonstrated for the first time in a direct way the effects of the regulation of PPII activity on one of the functions of TRH [89]. Intraperitoneal injection of HcPI (1, 5, 20, or 50 μg/g) in mice did not induce any mortality, obvious motor effect, or weight change for up to 15 days. The effect of different doses of HcPI injected intraperitoneally was tested on mouse PPII specific activity. Compared to saline injected animals, PPII activity was significantly decreased 45 min after injection in most of the tissues analyzed; the effect was dose-dependent. Less than 1 mg of the inhibitor per g of animal weight was sufficient to decrease activity by more than 50% in hypophysis; the maximum dose used (5 μg/g) almost completely abolished the activity. The order of potency was as follows: hypophysis > hypothalamus > cerebellum > olfactory bulb (Figure 9) [49]. Other experiments related to the role of PPII in TRH communication within the hypothalamic–adenohypophysis–thyroid axis were continued with the use of animal models. In these studies, HcPI was injected at the beginning of the experiment at a dose of 50 μg/g of animal weight to Wistar rats, dissolved in physiological saline (doses of 5–10 μg/g of animal weight strongly reduce PPII activity in the adenohypophysis and decrease it in CNS regions). The controls received only saline. Four groups of animals were subsequently treated with 1 ng/g animal weight TRH in saline or saline only and slaughtered by decapitation 15 min after the second treatment. Two additional groups were transferred to a cold room kept at 4 °C for 30 min and similarly sacrificed after the end of the experiment. Since cold stress rapidly activates the hypothalamic–adenohypophysis–thyroid axis by increasing concentrations of TRH in the portal hypothalamus–pituitary vessels, this paradigm was used in addition to exogenous administration of TRH, with the objective of evaluating the effects of inhibition of TRH-DE by HcPI on a naturally occurring surge of circulating TSH concentration. Compared to animals that received a single injection of saline, TRH-DE activity is significantly decreased in the hypothalamus and in the pituitary of animals that receive a single dose of HcPI. Similar changes are observed in the activity of serum thyroliberinase. Inhibition of TRH-DE activity by HcPI has no effect on baseline TSH levels, as observed in primary adenohypophyseal cell cultures. However, in animals injected with exogenous TRH or exposed to ambient cold, inhibition of TRH-DE activity by HcPI is associated with a significant increase in serum TSH concentration when compared to control groups that only received saline (Sánchez-Jaramillo et al. 2009). These results demonstrated for the first time the role that TRH-DE exerts on TRH activity and TSH secretion by adenohypophysis and made HcPI a very useful tool for further studies and potential biomedical applications in diseases such as Non-Thyroidal Illness Syndrome (NTIS) in which the levels of thyroid hormones are reduced [90].

2.4.2. Inhibitors of Aminopeptidase N Isolated from Marine Organisms

Neutral aminopeptidases are enzymes that catalyze the cleavage of neutral amino acids from the N-terminus of protein or peptide substrates. They have been classified in several metallopeptidase families, such M1 and M17 [1,8,9]. These enzymes are present in all living organisms, but the diversity of the functions in which they are involved is far from being entirely deciphered. Mammalian neutral aminopeptidase (APN, EC 3.4.11.2,

M1 family) is the most extensively studied member of the M1 family of zinc-dependent aminopeptidases; it is noteworthy that it catalyzes the cleavage of not only neutral but also basic N-terminal residues. This enzyme, also known as CD13, is widely expressed on cell surfaces of tissues, such as intestinal epithelia and the nervous system. Mammalian APN is a type II membrane protein generally found as a homodimer in several mammalian species. Full-length human APN consists of 967 amino acids with a short N-terminal cytoplasmic domain, a single transmembrane segment, and a large ectodomain containing two catalytic motifs highly conserved across the M1 family: the zinc-binding motif HEXXHX18E and the exopeptidase signature GAMEN [70]. APN plays pivotal roles in many physiological processes, such as pain sensation, sperm motility, cell–cell adhesion, and blood pressure regulation (Figure 10) [8,18]. This enzyme is also up-regulated in human pathologies, such as coronavirus entry, inflammation, immune cell chemotaxis, tumor angiogenesis, and metastasis in several types of cancer, with a strong correlation between the level of APN expression of a cell and its resultant invasive capacity (Figure 10). Dysregulation of APN expression evolves in almost all types of human malignancies, including breast cancer, cervical cancer, ovarian cancer, prostate cancer, non-small-cell lung cancer (NSCLC), liver cancer, colon cancer, cirrhosis gastric cancer, pancreatic cancer, renal cell carcinoma (RCC), hepatocellular carcinoma (HCC), head and neck squamous cell carcinoma (SCC), melanoma, osteosarcoma, and thyroid cancer [19,91]. This makes human APN an attractive target for the treatment of diseases, including cancers (Figure 11) [8,18,19,91–93]. Accordingly, strategies for its inhibition have been developed primarily for the treatment of pain [94,95]. Only Ubenimex (bestatin), a drug inhibitor, is currently approved by the FDA for its uses in human pathologies, mainly in cancer [91].

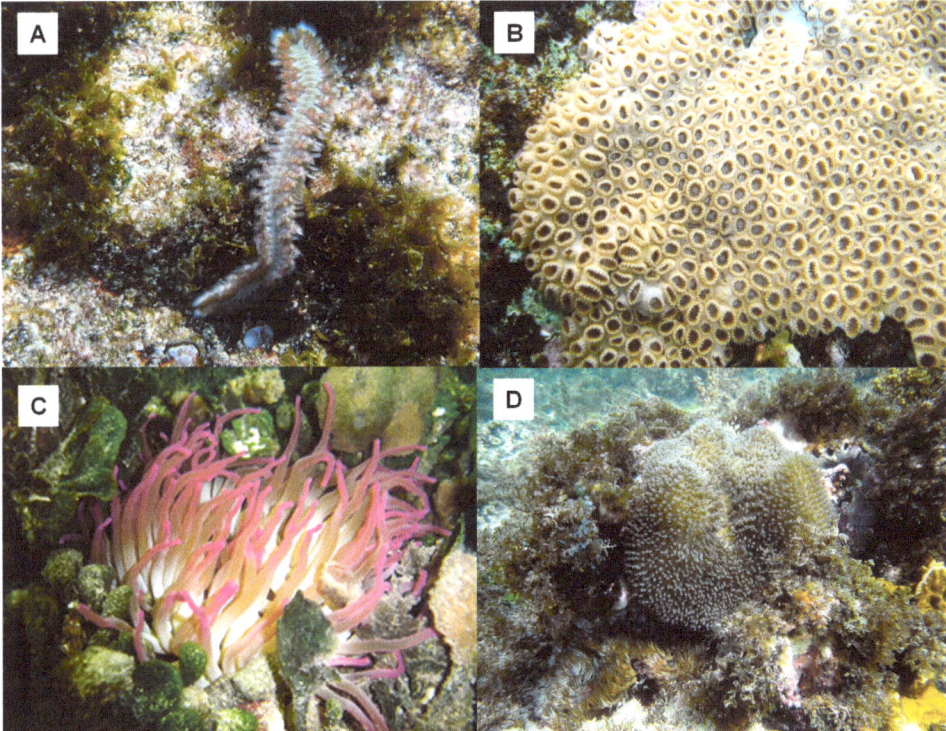

Figure 8. Some of the marine organisms screened for inhibitory activity of TRH-DE and DPP-IV. (**A**) *Hermodice carunculata*, (**B**) *Palythoa caribaeorum*, (**C**) *Condylactis gigantea*, and (**D**) *Stichodactyla helianthus*. Pictures courtesy of Professor José Espinosa, PhD, ICIMAR, CITMA, Cuba.

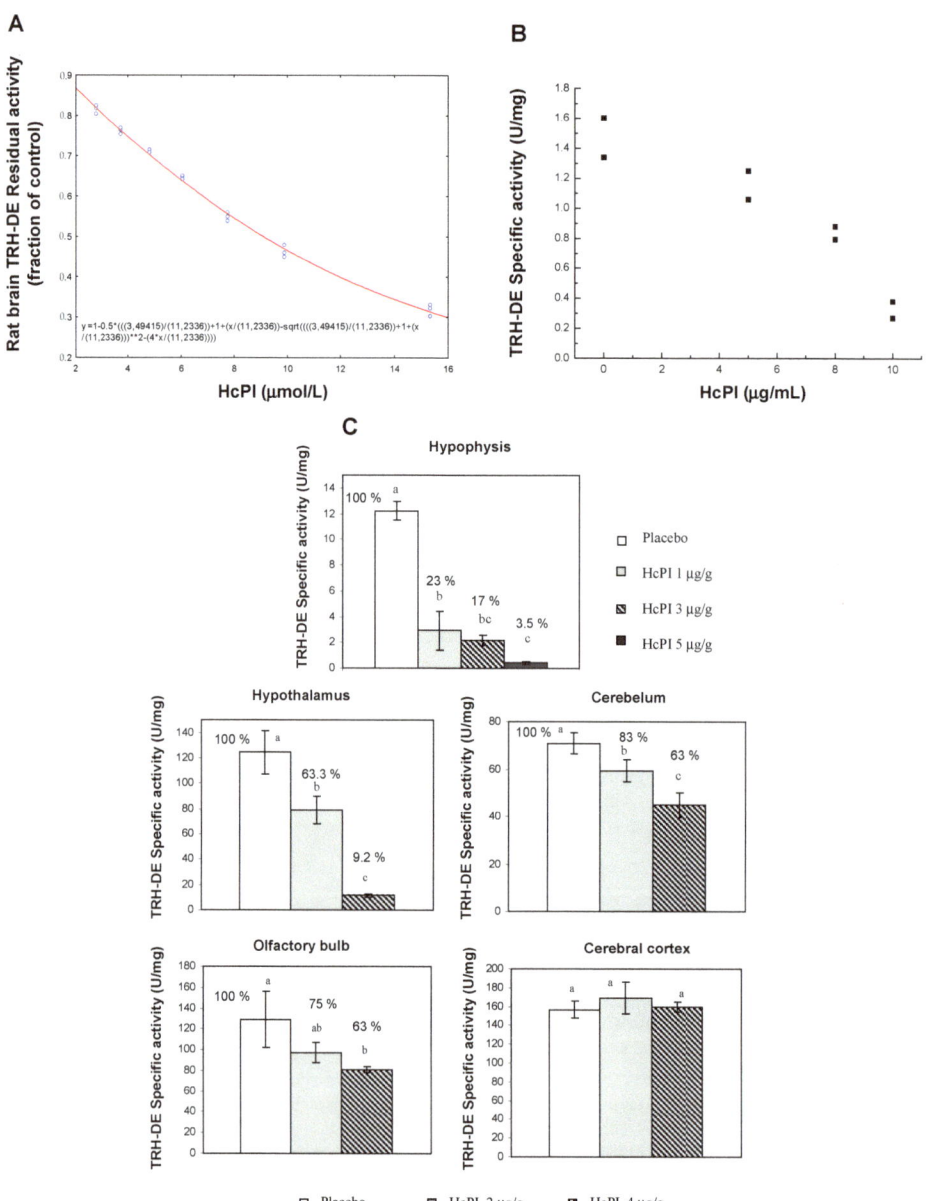

Figure 9. TRH-DE inhibition by HcPI in different enzyme models. (**A**) Ki determination of HcPI effect on TRH-DE activity in rat brain membranes, (**B**) inhibition effect of HcPI on TRH-DE activity in primary cultures of rat adepnohypophysis, and (**C**) effect of intraperitoneal injection of different doses of HcPI on mouse TRH-DE specific activity in brain [49]; Different letters indicate a significant difference between treatment groups, with *p* < 0.001.

Natural inhibitors of human and mammalian APN in general are scarce and have mainly been described from microorganisms [18,96], plants [97], marine invertebrates [36,48,98,99], and more recently from Cuban toad secretions [100,101] (Figure 12). Several compounds from marine organisms have been described with anticancer activities; however, very few of them have been linked with APN inhibition or interaction [102–106]. In the next section, we review the information available regarding marine invertebrates as a promissory and still unexplored source of inhibitors of APN with biomedical relevance mainly in cancer.

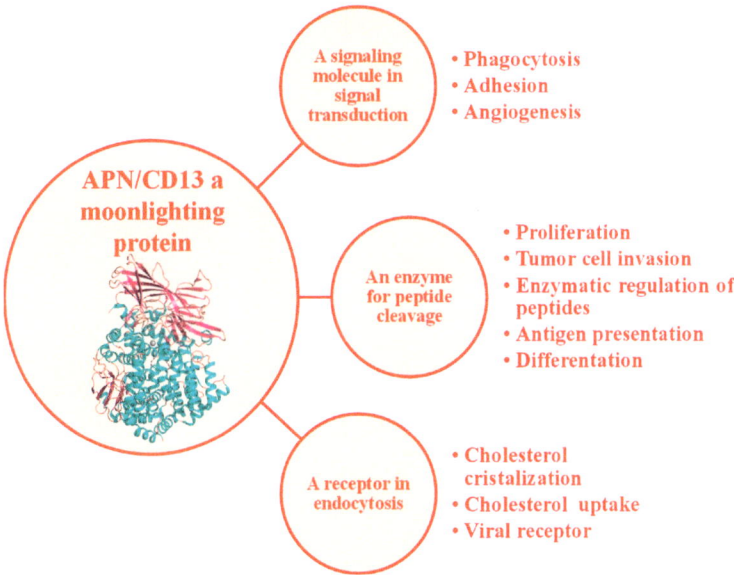

Figure 10. Functions of human APN/CD13 (adapted from Amin et al. [19]).

Different type of cancer with high activity of APN

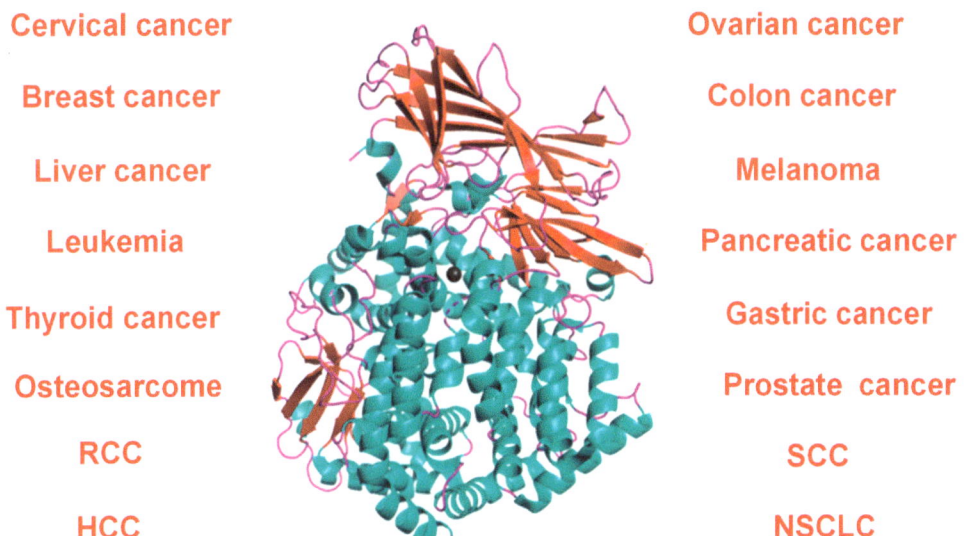

Figure 11. Up-regulation of human APN in different cancers. Abbreviations: renal cell cancer (RCC), hepatocellular carcinoma (HCC), squamous cell carcinoma (SCC), non-small-cell lung carcinoma (NSCLC).

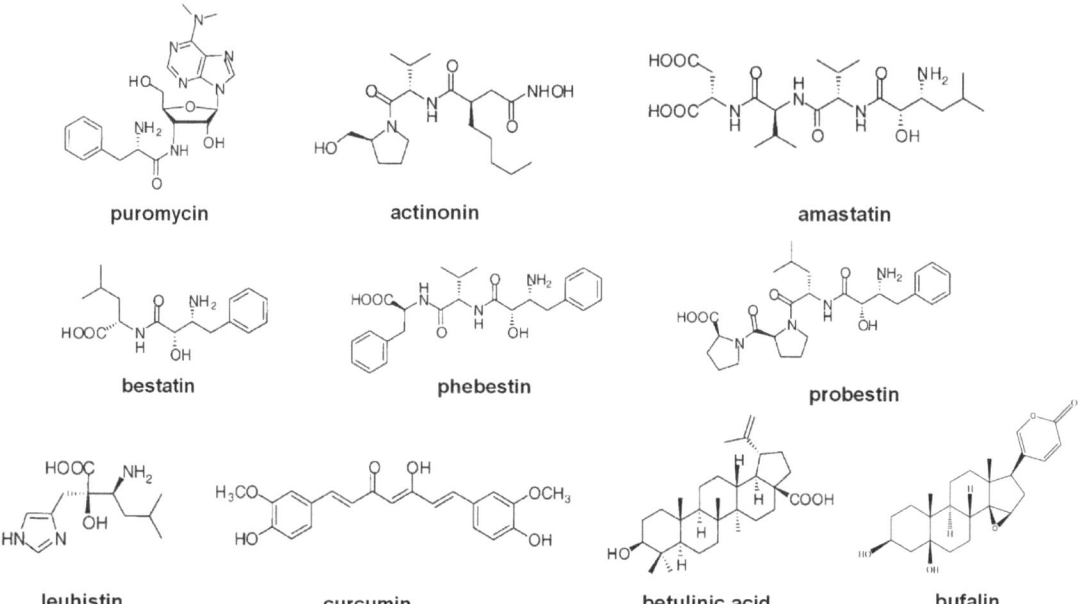

Figure 12. Natural inhibitors of Aminopeptidase N.

Psammaplin A

Psammaplin A (PsA) is a natural bromothyrosine compound belonging to the open-chain-oximinoamidesis bromo-derivates group (Figure 13), isolated from the association between two sponges, *Poecillastra* sp. and *Jaspis* sp. [107], which represents the first isolated natural product containing oxime and disulfide moieties from marine sponges. Subsequently, other natural derivatives, such as biprasin, psammaplin C, psammaplin E, psammaplin F, psammaplin G, and psammaplin K (Figure 13), were also isolated and described [108–112].

Several biological activities have been described for PsA; it is an antibacterial mainly against Staphylococcus aureus (SA) and methicillin-resistant *Staphylococcus aureus* (MRSA) due to DNA gyrase inhibition and bacterial DNA synthesis arrest [113]. PsA also inhibits chitinases that are common in fungi and are crucial for the control of ecdysis in insects [114]. In mammalian cells, PsA inhibits topoisomerase II, an enzyme catalyzing DNA relaxation, with a high IC_{50} of 18.8 mM [114]. In 2004, almost at the same time our group described HcPI as an inhibitor of TRH-DE, Shim et al. [48] found that PsA inhibits mammalian APN with a K_i value of 15 µM in a non-competitive way. Structural analogues of PsA, in which phenolic hydroxyl groups were replaced, did not inhibit human or porcine APN, indicating that these groups are crucial in the recognition and inhibition of this enzyme in mammals. This finding perfectly agreed with the effectiveness of bulky and hydrophobic groups in molecules targeting APN [115]. However, no other in-depth structure–activity or docking studies of aminopeptidase N inhibition by PsA have been carried out.

Psammaplin A possesses antiproliferative activities against various cancer cell lines, including triple-negative breast (TNBC, MDA-MB-231), doxorubicin-resistant human breast (MCF-7/adr), colon (HCT15), ovarian (SK-OV-3), lung (A549, LM4175), bone (BoM1833), skin (SK-MEL-2), central nervous system (BrM-2a, XF498) [116–118], and Ishikawa endometrial cells [119]. Some of the mechanisms described to explain the antiproliferative effects of this compound are the induction of cell cycle arrest and apoptosis associated with different factors [119,120]. Pretreatment with PsA was also shown to increase the sensitivity of human lung and glioblastoma cancer cells to radiation in vitro [120]. Moreover, this compound showed suppressive effects of the invasion and tube formation of endothelial cells stimulated by the basic fibroblast growth factor [48]. These results demonstrate that PsA is a new APN inhibitor that can be developed as a new antiangiogenic agent.

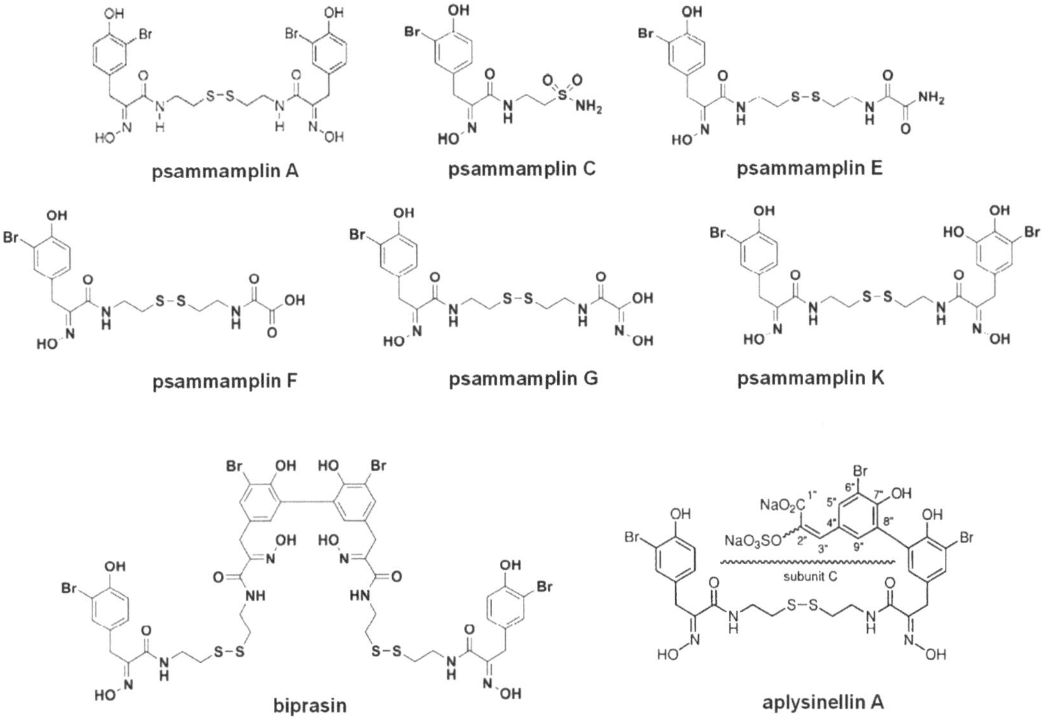

Figure 13. The chemical structure of psammaplin compounds, biprasin, and aplysinellin A.

PsA has also been described as a histone deacetylase (HDAC) inhibitor [119,121]. The mechanism of action underlying the HDAC inhibitory effect of PsA involves a change in the redox state of the disulfide bond. Replacement of the sulfur atom leads to the formation of a mercaptan, which in turn chelates the Zn^+ ion present in the characteristic active site of the HDAC enzyme, modifying its conformational state and thus preventing its accessibility to the natural substrate. This new conformational state determines an increase in acetylation levels of histone H3, a well-known epigenetic marker of chromatin structure and function, suggesting selectivity for HDACs. Moreover, PsA also exhibits potent enzyme inhibitory and antiproliferative activities under reduced conditions in cells, which indicates that PsA could be used as a natural prodrug [121].

Although PsA possesses a broad spectrum of bioactivities, its in-depth study has been hindered due to the limited amount of the compound that can be isolated from marine sources as well as its poor physiological stability. For these reasons, homodimeric or heterodimeric analogs of PsA have been obtained by chemical synthesis through a disulfide exchange strategy (Figure 14) [122]. Some of the new synthetic compounds, particularly heterodimeric derivatives, displayed higher antibacterial activity than psammaplin A, comparable to clinically used drugs vancomycin and ciprofloxacin [123,124]. However, the APN inhibitory activity of all the synthetic psammaplin derivatives (examples in Figures 13 and 14) has not been evaluated, being a still unexplored source of new aminopeptidase N inhibitors with biomedical potentialities taking into account the promissory effects of these compounds on several biomedical models [122].

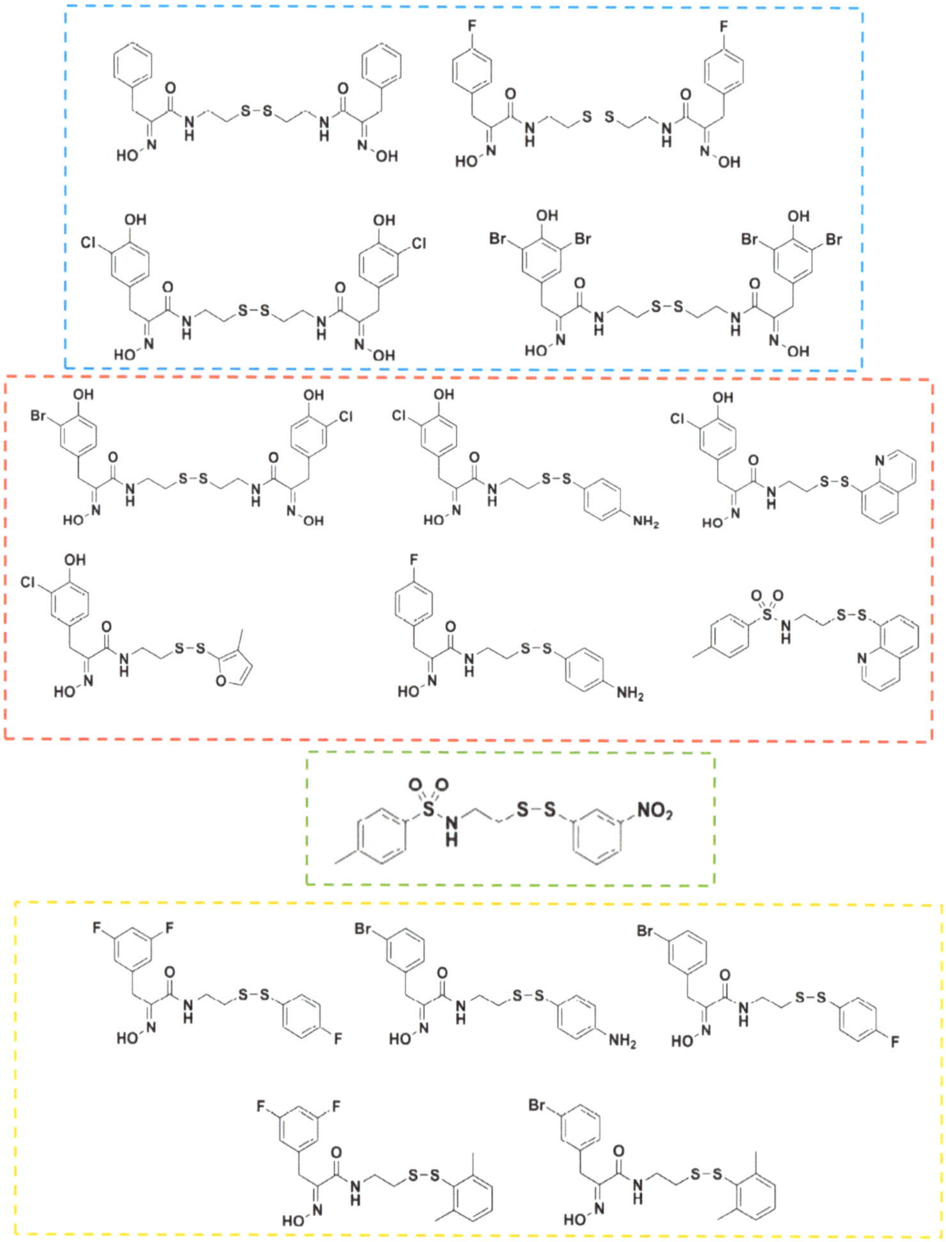

Figure 14. Examples of synthetic homo- and hetero-derivatives of psammaplin A. The blue dashed line box highlights derivatives that showed significant antibacterial effects against methicillin-resistant *Staphylococcus aureus* (MRSA) due to DNA gyrase inhibition and bacterial DNA synthesis arrest. The red dashed line box highlights derivatives that showed higher antibacterial activity than psammaplin A. The green dashed line box highlights a derivative that showed similar antibacterial activity to clinically used drugs vancomycin and ciprofloxacin. The yellow dashed line box highlights derivatives that possessed 50-fold higher activities than psammaplin A vs. *Staphylococcus aureus* and MRSA, in this case mainly by a nonspecific redox-based mechanism (reviewed in [122]).

Identification of Inhibitory Activity of Mammalian APN in Marine Invertebrates from Cuban Coastline

Considering the identification of a highly specific inhibitor of TRH-DE in the marine annelide *Hermodice carunculata* in aqueous extracts from Cuban marine invertebrates, our group extended the screening to porcine and human APN as targets. As part of a first study carried out in 2011–2015 in aqueous extracts from marine invertebrates belonging to the phyla (Table 4), an APN inhibitory activity is detected in all the extracts evaluated except for *Lebrunia danae* and *Hermodice carunculata*, whose extracts display values of enzymatic activity higher than those of the control test of porcine APN (pAPN) (Table 4, Figure 15). The L-Leu-pNA substrate is also hydrolyzed when the assay is performed only in the presence of the extract and activity buffer, indicating the possible presence of a neutral aminopeptidase type activity in these two species. The extracts of the species *Bryozoo* sp. 2, *Diplosoma listerianum*, *Lisoclinum verrilli*, *Eucidaris tribuloides*, and *Ophiocoma echinata* were selected as the most promising in terms of the specific inhibitory activity of porcine APN as well as a dose-dependent inhibition behavior [125]. The extracts of the *Phallusia nigra*, *Ascidia sidneyense*, *Microcosmus guanus*, *Steinacidia turbinata*, and *Poticlenum constellatum* species do not show inhibition at increasing concentrations, indicating that the initial result is probably due to a component of the extract that interferes with the correct determination of the enzyme activity. All the selected extracts, except that of *Lisoclinum verrilli*, show slow inhibition, in the order of minutes. On the other hand, for the latter, equilibrium is reached within 1 min of preincubation time, suggesting a fast interaction of the inhibitory components of the extract with the porcine APN. The IC_{50} values are in the range of 0.11–2.39 mg/mL (Table 4), with the highest efficiency being for the extracts of the two sea squirts (*Diplosoma listerianum* and *Lisoclinum verrilli*) and that of *Bryiozoo sp2*. The active extracts were submitted to clarification treatments (such as 2.5% trichloroacetic acid and heat treatments) to eliminate contaminants (mainly proteins) and to promote dissociation from endogenous inhibitor–target complexes. Clarification increases the specific inhibitory activity of the extracts, suggesting that the procedure should be useful in future works dealing with the isolation of the inhibitory molecules [98].

Table 4. Summary of the preliminary characterization of the porcine APN inhibitory activity detected in crude extracts of marine invertebrate species (screening in the period 2011–2015) (adapted from Pascual et al. [125]).

Species	Phylum	pAPN Inhibitory Activity (U/mL)	pAPN Specific Inhibitory Activity (U/mg)	Pre-Incubation Time (min)	IC_{50} (mg/mL)
Phallusia nigra	Chordata	2.3060	0.8363	-	-
Lisoclinum verrilli	Chordata	7.8770	0.7361	1	0.11 ± 0.06
Ascidia sidneyensis	Chordata	3.1760	0.6481	-	-
Microcosmus guanus	Chordata	7.1368	0.5366	-	-
Esteinacidia turbinata	Chordata	3.6340	0.5344	-	-
Diplosoma listerianum	Chordata	8.1300	0.4394	30	0.11 ± 0.26
Poticlenum constellatum	Chordata	3.2230	0.2984	-	-
Eucidaris tribuloides	Echinodermata	6.2526	0.3206	5	1.35 ± 0.19
Ophiocoma echinata	Echinodermata	8.2337	0.0874	60	2.39 ± 1.09
Lebrunia danae	Echinodermata	-	-	-	-
Bryozoo sp1	Bryozoa	5.7240	0.0560	-	-
Bryozoo sp2	Bryozoa	6.7600	1.1266	30	0.29 ± 0.05
Hermodice carunculata	Annelida	-	-	-	-

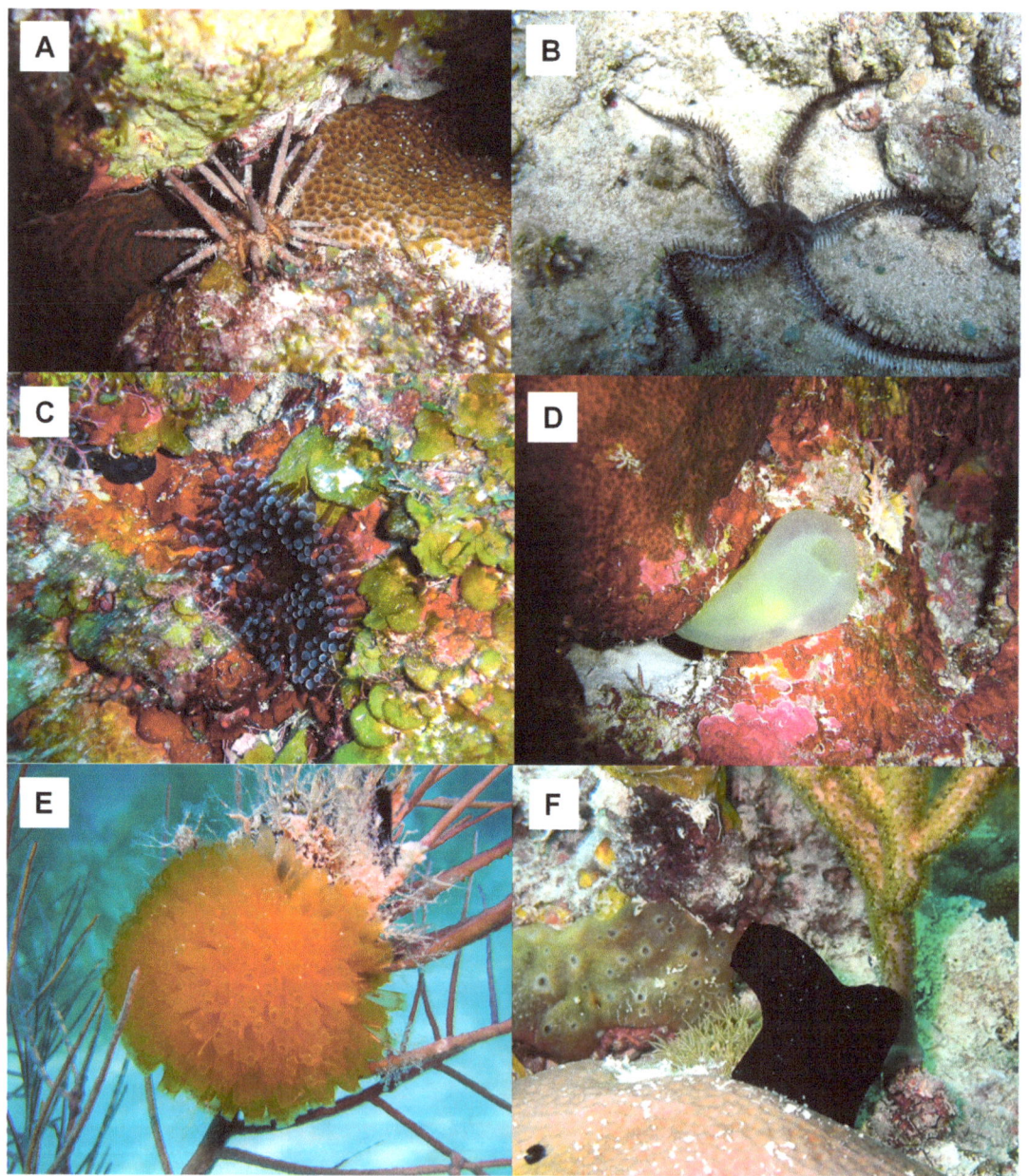

Figure 15. Some of the marine invertebrates screened for inhibitory activity of porcine APN. (**A**) *Eucidiaris tribuloides*, (**B**) *Ophiocoma echinata*, (**C**) *Lebrunia danae*, (**D**) *Ascidia sydneiensis*, (**E**) *Esteinacidia turbinata*, and (**F**) *Phallusia nigra*. Pictures courtesy of Professor José Espinosa, PhD from ICIMAR, CITMA, Cuba.

In a second study performed in 2015–2019, aqueous extracts from species belonging to the phyla Mollusca, Poriphera, Echinodermata, and Cnidaria (Figure 16) were screened using human placental APN as the target (Table 5). The initial evaluations allowed detection of an inhibitory activity of hAPN only from the species *Cenchritis muricatus* and *Isostichopus badionotus*. Increased L-Leu-AMC hydrolysis rates over the control value are found instead of inhibitory activities for the rest of the species. These results suggest either the presence of an activator of the target enzymes used in the assays or neutral aminopeptidase-like enzymes hydrolyzing L-Leu-AMC in the corresponding aqueous extracts. The clarification of all aqueous crude extracts (2.5% TCA treatment) increased, in all cases, the recovery of specific inhibitory activities as compared to their detection in positive crude extracts. The treatment also allowed the identification of inhibitory activities from species that were negative after screening using aqueous crude extracts. This result indicated that clarification eliminates contaminants and/or induces dissociation from endogenous inhibitor–target complexes that do not allow the detection of inhibitory components in crude extracts.

Table 5. Summary of the screening of phyla Mollusca, Poriphera, Echinodermata, and Cnidaria for inhibitory activity against human APN (hAPN) (see note below). Adapted from [98].

Species	Phylum	NA-like Activity ($\times 10^4$ U/mg)	Crude Extracts hAPN sIA (U/mg)	2.5% TCA Treated Extracts hAPN sIA (U/mg)
Cenchritis muricatus	Mollusca	ND	0.46	5.20
Nerita peloronta	Mollusca	6.95 ± 2.84	ND	5.06
Nerita versicolor	Mollusca	12.56 ± 1.70	ND	2.21
Lissodendoryx (Lissodendoryx) isodictyalis	Porifera	1.51 ± 0.49	ND	171.92
Tripneustes ventricosus	Echinodermata	6.39 ± 0.07	ND	56.86
Echinaster (Othilia) echinophorus	Echinodermata	58.87 ± 12.62	ND	10.82
Isostichopus badionotus	Echinodermata	ND	1.56	33.81
Stichodactyla helianthus	Cnidaria	9.63 ± 2.68	ND	32.81
Bunodosoma granuliferum	Cnidaria	39.44 ± 5.45	ND	4.31
Physalia physalis	Cnidaria	2.04 ± 0.52	ND	13.13

NOTE: hAPN inhibitory activities in aqueous crude and 2.5% TCA extracts are expressed as specific Inhibitory Activity (sIA) in U/mg. One unit of enzyme activity was defined as the amount of enzyme needed to produce one arbitrary unit of fluorescence per minute, and inhibitory activities are expressed per mg of extract. The first column indicates tested species, the second column shows neutral aminopeptidase-like activity (NA) detected in aqueous crude extracts using L-Leu-AMC as substrate, and the remaining columns refer to sIA. (ND): not detected.

The clarified extracts (2.5% TCA) from the species *Cenchritis muricatus, Nerita peloronta, Nerita versicolor, Lissodendoryx (Lissodendoryx) isodictyalis, Tripneustes ventricosus, Echinaster (Othilia) echinophorus, Isostichopus badionotus, Stichodactyla helianthus, Bunodosoma granuliferum*, and *Physalia physalis* were used to continue the inhibition studies vs. human APN (hAPN) [98]. Additionally, the enhanced activities over the control detected in some extracts were lost, in all cases, after the 2.5% TCA treatments, suggesting susceptibility of the active molecules to the chaotropic agent and/or to the acidic pH of the molecule(s) responsible for these effects (Table 5).

To test the presence of neutral aminopeptidase-like enzymes in aqueous crude extracts, preliminary enzymatic assays were performed using different amounts of the samples (in absence of the initial target hAPN) in the presence of L-Leu-AMC. A linear dependence of the initial rate versus the amount of crude extract in the assays was detected for the species *Nerita peloronta, Nerita versicolor, Lissodendoryx (Lissodendoryx) isodictyalis, Tripneustes ventricosus, Echinaster (Othilia) echinophorus, Stichodactyla helianthus, Bunodosoma granuliferum*, and *Physalia physalis*. These neutral aminopeptidase-like activities were recently characterized by a kinetic approach combining substrates, inhibitors, and cations, showing for the first time a biochemical behavior indicative of the presence of M1 and M17 enzymes in these species [30].

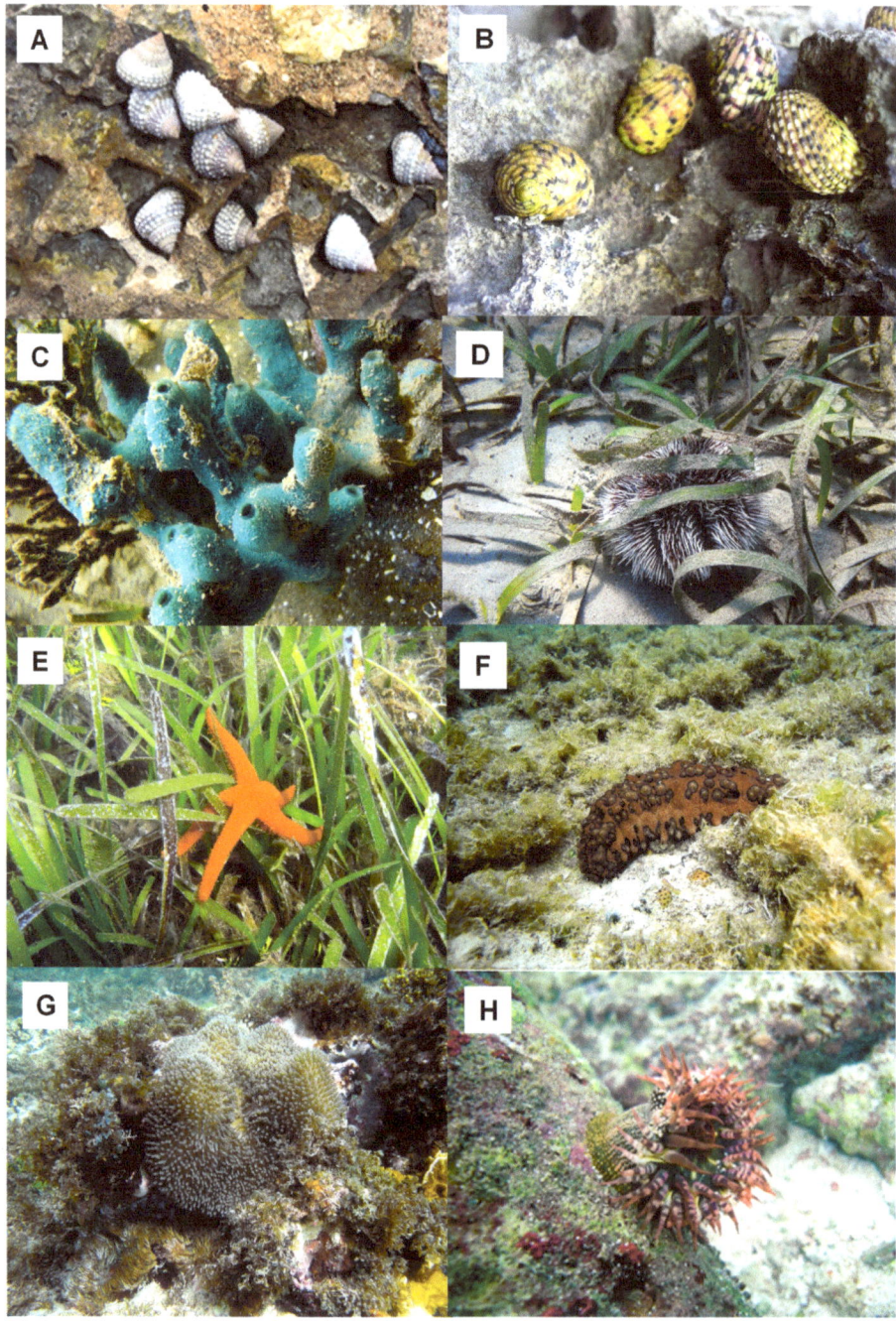

Figure 16. Some of the marine invertebrates which show inhibitory activity of pAPN, pAPA, hAPN, and rPfA-M17. (**A**) *Cenchritis muricatus,* (**B**) *Nerita versicolor,* (**C**) *Lissodendoryx (Lissodendoryx) iso-dictyalis,* (**D**) *Tripneustes ventricosus,* (**E**) *Echinaster (Othilia) echinophorus,* (**F**) *Isostichopus badionotus,* (**G**) *Stichodactyla helianthus,* and (**H**) *Bunodosoma granuliferum.* Pictures courtesy of Professor José Espinosa, PhD from ICIMAR, CITMA, Cuba.

The clarified extracts inhibit hAPN activity in a dose-dependent manner, and the inhibition was characterized by a concave behavior, indicating the reversibility of the inhibition and corroborating the presence of inhibitory molecules in the samples (and not artifacts interfering with the enzyme activity). The IC_{50} values are in the range of 11.7–567.6 μg/mL [98]. As a promissory result, hAPN is inhibited with IC_{50} values around or less than 100 μg/mL in four of the ten species tested (*Lissodendoryx (Lissodendoryx) isodictyalis, Tripneustes ventricosus, Isostichopus badionotus*, and *Stichodactyla helianthus*); this inhibition is stronger than that produced by bestatin or amastatin (pure compounds) assayed in parallel as controls (Table 5) [98].

Taking into account that the effect of the inhibition of hAPN was corroborated, the effect of each treated extract on the viability of two APN+ cancer cell lines PC3 and 3LL was evaluated [98]. All treated extracts, and bestatin used as a positive control, have a dose-dependent effect on PC3 and 3LL cell viability. The higher effects on both cell lines, with IC_{50} values below 100 μg/mL, are observed for the species showing the strongest hAPN inhibition. An IC_{50} value under 5 μg/mL for *L. isodictyalis* extract vs. both cancer cells lines, similar to the effect displayed by bestatin, indicates that this species is promissory for the isolation of hAPN inhibitors. In this work, the IC_{50} values for cell viability are in good agreement with the IC_{50} values for hAPN inhibition, including the bestatin results. To the best of our knowledge, this work was the first to show concomitantly natural inhibitor potency on hAPN and indications of activity on hAPN-expressing cells [98].

Inhibitors of Aminopeptidase A Isolated from Marine Organisms

Membrane glutamyl aminopeptidase, also known as acidic aminopeptidase (APA, EC 3.4.11.7), is a type II membrane protein of the M1 family, MA subclade (E), of metallopeptidases [8] (Figure 1B). This enzyme is widely distributed in mammalian tissues. Aminopeptidase A (APA) has been reported to have molecular weights around 109 kDa for the human and 108 kDa for the porcine enzyme [1]. APA's S1 pocket accommodates acid residue side chains, whereby this enzyme hydrolyzes aspartic and glutamic residues from the peptide N-terminus [77]. APA performs fundamental functions in a wide range of physiological processes, since it participates in the metabolism of angiotensin II, involved in the renin–angiotensin system in the central nervous system and other anatomical locations, making it an important regulator of blood pressure (Figure 17) [126]. In addition, it is involved in the development of Alzheimer's disease and glomerulosclerosis and in the progression of cancer. It is associated with the development of renal neoplasms, malignant trophoblasts, renal choriocarcinoma, and colorectal cancer [126–130]. APA plays a key role in blood pressure regulation, which has made it a promising therapeutic target for the development of antihypertensive agents (Figure 17) [30,126,131].

Recently, we extended the screening of marine organism extracts to porcine aminopeptidase A (pAPA). We observed that extracts from the species *Nerita peloronta, Nerita versicolor, Lissodendoryx (Lissodendoryx) isodictyalis, Tripneustes ventricosus, Echinaster (Othilia) echinophorus, Isostichopus badionotus*, and *Stichodactyla helianthus* displayed dose-dependent inhibition of porcine APA activity, with IC_{50} values in the range of 11.00–1005.00 μg/mL (Table 6), showing that *Nerita versicolor* has a certain selectivity for pAPA rather than for hAPN. These results strongly support the exploration of marine fauna of invertebrates as promissory sources of inhibitors of M1 family enzymes with potential biomedical applications, such as APN and APA.

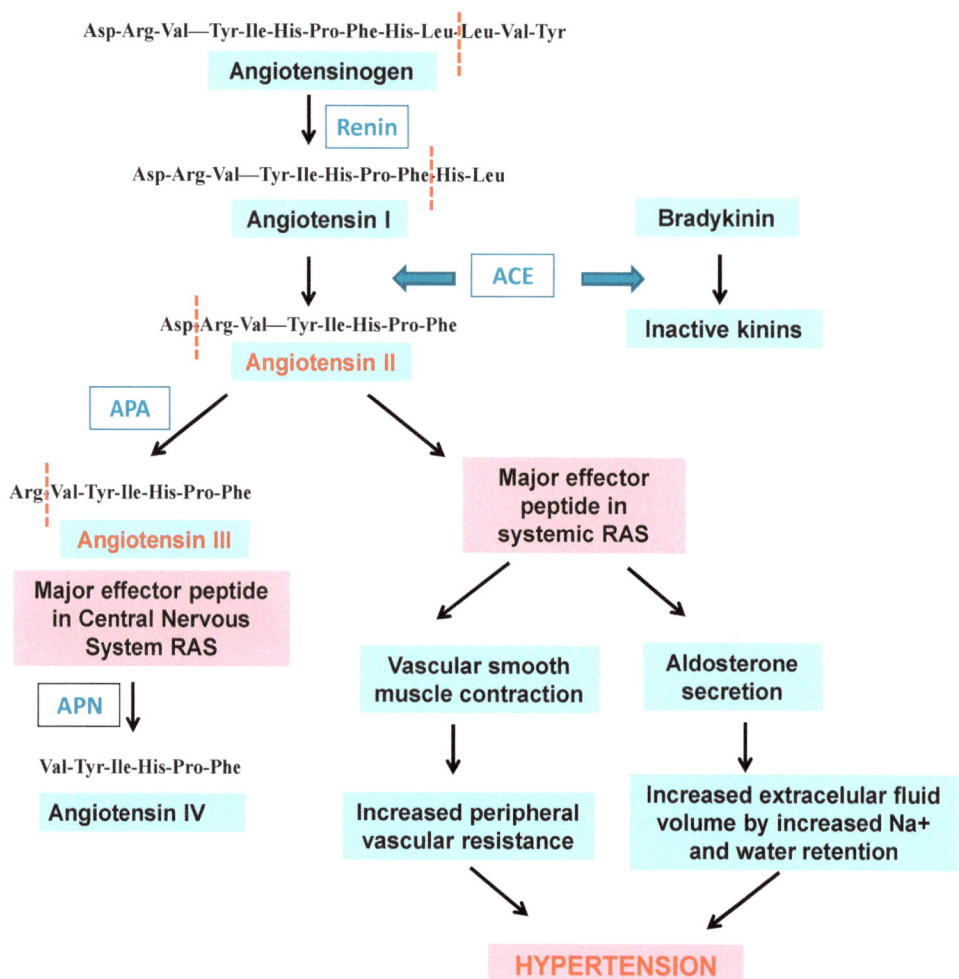

Figure 17. Role of aminopeptidase A and aminopeptidase N in the renin–angiotensin systems.

2.5. Clan MF: Family M17

Clan MF contains aminopeptidases that require cocatalytic metal ions for activity. The clan contains only the single family M17, a family of leucyl aminopeptidases [1], summarized in Table 7. The M17 aminopeptidases utilize two divalent metal ion cofactors to catalyze the removal of selected N-terminal amino acids from short peptide chains. M17 aminopeptidases are found in all kingdoms (Figure 18), wherein they possess a characteristic homo-hexameric three-dimensional arrangement of their monomers (Figure 19) and play roles in a wide range of cellular processes [9]. The proteolytic reaction contributes to intracellular protein turnover, a fundamental housekeeping process across all living organisms [132] (Figure 18). However, a wide range of additional functions beyond aminopeptidase activity have also been attributed to M17 family members. M17 aminopeptidases from plants possess chaperone activity [133], which might contribute to their function in the stress response pathway [134], while in bacteria they play roles in site-specific DNA recombination [135], and further, can moderate transcription of key virulence factors [136]. Therefore, the family of M17 aminopeptidases is multifunctional, capable of performing diverse organism-specific functions far beyond peptide hydrolysis (Figure 18).

Table 6. Summary of the preliminary characterization of inhibitory activities against porcine APA, porcine APN, and human APN in TCA 2.5% treated crude extracts from marine invertebrates (screening in the period 2015–2019). Effect on 3LL and PC3 tumor cell viability (adapted from [98]). ND: not determined.

Species	Phylum	IC$_{50}$ vs. pAPA (µg/mL)	IC$_{50}$ vs. pAPN (µg/ML)	IC$_{50}$ vs. hAPN (µg/mL)	IC$_{50}$ vs. 3LL Viability (µg/mL)	IC$_{50}$ vs. PC3 Viability (µg/mL)
Cenchritis muricatus	Mollusca	ND	ND	450.20 ± 77.40	214.00 ± 46.50	352.90 ± 65.00
Nerita peloronta	Mollusca	487 ± 11.03	287.03 ± 12.00	237.80 ± 20.90	273.30 ± 78.80	299.10 ± 31.70
Nerita versicolor	Mollusca	92.23 ± 12.34	132.11 ± 22.05	370.00 ± 50.00	358.80 ± 70.20	289.70 ± 39.70
Lissodendoryx (Lissodendoryx) isodictyalis	Porifera	659.87 ± 10.65	613.24 ± 10.76	11.70 ± 2.70	<5.00	<5.00
Tripneustes ventricosus	Echinodermata	11.03 ± 0.12	13.35 ± 3.91	25.00 ± 3.10	39.90 ± 2.00	77.00 ± 3.90
Echinaster (Othilia) echinophorus	Echinodermata	182.01 ± 67.12	112.55 ± 23.21	198.20 ± 27.20	265.70 ± 29.60	405.60 ± 50.40
Isostichopus badionotus	Echinodermata	1005.12 ± 293.32	11.08 ± 0.27	69.70 ± 10.00	57.10 ± 2.70	83.10 ± 3.00
Stichodactyla helianthus	Cnidaria	256.3 ± 10.00	136.56 ± 22.87	103.60 ± 20.60	110.80 ± 13.20	58.10 ± 7.50
Bunodosoma granuliferum	Cnidaria	ND	98.02 ± 18.05	567.60 ± 88.00	786.80 ± 37.10	711.30 ± 29.30
Physalia physalis	Cnidaria	ND	198.92 ± 10.76	123.10 ± 21.30	257.30 ± 6.70	234.50 ± 5.00
Bestatin (positive control)	-	25.50 ± 2.35	6.54 ± 0.82	6.70 ± 1.90	0.54 ± 0.01	3.15 ± 0.72
Amastatin (positive control)	-	75.45 ± 4.55	58.32 ± 3.34	63.45 ± 7.61	ND	ND

Table 7. Some members of the M17 family of the MF clan of metallopeptidases. (Compiled from https://www.ebi.ac.uk/merops/cgi-bin/, accessed on 11 January 2023).

Enzyme	IUBMB * Nomenclature	Merops ID	Sources
Leucyl aminopeptidase 3	3.4.11.1	M17.001	*Homo sapiens, Haemaphysalis longicornis, Mus musculus*
Leucyl aminopeptidase (plant-type)	3.4.11.1	M17.002	*Solanum lycopersicum*
PepA aminopeptidase	3.4.11.10	M17.003	*Escherichia coli, Pseudomonas aeruginosa*
PepB aminopeptidase	3.4.11.23	M17.004	*Escherichia coli, Salmonella typhimurium*
Mername-AA040 peptidase	-	M17.005	*Homo sapiens*
Leucyl aminopeptidase-1 (*Caenorhabditis*-type)	-	M17.006	*Caenorhabditis elegans*
M17 aminopeptidase (*Plasmodium* spp.)	3.4.11.1	M17.008	*Plasmodium* spp.
Aminopeptidase yspII (*Schizosaccharomyces* sp.)	-	M17.009	*Schizosaccharomyces* sp.
Leucyl aminopeptidase (*Bacillus*-type)	-	M17.010	*Geobacillus kaustophilus*
Leucyl aminopeptidase (*Fasciola*-type)	-	M17.011	*Fasciola hepática*
PwLAP aminopeptidase	-	M17.012	*Paragonimus westermani*
Cysteinylglycinase (*Treponema denticola*)-like peptidase	-	M17.013	*Treponema denticola*
LAPTc aminopeptidase	-	M17.014	*Trypanosoma cruzi, Leishmania major*
Aminopeptidase pepZ (*Staphylococcus* sp.)	-	M17.015	*Staphylococcus aureus*
Aminopeptidase A/I (*Helicobacter*-type)	-	M17.016	*Helicobacter pylori*
similar to cytosol aminopeptidase (*Rattus norvegicus*)	-	M17.950	*Rattus norvegicus*
At4g30920 (*Arabidopsis thaliana*)	-	M17.A01	*Arabidopsis thaliana*
At4g30910 (*Arabidopsis thaliana*)	-	M17.A02	*Arabidopsis thaliana*
At2g24200 (*Arabidopsis thaliana*)	-	M17.A03	*Arabidopsis thaliana*
CG7340 g.p. (*Drosophila melanogaster*)	-	M17.A04	*Drosophila melanogaster*
ZK353.6 (*Caenorhabditis elegans*)	-	M17.A05	*Caenorhabditis elegans*

* IUBMB: International Union of Biochemistry and Molecular Biology.

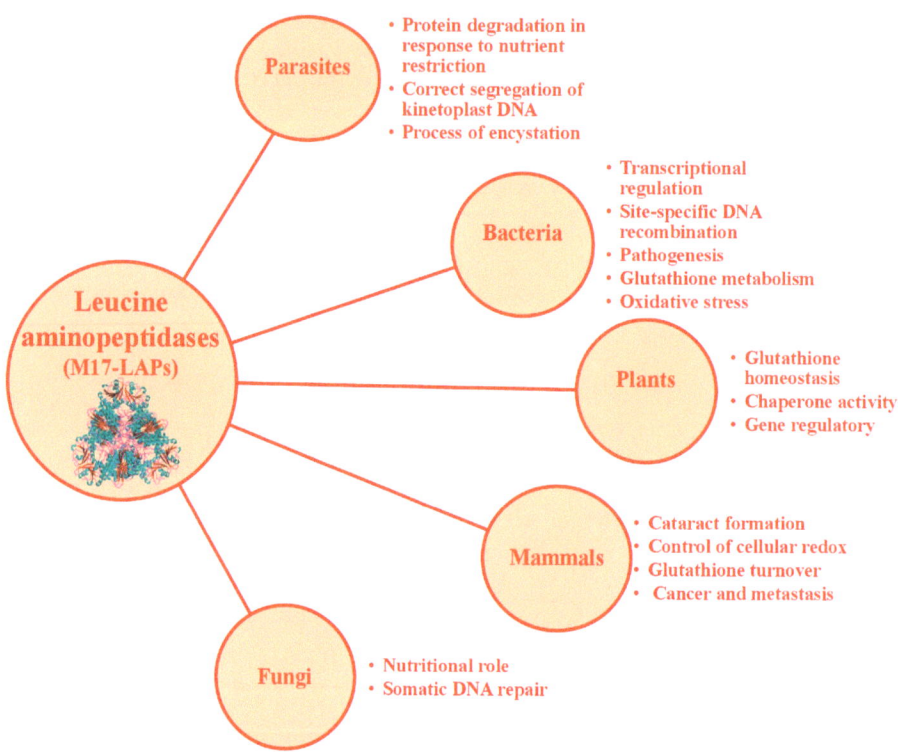

Figure 18. Functions of M17 aminopeptidases from different life groups.

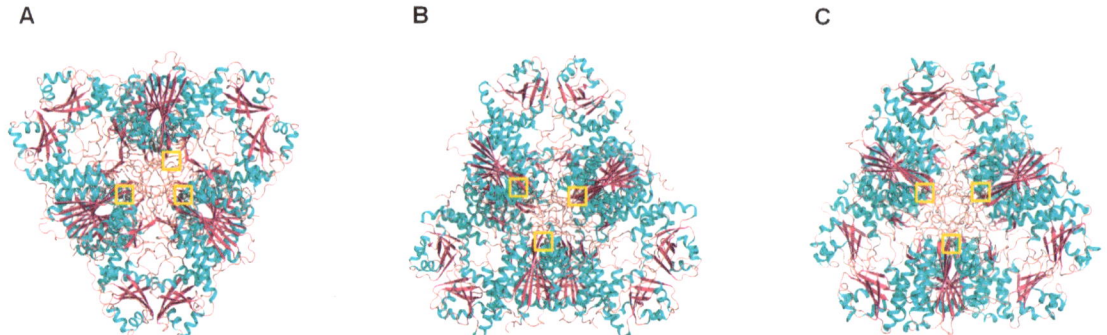

Figure 19. Cartoon representation of different M17 family aminopeptidases: (**A**) *Bos taurus* leucyl aminopeptidase 3 (PDB ID: 1bll), (**B**) *Escherichia coli* PepA aminopeptidase (PDB ID: 1gyt), and (**C**) ZK353.6 (*Caenorhabditis elegans*) (PDB ID: 42hc9). Colors: alpha-helices (cyan), beta sheets (warm pink), and loops (salmon). The zinc atoms are shown as gray spheres highlighted in a yellow box.

Leucyl aminopeptidases are also distributed in Apicomplexan protist parasites such as *Plasmodium falciparum*, the main agent of malaria in humans. The most important clinical stage of the complex *P. falciparum* life cycle [137], which has attracted the highest attention for the development of antimalarials, takes place in the human erythrocyte, where significant hemoglobin degradation occurs under the concerted action of endo- and exopeptidases [138]. PfA-M17 is involved in the final steps of hemoglobin digestion [139] and is currently a promising chemotherapeutic target as its inhibitors can kill parasites in vitro and in vivo (Figure 1) [9,140,141].

Through the technique of crystallography and X-ray diffraction, the three-dimensional structure of several members of this family has been elucidated, such as leucyl aminopeptidase 3 *from Bos taurus*, leucyl aminopeptidase (plant-type) from *Solanum lycopersicum*, PepA aminopeptidasa from *Escherichia coli* and other bacteria, and PfA-M17 from *Plasmodium falciparum* among others, being PfA-M17, joint with the mammalian enzyme, the more representative in tridimensional structure available at PDB, supporting the relevance of the search for new inhibitors as potential new antimalarial chemotherapy agents (Table 8, Figure 19).

Table 8. Crystallographic structures reported for members of the M17 family of metallopeptidases (Compiled from https://www.ebi.ac.uk/merops/cgi-bin/, accessed on 11 January 2023).

Enzyme	Source	Crystallographic Codes of the Structures at Protein Data Bank (PDB)
Leucyl aminopeptidase 3	*Bos taurus*	1BLL, 1BPM, 1BPN, 1LAM, 1LAN, 1LAP, 1LCP, 2EWB, 2J9A
Leucyl aminopeptidase (plant-type)	*Solanum lycopersicum*	4KSI, 5D8N
PepA aminopeptidase	*Escherichia coli*	1GYT
	Francisella tularensis	3PEI
	Pseudomonas putida	3H8E, 3H8F, 3H8G
	Xanthomonas oryzae	3JRU
PepB aminopeptidase	*Escherichia coli*	6OV8
	Yersinia pestis	6CXD
M17 aminopeptidase (*Plasmodium* spp.)	*Plasmodium falciparum*	3KQX, 3KQZ, 3KR4, 3KR5, 3T8W, 4K3N, 4R6T, 4R7M, 4X2T
LAPTc aminopeptidase	*Leishmania major*	5NTH
	Trypanosoma brucei	5NSK, 5NSM, 5NSQ, 5NTD
Aminopeptidase A/I (*Helicobacter*-type)	*Helicobacter pylori*	4ZI6, 4ZLA
ZK353.6 (*Caenorhabditis elegans*)	*Caenorhabditis elegans*	2HB6, 2HC9

Natural inhibitors of leucine aminopeptidases are scarce and have mainly been described from microorganisms sharing unspecific inhibition of APN and other M1 family inhibitors, such as actinonin, amastatin, bestatin, and various bestatin derivates (Figures 12 and 20) [18,139,142]. Several compounds from marine organisms have been described with anticancer and antiplasmodial activities [103,106,143–146]; however, only two of them have been linked with LAP inhibition or interaction [102,104,105]. In the next section, we review the information available regarding marine organisms as a promissory and still unexplored source of inhibitors of M17 enzyme inhibitors with biomedical relevance, mainly in cancer and malaria.

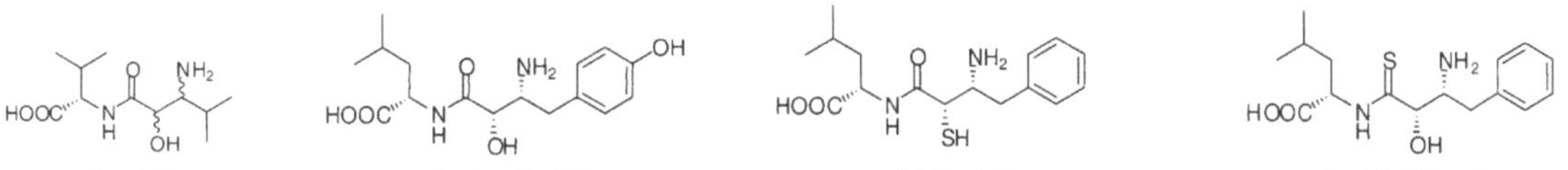

Figure 20. Examples of natural inhibitors of M17 enzymes.

2.6. Inhibitors of M17 Leucyl Aminopeptidases from Marine Organisms

In the work of Pascual et al. [98], the screening of inhibitory activities in aqueous extracts from species belonging to the phyla Mollusca, Poriphera, Echinodermata, and Cnidaria from the Cuban coastline involved human LAP (hLAP) and a recombinant form of PfA-M17 (rPfA-M17), both leucil aminopeptidases. As a result of preliminary assays, inhibitory activity vs. hLAP was detected in the species *Cenchritis muricatus, Lissodendoryx (Lissodendoryx) isodyctialis, Isostichopus badionotus*, and *Stichodactyla helianthus*. Inhibitory activity against rPfA-M17 was detected in the species *Cenchritis muricatus, Echinaster (Othilia) echinophorus, Isostichopus badionotus, Physalia physalis, Stichodactyla helianthus*, and *Buno-*

dosoma granuliferum (specific inhibitory activity values are summarized in Table 9, Figure 16), i.e., in four different phyla. The clarification of all aqueous crude extracts with a 2.5% TCA treatment increased the recovery of specific inhibitory activities as compared to their detection in positive crude extracts. The treatment also allowed the identification of inhibitory activities from species that were negative after screening using aqueous crude extracts. This result indicated that this clarification step was useful in the elimination of contaminants and/or induced dissociation from endogenous inhibitor–target complexes that did not allow the detection of inhibitory components in crude extracts.

Table 9. Summary of the screening of inhibitory activity against malarial rPfA-M17 and hLAP in aqueous extracts from marine invertebrates from the Cuban coastline (see note below). (adapted from Pascual et al. [98]).

Species	Phyla	Crude Extract rPfA-M17 sIA (U/mg)	Crude Extract hLAP sIA (U/mg)	2.5% TCA Treated Extracts rPfA-M17 sIA (U/mg)	2.5% TCA Treated Extracts hLAP sIA (U/mg)
Cenchritis muricatus	Mollusca	0.40	0.16	7.56	4.30
Nerita peloronta	Mollusca	ND	ND	10.61	6.48
Nerita versicolor	Mollusca	ND	ND	7.17	5.58
Lissodendoryx (Lissodendoryx) isodictyalis	Porifera	ND	0.27	256.13	312.01
Tripneustes ventricosus	Equinodermata	ND	ND	41.85	43.31
Echinaster (Othilia) echinophorus	Equinodermata	0.11	ND	9.10	7.85
Isostichopus badionotus	Equinodermata	0.18	1.24	55.83	27.86
Stichodactyla helianthus	Cnidaria	0.55	0.68	38.15	18.67
Bunodosoma granuliferum	Cnidaria	0.19	ND	5.45	4.08
Physalia physalis	Cnidaria	0.40	ND	19.21	11.00

NOTE: Inhibitory activities found in aqueous crude and 2.5% TCA extracts are expressed as specific Inhibitory Activity (sIA) in U/mg. One unit of enzyme activity was defined as the amount of enzyme needed to produce one arbitrary unit of fluorescence (AUF) per minute, and inhibitory activities are expressed per mg of extracts. The first column indicates the species, and the remaining columns refer to specific sIA. (ND): not detected.

All the clarified extracts showed inhibitory activity against both peptidases: malarial rPfA-M17 and native human LAP (Table 10, Figure 16). These activities have a concave dose-response behavior, corroborating the presence of reversible inhibitory molecules with IC_{50} values in µg/mL for both enzymes tested (Table 10). Inhibition of rPfA-M17 with IC_{50} values up to ~100 µg/mL is detected for 6 of the 10 extracts (those of *Cenchritis muricatus*, *Nerita peloronta*, *Lissodendoryx (Lissodendoryx) isodictyalis*, *Tripneustes ventricosus*, *Isostichopus badionotus*, and *Stichodactyla helianthus*). Comparing the inhibitions on rPfA-M17 and hLAP, in all cases, the plasmodial enzyme was more susceptible than its human counterpart, with ratios of selectivity between 1.87 and 60 times. The most selective extract was from *Nerita versicolor*, an attractive result even if its IC_{50} value for the malarial enzyme is moderate. All of the treated extracts displayed a dose-dependent effect on a chloroquine-resistant *Plasmodium falciparum* strain (FcB1) cell's viability, with the exception of *Cenchritis muricatus*, *Stichodactyla helianthus*, and *Bunodosoma granuliferum*. The best effects were obtained for *Tripneustes ventricosus* and *Lissodendoryx (Lissodendoryx) isodictyalis*. Particularly attractive were the *T. ventricosus* extracts that displayed a 300 times more potent effect on the FcB1 strain of *P. falciparum* than the human cancer cells, indicating parasite effect specificity. Additionally, this effect of the *T. ventricosus* extract on the FcB1 strain was stronger than the effect of bestatin (a pure compound). Due to the fact that IC_{50} for *L. isodyctialis* and *T. ventricosus* were lower on the FcB1 strain of *P. falciparum* than on the PfA-M17 recombinant enzyme, it is very likely that these extracts may contain not only PfA-M17 inhibitors but also other compounds active on other malarial targets. For example, for *L. isodyctialis*, inhibition of subtilisin from *Bacillus licheniformes* with an IC_{50} value of 3 μg/mL was described by Gonzalez et al. [39]. Another interesting result is the selectivity for rPfA-M17 regarding hLAP of *Nerita versicolor* extract showing effects on parasite growth with IC_{50} in the same order of enzyme inhibition, indicating that this species is also attractive. These results are the first and still only report of inhibition of M17 enzymes (human and plasmodial) by marine invertebrate species aqueous extracts and supports that sponges as well as marine invertebrates from other phyla such as mollusks, echinoderms, and cnidarians are a good and still underexplored source of potential anticancer and antimalarials associated with the inhibition of neutral aminopeptidases from the M1 and M17 families involved in these human pathologies.

Table 10. Summary of the IC_{50} determination for the 2.5% TCA clarified extracts against rPfA-M17 and hLAP. Preliminarndicates position with high degree of conservation of the resy inhibitory analyses on the growth of *Plasmodium falciparum* FcB1 strain are included in the last column (adapted from Pascual et al. [98]).

Species	IC_{50} Value vs. rPfA-M17 (μg/mL)	IC_{50} vs. hLAP (μg/mL)	IC_{50}hLAP/ IC_{50}rPfA-M17	IC_{50} Pf FcB1 (μg/mL)
Cenchritis muricatus	113.40 ± 3.00	341.00 ± 110.00	3.00	>400
Nerita peloronta	22.20 ± 2.70	329.50 ± 100.00	14.80	291.80 ± 38.50
Nerita versicolor	207.00 ± 30.60	12 429.60 ± 633.00	60.00	325.50 ± 0.80
Lissodendoryx (Lissodendoryx) isodictyalis	27.30 ± 9.40	66.30 ± 27.60	2.42	2.60 ± 0.60
Tripneustes ventricosus	84.80 ± 7.30	607.70 ± 300.50	7.16	0.24 ± 0.01
Echinaster (Othilia) echinophorus	127.50 ± 82.10	308.70 ± 100.00	2.42	201.60 ± 162.10
Isostichopus badionotus	86.70 ± 32.60	272.70 ± 63.50	3.13	183.70 ± 155.70
Stichodactyla helianthus	15.30 ± 6.20	234.90 ± 34.60	15.35	>400
Bunodosoma granuliferum	509.20 ± 100.90	1171.00 ± 92.10	2.29	>400
Physalia physalis	293.70 ± 100.00	550.00 ± 85.00	1.87	206.00 ± 84.00
Bestatin (positive control)	0.15 ± 0.02	11.83 ± 2.61	78.86	1.14 ± 0.27
Amastatin (positive control)	60.70 ± 19.84	158.05 ± 28.44	2.60	ND

M17 enzymes are not only a very well established target for malaria and other parasitic diseases but also for bacterial infections and chronic pathologies such as cancer. Bacterial LAPs (from gram-negative or -positive bacteria such as *Escherichia coli*, *Aeromonas proteolytica*, *Streptomyces lividans*, and *Pseudomonas aeruginosa*, among others) are important virulence factors [147]. Leucine aminopeptidase 3 in humans (LAP3) is associated with various diseases and cancers, such as breast cancer and ovarian cancer [148]. Recently, Yang et al. [149] identified two compounds named compounds 5 and 6 (Figure 21) from 43 natural marine products screened as new inhibitors of LAP3 (from K562 cells with overexpression of LAP3). The inhibition of LAP3 at 30 μM by these two compounds was stronger than that of bestatin used as a control of inhibition in the same conditions. The authors explored the anticancer properties of these new compounds in different models of breast cancer. The results showed that compounds 5 and 6 displayed stronger antiproliferative activity of the breast cancer tumor cells MDA-MB-231 at 30 μM than bestatin. Additionally, both compounds 5 and 6 displayed a more potent suppression effect on the migration of MDA-MB-231 cells than bestatin (the effect of compound **5** was stronger than that of compound **6**). It is well established that LAP3 plays an important role in the metastasis of breast cancer; hence LAP3 inhibitors may have a remarkable effect on the treatment of breast cancer [149].

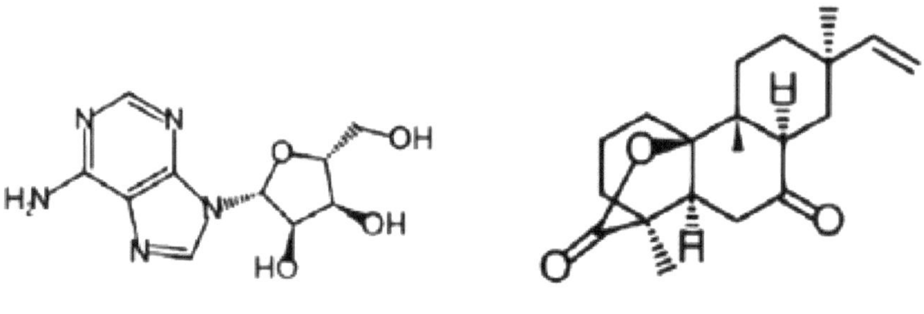

compound 5   **compound 6**

Figure 21. Compounds **5** and **6** as new inhibitors of LAP3 (adapted from Yang et al. [149]).

3. Conclusions

Marine biodiversity is an important and promising source of inhibitors of metalloexopeptidases from different families, in particular M1 and M17 enzymes with biomedical applications in human diseases. The results reviewed in the present contribution support and encourage further fundamental applicative studies with inhibitors isolated from marine species in different biomedical models associated with the activity of these families of exopeptidases.

Author Contributions: Conceptualization, I.P.A. and F.X.A.; writing—original draft preparation I.P.A., F.A.G., M.E.V.T., Y.A.S., D.O.d.S., B.S.R., I.F., M.S. and F.X.A.; writing—review and editing, I.P.A., F.A.G. and F.X.A.; visualization, I.P.A. and M.E.V.T. All authors have read and agreed to the published version of the manuscript.

Funding: This research was funded by the French ANR-12-BS07-0020 project MAMMAMIA: "design of potential anti MAlarial M1/M17 AMinopeptIdase Agents" and UH-CIM project: "New inhibitors of aminopeptidases with potential applications in cancer" (2020–2023).

Data Availability Statement: Not applicable.

Acknowledgments: This contribution is dedicated to María de los Angeles Chávez, renowned Cuban Biochemistry Professor, founder of the teaching of Biochemistry in Cuba and the Center for Protein Studies at the University of Havana. She significantly contributed to the knowledge in the field of peptidase inhibitors of different mechanistic classes isolated from Cuban marine biodiversity. To Jean Louis Charli, IBT-UNAM, Cuernavaca, Mexico, for the revision of the manuscript and useful comments. To Aymara Cabrera Munoz, from the Center for Protein Studies, Faculty of Biology, University of Havana, who kindly supplied images for Figure 4. To José Espinosa, PhD from ICIMAR, CITMA, Cuba, who kindly supplied the pictures of the marine species. To IFS-OPCW research grants 3276/1, 3276/2, 3276/3, to Isel Pascual Alonso. To IUBMB mid-career fellowship program for supporting the research stay of Isel Pascual Alonso at Laboratory MCAM, UMR 7245, MNHN, Paris, in 2014 and in Instituto de Biotecnología, UNAM, Cuernavaca, Mexico, in 2017. To the French ANR-12-BS07-0020 project MAMMAMIA: "design of potential anti MAlarial M1/M17 AMinopeptIdase Agents". To UH-CIM project: "New inhibitors of aminopeptidases with potential applications in cancer" (2020–2023).

Conflicts of Interest: The authors declare no conflict of interest.

References

1. Rawlings, N.D.; Barrett, A.J.; Thomas, P.D.; Huang, X.; Bateman, A.; Finn, R.D. The Merops Database of Proteolytic Enzymes, Their Substrates and Inhibitors in 2017 and a Comparison with Peptidases in the Panther Database. *Nucleic Acids Res.* **2018**, *46*, D624–D632. [CrossRef] [PubMed]
2. Drag, M.; Salvesen, G.S. Emerging Principles in Protease-Based Drug Discovery. *Nat. Rev. Drug Discov.* **2010**, *9*, 690–701. [CrossRef] [PubMed]

3. Deu, E.; Verdoes, M.; Bogyo, M. New Approaches for Dissecting Protease Functions to Improve Probe Development and Drug Discovery. *Nat. Struct. Mol. Biol.* **2012**, *19*, 9–16. [CrossRef] [PubMed]
4. Kryvalap, Y.; Czyzyk, J. The Role of Proteases and Serpin Protease Inhibitors in Β-Cell Biology and Diabetes. *Biomolecules* **2022**, *12*, 67. [CrossRef]
5. Rai, M.; Curley, M.; Coleman, Z.; Demontis, F. Contribution of Proteases to the Hallmarks of Aging and to Age-Related Neurodegeneration. *Aging Cell* **2022**, *21*, e13603. [CrossRef]
6. Verhulst, E.; Garnier, D.; De Meester, I.; Bauvois, B. Validating Cell Surface Proteases as Drug Targets for Cancer Therapy: What Do We Know, and Where Do We Go? *Cancers* **2022**, *14*, 624. [CrossRef]
7. Newman, D.J.; Cragg, G.M. Drugs and Drug Candidates from Marine Sources: An Assessment of the Current State of Play. *Planta Med.* **2016**, *82*, 775–789. [CrossRef]
8. Drinkwater, N.; Lee, J.; Yang, W.; Malcolm, T.R.; McGowan, S. M1 Aminopeptidases as Drug Targets: Broad Applications or Therapeutic Niche? *FEBS J.* **2017**, *284*, 1473–1488. [CrossRef]
9. Drinkwater, N.; Malcolm, T.R.; McGowan, S. M17 Aminopeptidases Diversify Function by Moderating Their Macromolecular Assemblies and Active Site Environment. *Biochimie* **2019**, *166*, 38–51. [CrossRef]
10. Hammers, D.; Carothers, K.; Lee, S. The Role of Bacterial Proteases in Microbe and Host-Microbe Interactions. *Curr. Drug Targets* **2022**, *23*, 222–239. [CrossRef]
11. Carvalho, L.A.; Bernardes, G.J. The Impact of Activity-Based Protein Profiling in Malaria Drug Discovery. *ChemMedChem* **2022**, *17*, e202200174. [CrossRef] [PubMed]
12. Beltran-Hortelano, I.; Alcolea, V.; Font, M.; Pérez-Silanes, S. Examination of Multiple *Trypanosoma cruzi* Targets in a New Drug Discovery Approach for Chagas Disease. *Bioorganic Med. Chem.* **2022**, *58*, 116577. [CrossRef] [PubMed]
13. Vermelho, A.B.; Cardoso, V.; Mansoldo, F.R.P.; Supuran, C.T.; Cedrola, S.M.L.; Rodrigues, I.A.; Rodrigues, G.C. Chagas Disease: Drug Development and Parasite Targets. In *Antiprotozoal Drug Development and Delivery*; Springer: Berlin/Heidelberg, Germany, 2022; pp. 49–81.
14. Mukherjee, R.; Dikic, I. Regulation of Host-Pathogen Interactions Via the Ubiquitin System. *Annu. Rev. Microbiol.* **2022**, *76*, 211–233. [CrossRef] [PubMed]
15. Salomon, E.; Schmitt, M.; Marapaka, A.K.; Stamogiannos, A.; Revelant, G.; Schmitt, C.; Alavi, S.; Florent, I.; Addlagatta, A.; Stratikos, E.; et al. Aminobenzosuberone Scaffold as a Modular Chemical Tool for the Inhibition of Therapeutically Relevant M1 Aminopeptidases. *Molecules* **2018**, *23*, 2607. [CrossRef] [PubMed]
16. Albiston, A.L.; Ye, S.; Chai, S.Y. Membrane Bound Members of the M1 Family: More Than Aminopeptidases. *Protein Pept. Lett.* **2004**, *11*, 491–500. [CrossRef] [PubMed]
17. Carl-McGrath, S.; Lendeckel, U.; Ebert, M.; Röcken, C. Ectopeptidases in Tumour Biology: A Review. *Histol. Histopathol.* **2006**, *12*, 1339–1353.
18. Mucha, A.; Drag, M.; Dalton, J.P.; Kafarski, P. Metallo-Aminopeptidase Inhibitors. *Biochimie* **2010**, *92*, 1509–1529. [CrossRef] [PubMed]
19. Amin, S.A.; Adhikari, N.; Jha, T. Design of Aminopeptidase N Inhibitors as Anti-Cancer Agents. *J. Med. Chem.* **2018**, *61*, 6468–6490. [CrossRef]
20. Alvarez, C.; Pazos, F.; Soto, C.; Laborde, R.; Lanio, M.E. Pore-Forming Toxins from Sea Anemones: From Protein-Membrane Interaction to Its Implications for Developing Biomedical Applications. In *Advances in Biomembranes and Lipid Self-Assembly*; Elsevier: Amsterdam, The Netherlands, 2020; pp. 129–183.
21. Alvarez, C.; Soto, C.; Cabezas, S.; Alvarado-Mesén, J.; Laborde, R.; Pazos, F.; Ros, U.; Hernández, A.M.; Lanio, M.E. Panorama of the Intracellular Molecular Concert Orchestrated by Actinoporins, Pore-Forming Toxins from Sea Anemones. *Toxins* **2021**, *13*, 567. [CrossRef]
22. Martell, E.M.; González-Garcia, M.; Ständker, L.; Otero-González, A.J. Host Defense Peptides as Immunomodulators: The Other Side of the Coin. *Peptides* **2021**, *146*, 170644. [CrossRef]
23. Rodríguez, A.A.; Otero-González, A.; Ghattas, M.; Ständker, L. Discovery, Optimization, and Clinical Application of Natural Antimicrobial Peptides. *Biomedicines* **2021**, *9*, 1381. [CrossRef] [PubMed]
24. Riccio, G.; Ruocco, N.; Mutalipassi, M.; Costantini, M.; Zupo, V.; Coppola, D.; De Pascale, D.; Lauritano, C. Ten-Year Research Update Review: Antiviral Activities from Marine Organisms. *Biomolecules* **2020**, *10*, 1007. [CrossRef] [PubMed]
25. Nakao, Y.; Fusetani, N. Enzyme Inhibitors from Marine Invertebrates. *J. Nat. Prod.* **2007**, *70*, 689–710. [CrossRef]
26. Pujiastuti, D.Y.; Amin, M.N.G.; Alamsjah, M.A.; Hsu, J.-L. Marine Organisms as Potential Sources of Bioactive Peptides That Inhibit the Activity of Angiotensin I-Converting Enzyme: A Review. *Molecules* **2019**, *24*, 2541. [CrossRef]
27. Tischler, D. A Perspective on Enzyme Inhibitors from Marine Organisms. *Mar. Drugs* **2020**, *18*, 431. [CrossRef] [PubMed]
28. Moodie, L.W.K.; Sepčić, K.; Turk, T.; Frangež, R.; Svenson, J. Natural Cholinesterase Inhibitors from Marine Organisms. *Nat. Prod. Rep.* **2019**, *36*, 1053–1092. [CrossRef]
29. Alonso-del-Rivero, M.; Trejo, S.A.; Rodriguez de la Vega, M.; González, Y.; Bronsoms, S.; Canals, F.; Delfín, J.; Diaz, J.; Aviles, F.X.; Chávez, M.A. A Novel Metallocarboxypeptidase-Like Enzyme from the Marine Annelid *Sabellastarte magnifica*–a Step into the Invertebrate World of Proteases. *FEBS J.* **2009**, *276*, 4875–4890. [CrossRef]

30. Alonso, I.P.; Méndez, L.R.; Almeida, F.; Tresano, M.E.V.; Sánchez, Y.A.; Hernández-Zanuy, A.; Álvarez-Lajonchere, L.; Díaz, D.; Sánchez, B.; Florent, I. Marine Organisms: A Source of Biomedically Relevant Metallo M1, M2 and M17 Exopeptidase Inhibitors. *Rev. Cuba. Cienc. Biológicas* **2020**, *8*, 1–36.

31. Chávez, M.; Delfín, J.; Díaz, J.; Pérez, U.; Martínez, J.; González, J.; Márquez, M.; Más, R. Caracterización de un Inhibidor de Proteasas Obtenido de la Anémona *S. helianthus*. *Rev. CENIC* **1988**, *19*, 82.

32. Delfin, J.; Gonzalez, Y.; Diaz, J.; Chavez, M. Proteinase Inhibitor from *Stichodactyla helianthus*: Purification, Characterization and Immobilization. *Arch. Med. Res.* **1994**, *25*, 199–204.

33. Delfin, J.; Martinez, I.; Antuch, W.; Morera, V.; Gonzalez, Y.; Rodriguez, R.; Marquez, M.; Saroyan, A.; Larionova, N.; Diaz, J. Purification, Characterization and Immobilization of Proteinase Inhibitors from *Stichodactyla helianthus*. *Toxicon* **1996**, *34*, 1367–1376. [CrossRef] [PubMed]

34. Lenarčič, B.; Ritonja, A.; Štrukelj, B.; Turk, B.; Turk, V. Equistatin, a New Inhibitor of Cysteine Proteinases from *Actinia equina*, Is Structurally Related to Thyroglobulin Type-1 Domain. *J. Biol. Chem.* **1997**, *272*, 13899–13903. [CrossRef] [PubMed]

35. González, Y.; Araujo, M.; Oliva, M.; Sampaio, C.; Chávez, M. Purification and Preliminary Characterization of a Plasma Kallikrein Inhibitor Isolated from Sea Hares *Aplysia dactylomela* Rang, 1828. *Toxicon* **2004**, *43*, 219–223. [CrossRef] [PubMed]

36. Reytor, M.L.; González, Y.; Pascual, I.; Hernández, A.; Chávez M, Á.; Alonso del Rivero, M. Screening of Protease Inhibitory Activity in Extracts of Five Ascidian Species from Cuban Coasts. *Biotecnol. Apl.* **2011**, *28*, 77–82.

37. Alonso-Del-Rivero, M.; Trejo, S.; Reytor, M.L.; Rodriguez-De-La-Vega, M.; Delfin, J.; Diaz, J.; Gonzalez, M.L.R.; Canals, F.; Chavez, M.A.; Aviles, F.X. Tri-Domain Bifunctional Inhibitor of Metallocarboxypeptidases a and Serine Proteases Isolated from Marine Annelid *Sabellastarte magnifica*. *J. Biol. Chem.* **2012**, *287*, 15427–15438. [CrossRef] [PubMed]

38. Salas-Sarduy, E.; Cabrera-Muñoz, A.; Cauerhff, A.; González-González, Y.; Trejo, S.A.; Chidichimo, A.; de los Angeles Chávez-Planes, M.; José Cazzulo, J. Antiparasitic Effect of a Fraction Enriched in Tight-Binding Protease Inhibitors Isolated from the Caribbean Coral *Plexaura homomalla*. *Exp. Parasitol.* **2013**, *135*, 611–622. [CrossRef]

39. González, L.; Sánchez, R.E.; Rojas, L.; Pascual, I.; García-Fernández, R.; Chávez, M.A.; Betzel, C. Screening of Protease Inhibitory Activity in Aqueous Extracts of Marine Invertebrates from Cuban Coast. *Am. J. Anal. Chem.* **2016**, *7*, 319–331. [CrossRef]

40. Salas-Sarduy, E.; Guerra, Y.; Covaleda Cortés, G.; Avilés, F.X.; Chávez Planes, M.A. Identification of Tight-Binding Plasmepsin Ii and Falcipain 2 Inhibitors in Aqueous Extracts of Marine Invertebrates by the Combination of Enzymatic and Interaction-Based Assays. *Mar. Drugs* **2017**, *15*, 123. [CrossRef]

41. Covaleda, G.; Trejo, S.A.; Salas-Sarduy, E.; del Rivero, M.A.; Chavez, M.A.; Aviles, F.X. Intensity Fading Maldi-Tof Mass Spectrometry and Functional Proteomics Assignments to Identify Protease Inhibitors in Marine Invertebrates. *J. Proteom.* **2017**, *165*, 75–92. [CrossRef]

42. Hong, T.T.; Dat, T.T.H.; Cuong, P.V.; Cuc, N.T.K. Protease Inhibitors from Marine Sponge and Sponge-Associated Microorganisms. *Vietnam. J. Sci. Technol.* **2018**, *56*, 405–423. [CrossRef]

43. Ikegami, S.; Kobayashi, H.; Myotoishi, Y.; Ohta, S.; Kato, K.H. Selective Inhibition of Exoplasmic Membrane Fusion in Echinoderm Gametes with Jaspisin, a Novel Antihatching Substance Isolated from a Marine Sponge. *J. Biol. Chem.* **1994**, *269*, 23262–23267. [CrossRef] [PubMed]

44. Kato, K.H.; Takemoto, K.; Kato, E.; Miyazaki, K.; Kobayashi, H.; Ikegami, S. Inhibition of Sea Urchin Fertilization by Jaspisin, a Specific Inhibitor of Matrix Metalloendoproteinase. *Dev. Growth Differ.* **1998**, *40*, 221–230. [CrossRef] [PubMed]

45. Fusetani, N.; Fujita, M.; Nakao, Y.; Matsunaga, S.; van Soest, R.W. Tokaramide a, a New Cathepsin B Inhibitor from the Marine Sponge *Theonella* Aff. *mirabilis*. *Bioorganic Med. Chem. Lett.* **1999**, *9*, 3397–3402. [CrossRef] [PubMed]

46. Fujita, M.; Nakao, Y.; Matsunaga, S.; van Soest, R.W.; Itoh, Y.; Seiki, M.; Fusetani, N. Callysponginol Sulfate a, an Mt1-Mmp Inhibitor Isolated from the Marine Sponge *Callyspongia truncata*. *J. Nat. Prod.* **2003**, *66*, 569–571. [CrossRef] [PubMed]

47. Fujita, M.; Nakao, Y.; Matsunaga, S.; Seiki, M.; Itoh, Y.; Yamashita, J.; Van Soest, R.W.; Fusetani, N. Ageladine A: An Antiangiogenic Matrixmetalloproteinase Inhibitor from the Marine Sponge *Agelas* N *Akamurai*. *J. Am. Chem. Soc.* **2003**, *125*, 15700–15701. [CrossRef]

48. Shim, J.S.; Lee, H.-S.; Shin, J.; Kwon, H.J. Psammaplin a, a Marine Natural Product, Inhibits Aminopeptidase N and Suppresses Angiogenesis in Vitro. *Cancer Lett.* **2004**, *203*, 163–169. [CrossRef]

49. Pascual, I.; Gil-Parrado, S.; Cisneros, M.; Joseph-Bravo, P.; Dıaz, J.; Possani, L.D.; Charli, J.L.; Chávez, M. Purification of a Specific Inhibitor of Pyroglutamyl Aminopeptidase Ii from the Marine Annelide *Hermodice carunculata*: In Vivo Effects in Rodent Brain. *Int. J. Biochem. Cell Biol.* **2004**, *36*, 138–152. [CrossRef]

50. Thomas, N.V.; Kim, S.-K. Metalloproteinase Inhibitors: Status and Scope from Marine Organisms. *Biochem. Res. Int.* **2010**, *2010*, 845975. [CrossRef]

51. del Rivero, M.A.; Reytor, M.L.; Trejo, S.A.; Chávez, M.A.; Avilés, F.X.; Reverter, D. A Noncanonical Mechanism of Carboxypeptidase Inhibition Revealed by the Crystal Structure of the Tri-Kunitz Smci in Complex with Human Cpa4. *Structure* **2013**, *21*, 1118–1126.

52. Covaleda, G.; del Rivero, M.A.; Chávez, M.A.; Avilés, F.X.; Reverter, D. Crystal Structure of Novel Metallocarboxypeptidase Inhibitor from Marine Mollusk *Nerita versicolor* in Complex with Human Carboxypeptidase A4. *J. Biol. Chem.* **2012**, *287*, 9250–9258. [CrossRef]

53. Cabrera-Muñoz, A.; Valiente, P.A.; Rojas, L.; Antigua, M.A.D.R.; Pires, J.R. Nmr Structure of Cmpi-Ii, a Non-Classical Kazal Protease Inhibitor: Understanding Its Conformational Dynamics and Subtilisin a Inhibition. *J. Struct. Biol.* **2019**, *206*, 280–294. [CrossRef] [PubMed]

54. Pascual Alonso, I.; Rivera Méndez, L.; Valdés-Tresanco, M.E.; Bounaadja, L.; Schmitt, M.; Arrebola Sánchez, Y.; Alvarez Lajonchere, L.; Charli, J.L.; Florent, I. Biochemical Evidences for M1-, M17- and M18-Like Aminopeptidases in Marine Invertebrates from Cuban Coastline. *Z. Für Nat. C* **2020**, *75*, 397–407. [CrossRef] [PubMed]

55. Sarfaraj, H.M.; Sheeba, F.; Saba, A.; Khan, M. *Marine Natural Products: A Lead for Anti-Cancer*; NISCAIR-CSIR: New Delhi, India, 2012.

56. Nakao, Y.; Oku, N.; Matsunaga, S.; Fusetani, N. Cyclotheonamides E2 and E3, New Potent Serine Protease Inhibitors from the Marine Sponge of the Genus *Theonella*. *J. Nat. Prod.* **1998**, *61*, 667–670. [CrossRef] [PubMed]

57. Hanessian, S.; Tremblay, M.; Petersen, J.F. The N-Acyloxyiminium Ion Aza-Prins Route to Octahydroindoles: Total Synthesis and Structural Confirmation of the Antithrombotic Marine Natural Product Oscillarin. *J. Am. Chem. Soc.* **2004**, *126*, 6064–6071. [CrossRef]

58. Gunasekera, S.P.; McCarthy, P.J.; Longley, R.E.; Pomponi, S.A.; Wright, A.E.; Lobkovsky, E.; Clardy, J. Discorhabdin P, a New Enzyme Inhibitor from a Deep-Water Caribbean Sponge of the Genus *Batzella*. *J. Nat. Prod.* **1999**, *62*, 173–175. [CrossRef]

59. Gunasekera, S.P.; McCarthy, P.J.; Longley, R.E.; Pomponi, S.A.; Wright, A.E. Secobatzellines a and B, Two New Enzyme Inhibitors from a Deep-Water Caribbean Sponge of the Genus *Batzella*. *J. Nat. Prod.* **1999**, *62*, 1208–1211. [CrossRef] [PubMed]

60. Hu, J.F.; Schetz, J.A.; Kelly, M.; Peng, J.N.; Ang, K.K.; Flotow, H.; Leong, C.Y.; Ng, S.B.; Buss, A.D.; Wilkins, S.P. New Antiinfective and Human 5-Ht2 Receptor Binding Natural and Semisynthetic Compounds from the Jamaican Sponge *Smenospongia aurea*. *J. Nat. Prod.* **2002**, *65*, 476–480. [CrossRef] [PubMed]

61. Fujita, M.; Nakao, Y.; Matsunaga, S.; Nishikawa, T.; Fusetani, N. Sodium 1-(12-Hydroxy) Octadecanyl Sulfate, an Mmp2 Inhibitor, Isolated from a Tunicate of the Family *Polyclinidae*. *J. Nat. Prod.* **2002**, *65*, 1936–1938. [CrossRef]

62. Joe, M.-J.; Kim, S.-N.; Choi, H.-Y.; Shin, W.-S.; Park, G.-M.; Kang, D.-W.; Kim, Y.K. The Inhibitory Effects of Eckol and Dieckol from *Ecklonia stolonifera* on the Expression of Matrix Metalloproteinase-1 in Human Dermal Fibroblasts. *Biol. Pharm. Bull.* **2006**, *29*, 1735–1739. [CrossRef]

63. Harper, J.W.; Powers, J.C. Inhibitors of Metallo-Proteases. In *Proteinase Inhibitors*; Elsevier: Amsterdam, The Netherlands, 1986; pp. 219–298.

64. Rawlings, N.D.; Barrett, A.J. Evolutionary Families of Peptidases. *Biochem. J.* **1993**, *290*, 205–218. [CrossRef]

65. Rawlings, N.D.; Barrett, A.J. [13] Evolutionary Families of Metallopeptidases. In *Methods in Enzymology*; Elsevier: Amsterdam, The Netherlands, 1995; pp. 183–228.

66. Reeck, G.R.; de Haën, C.; Teller, D.C.; Doolittle, R.F.; Fitch, W.M.; Dickerson, R.E.; Chambon, P.; McLachlan, A.D.; Margoliash, E.; Jukes, T.H.; et al. Homology in Proteins and Nucleic Acids: A Terminology Muddle and a Way out of It. *Cell* **1987**, *50*, 667. [CrossRef] [PubMed]

67. Haeggström, J.Z.; Nordlund, P.; Thunnissen, M.M. Functional Properties and Molecular Architecture of Leukotriene A4 Hydrolase, a Pivotal Catalyst of Chemotactic Leukotriene Formation. *Sci. World J.* **2002**, *2*, 1734–1749. [CrossRef] [PubMed]

68. Fukasawa, K.M.; Fukasawa, K.; Harada, M.; Hirose, J.; Izumi, T.; Shimizu, T. Aminopeptidase B Is Structurally Related to Leukotriene-A4 Hydrolase but Is Not a Bifunctional Enzyme with Epoxide Hydrolase Activity. *Biochem. J.* **1999**, *339*, 497–502. [CrossRef] [PubMed]

69. Klinke, T.; Rump, A.; Pönisch, R.; Schellenberger, W.; Müller, E.C.; Otto, A.; Klimm, W.; Kriegel, T.M. Identification and Characterization of Caape2–a Neutral Arginine/Alanine/Leucine-Specific Metallo-Aminopeptidase from *Candida albicans*. *FEMS Yeast Res.* **2008**, *8*, 858–869. [CrossRef]

70. Wong, A.H.M.; Zhou, D.; Rini, J.M. The X-Ray Crystal Structure of Human Aminopeptidase N Reveals a Novel Dimer and the Basis for Peptide Processing. *J. Biol. Chem.* **2012**, *287*, 36804–36813. [CrossRef]

71. Thunnissen, M.M.; Nordlund, P.; Haeggström, J.Z. Crystal Structure of Human Leukotriene A4 Hydrolase, a Bifunctional Enzyme in Inflammation. *Nat. Struct. Biol.* **2001**, *8*, 131–135. [CrossRef]

72. Kyrieleis, O.J.; Goettig, P.; Kiefersauer, R.; Huber, R.; Brandstetter, H. Crystal Structures of the Tricorn Interacting Factor F3 from Thermoplasma Acidophilum, a Zinc Aminopeptidase in Three Different Conformations. *J. Mol. Biol.* **2005**, *349*, 787–800. [CrossRef]

73. Ito, K.; Nakajima, Y.; Onohara, Y.; Takeo, M.; Nakashima, K.; Matsubara, F.; Ito, T.; Yoshimoto, T. Crystal Structure of Aminopeptidase N (Proteobacteria Alanyl Aminopeptidase) from *Escherichia coli* and Conformational Change of Methionine 260 Involved in Substrate Recognition. *J. Biol. Chem.* **2006**, *281*, 33664–33676. [CrossRef]

74. McGowan, S.; Porter, C.J.; Lowther, J.; Stack, C.M.; Golding, S.J.; Skinner-Adams, T.S.; Trenholme, K.R.; Teuscher, F.; Donnelly, S.M.; Grembecka, J.; et al. Structural Basis for the Inhibition of the Essential Plasmodium Falciparum M1 Neutral Aminopeptidase. *Proc. Natl. Acad. Sci. USA* **2009**, *106*, 2537–2542. [CrossRef]

75. Harbut, M.B.; Velmourougane, G.; Dalal, S.; Reiss, G.; Whisstock, J.C.; Onder, O.; Brisson, D.; McGowan, S.; Klemba, M.; Greenbaum, D.C. Bestatin-Based Chemical Biology Strategy Reveals Distinct Roles for Malaria M1-and M17-Family Aminopeptidases. *Proc. Natl. Acad. Sci. USA* **2011**, *108*, E526–E534. [CrossRef]

76. Salomon, E.; Schmitt, M.; Mouray, E.; McEwen, A.G.; Bounaadja, L.; Torchy, M.; Poussin-Courmontagne, P.; Alavi, S.; Tarnus, C.; Cavarelli, J.; et al. Aminobenzosuberone Derivatives as Pfa-M1 Inhibitors: Molecular Recognition and Antiplasmodial Evaluation. *Bioorganic Chem.* **2020**, *98*, 103750. [CrossRef] [PubMed]
77. Yang, Y.; Liu, C.; Lin, Y.-L.; Li, F. Structural Insights into Central Hypertension Regulation by Human Aminopeptidase A. *J. Biol. Chem.* **2013**, *288*, 25638–25645. [CrossRef] [PubMed]
78. Kochan, G.; Krojer, T.; Harvey, D.; Fischer, R.; Chen, L.; Vollmar, M.; von Delft, F.; Kavanagh, K.L.; Brown, M.A.; Bowness, P.; et al. Crystal Structures of the Endoplasmic Reticulum Aminopeptidase-1 (Erap1) Reveal the Molecular Basis for N-Terminal Peptide Trimming. *Proc. Natl. Acad. Sci. USA* **2011**, *108*, 7745–7750. [CrossRef] [PubMed]
79. Chen, J.; Wang, Y.; Zhong, Q.; Wu, Y.; Xia, W. Purification and Characterization of a Novel Angiotensin-I Converting Enzyme (Ace) Inhibitory Peptide Derived from Enzymatic Hydrolysate of Grass Carp Protein. *Peptides* **2012**, *33*, 52–58. [CrossRef] [PubMed]
80. Gago, F. Computational Approaches to Enzyme Inhibition by Marine Natural Products in the Search for New Drugs. *Mar. Drugs* **2023**, *21*, 100. [CrossRef] [PubMed]
81. Omar, A.M.; Mohammad, K.A.; Sindi, I.A.; Mohamed, G.A.; Ibrahim, S.R.M. Unveiling the Efficacy of Sesquiterpenes from Marine Sponge *Dactylospongia elegans* in Inhibiting Dihydrofolate Reductase Using Docking and Molecular Dynamic Studies. *Molecules* **2023**, *28*, 1292. [CrossRef] [PubMed]
82. Joseph-Bravo, P.; Jaimes-Hoy, L.; Uribe, R.M.; Charli, J.L. 60 Years of Neuroendocrinology: TRH, the First Hypophysiotropic Releasing Hormone Isolated: Control of the Pituitary–Thyroid Axis. *J. Endocrinol.* **2015**, *226*, T85–T100. [CrossRef]
83. Kronenberg, H.M.; Shlomo Melmed, M.D.; Polonsky, K.S.; Wilson, J.D.; Foster, D.W.; Kronenberg, H.M. *Williams Textbook of Endocrinology*; Saunders: Philadelphia, PA, USA, 2002.
84. Charli, J.L.; Rodríguez-Rodríguez, A.; Hernández-Ortega, K.; Cote-Vélez, A.; Uribe, R.M.; Jaimes-Hoy, L.; Joseph-Bravo, P. The Thyrotropin-Releasing Hormone-Degrading Ectoenzyme, a Therapeutic Target? *Front. Pharm.* **2020**, *11*, 640. [CrossRef]
85. A Kelly, J. Thyrotropin-Releasing Hormone: Basis and Potential for Its Therapeutic Use. *Essays Biochem.* **1995**, *30*, 133.
86. Charli, J.-L.; Mendez, M.; Vargas, M.-A.; Cisneros, M.; Assai, M.; Joseph-Bravo, P.; Wilk, S. Pyroglutamyl Peptidase Ii Inhibition Specifically Increases Recovery of Trh Released from Rat Brain Slices. *Neuropeptides* **1989**, *14*, 191–196. [CrossRef]
87. Kelly, J.A.; Slator, G.R.; Tipton, K.F.; Williams, C.H.; Bauer, K. Kinetic Investigation of the Specificity of Porcine Brain Thyrotropin-Releasing Hormone-Degrading Ectoenzyme for Thyrotropin-Releasing Hormone-Like Peptides. *J. Biol. Chem.* **2000**, *275*, 16746–16751. [CrossRef] [PubMed]
88. Kelly, J.A.; Scalabrino, G.A.; Slator, G.R.; Cullen, A.A.; Gilmer, J.F.; Lloyd, D.G.; Bennett, G.W.; Bauer, K.; Tipton, K.F.; Williams, C.H. Structure–Activity Studies with High-Affinity Inhibitors of Pyroglutamyl-Peptidase Ii. *Biochem. J.* **2005**, *389*, 569–576. [CrossRef] [PubMed]
89. Cruz, R.; Vargas, M.A.; Uribe, R.M.; Pascual, I.; Lazcano, I.; Yiotakis, A.; Matziari, M.; Joseph-Bravo, P.; Charli, J.-L. Anterior Pituitary Pyroglutamyl Peptidase Ii Activity Controls Trh-Induced Prolactin Release. *Peptides* **2008**, *29*, 1953–1964. [CrossRef] [PubMed]
90. Sinko, R.; Mohácsik, P.; Kővári, D.; Penksza, V.; Wittmann, G.; Mácsai, L.; Fonseca, T.L.; Bianco, A.C.; Fekete, C.; Gereben, B. Different Hypothalamic Mechanisms Control Decreased Circulating Thyroid Hormone Levels in Infection and Fasting-Induced Non-Thyroidal Illness Syndrome in Male Thyroid Hormone Action Indicator Mice. *Thyroid* **2023**, *33*, 109–118. [CrossRef]
91. Barnieh, F.M.; Loadman, P.M.; Falconer, R.A. Is Tumour-Expressed Aminopeptidase N (Apn/Cd13) Structurally and Functionally Unique? *Biochim. Biophys. Acta (BBA)-Rev. Cancer* **2021**, *1876*, 188641. [CrossRef]
92. Wickström, M.; Larsson, R.; Nygren, P.; Gullbo, J. Aminopeptidase N (Cd13) as a Target for Cancer Chemotherapy. *Cancer Sci.* **2011**, *102*, 501–508. [CrossRef]
93. Ni, J.; Wang, X.; Shang, Y.; Li, Y.; Chen, S. Cd13 Inhibition Augments Dr4-Induced Tumor Cell Death in a P-Erk1/2-Independent Manner. *Cancer Biol. Med.* **2021**, *18*, 569. [CrossRef]
94. Schreiter, A.; Gore, C.; Labuz, D.; Fournie-Zaluski, M.C.; Roques, B.P.; Stein, C.; Machelska, H. Pain Inhibition by Blocking Leukocytic and Neuronal Opioid Peptidases in Peripheral Inflamed Tissue. *FASEB J.* **2012**, *26*, 5161–5171. [CrossRef]
95. Bonnard, E.; Poras, H.; Nadal, X.; Maldonado, R.; Fournié-Zaluski, M.C.; Roques, B.P. Long-Lasting Oral Analgesic Effects of N-Protected Aminophosphinic Dual Enk Ephalinase Inhibitors (Denki S) in Peripherally Controlled Pain. *Pharmacol. Res. Perspect.* **2015**, *3*, e0116. [CrossRef]
96. Arrebola, Y.; Rivera, L.; Pedroso, A.; McGuire, R.; Tresanco, M.E.V.; Bergado, G.; Charli, J.-L.; Sánchez, B.; Alonso, I.P. Bacitracin Is a Non-Competitive Inhibitor of Porcine M1 Family Neutral and Glutamyl Aminopeptidases. *Nat. Prod. Res.* **2021**, *35*, 2958–2962. [CrossRef]
97. Melzig, M.F.; Bormann, H. Betulinic Acid Inhibits Aminopeptidase N Activity. *Planta Med.* **1998**, *64*, 655–657. [CrossRef] [PubMed]
98. Pascual Alonso, I.; Bounaadja, L.; Sánchez, L.; Rivera, L.; Tarnus, C.; Schmitt, M.; Garcia, G.; Diaz, L.; Hernandez-Zanuy, A.; Sánchez, B.; et al. Aqueous Extracts of Marine Invertebrates from Cuba Coastline Display Neutral Aminopeptidase Inhibitory Activities and Effects on Cancer Cells and Plasmodium Falciparum Parasites. *Indian J. Nat. Prod. Resour.* **2017**, *8*, 107–119.
99. Pascual, I.; Valiente, P.A.; García, G.; Valdés-Tresanco, M.E.; Arrebola, Y.; Díaz, L.; Bounaadja, L.; Uribe, R.M.; Pacheco, M.C.; Florent, I.; et al. Discovery of Novel Non-Competitive Inhibitors of Mammalian Neutral M1 Aminopeptidase (Apn). *Biochimie* **2017**, *142*, 216–225. [CrossRef]

100. Pascual-Alonso, I.; Alonso-Bosch, R.; Cabrera-Muñoz, A.; Perera, W.H.; Charli, J.L. Methanolic Extracts of Paratoid Gland Secretions from Cuban *Peltophryne* Toads Contain Inhibitory Activities against Peptidases with Biomedical Relevance. *Biotecnol. Apl.* **2019**, *36*, 2221–2227.

101. Alonso, I.P.; Méndez, L.R.; García, F.A.; Valdés-Tresanco, M.E.; Bosch, R.A.; Perera, W.H.; Sánchez, Y.A.; Bergado, G.; Ramírez, B.S.; Charli, J.-L. Bufadienolides Preferentially Inhibit Aminopeptidase N among Mammalian Metallo-Aminopeptidases; Relationship with Effects on Human Melanoma Mewo Cells. *Int. J. Biol. Macromol.* **2023**, *229*, 825–837. [CrossRef] [PubMed]

102. Wang, E.; Sorolla, M.A.; Krishnan, P.D.G.; Sorolla, A. From Seabed to Bedside: A Review on Promising Marine Anticancer Compounds. *Biomolecules* **2020**, *10*, 248. [CrossRef] [PubMed]

103. Malla, R.R.; Farran, B.; Nagaraju, G.P. Understanding the Function of the Tumor Microenvironment, and Compounds from Marine Organisms for Breast Cancer Therapy. *World J. Biol. Chem.* **2021**, *12*, 15. [CrossRef]

104. Aldrich, L.N.; Burdette, J.E.; de Blanco, E.C.; Coss, C.C.; Eustaquio, A.S.; Fuchs, J.R.; Kinghorn, A.D.; MacFarlane, A.; Mize, B.K.; Oberlies, N.H.; et al. Discovery of Anticancer Agents of Diverse Natural Origin. *J. Nat. Prod.* **2022**, *85*, 702–719. [CrossRef]

105. Nuzzo, G.; Senese, G.; Gallo, C.; Albiani, F.; Romano, L.; D'ippolito, G.; Manzo, E.; Fontana, A. Antitumor Potential of Immunomodulatory Natural Products. *Mar. Drugs* **2022**, *20*, 386. [CrossRef]

106. Saeed, A.F.; Su, J.; Ouyang, S. Marine-Derived Drugs: Recent Advances in Cancer Therapy and Immune Signaling. *Biomed. Pharmacother.* **2021**, *134*, 111091. [CrossRef]

107. Jung, J.H.; Sim, C.J.; Lee, C.-O. Cytotoxic Compounds from a Two-Sponge Association. *J. Nat. Prod.* **1995**, *58*, 1722–1726. [CrossRef] [PubMed]

108. Shin, J.; Lee, H.-S.; Seo, Y.; Rho, J.-R.; Cho, K.W.; Paul, V.J. New Bromotyrosine Metabolites from the Sponge *Aplysinella rhax*. *Tetrahedron* **2000**, *56*, 9071–9077. [CrossRef]

109. Pina, I.C.; Gautschi, J.T.; Wang, G.Y.S.; Sanders, M.L.; Schmitz, F.J.; France, D.; Cornell-Kennon, S.; Sambucetti, L.C.; Remiszewski, S.W.; Perez, L.B.; et al. Psammaplins from the Sponge Pseudoceratina P Urpurea: Inhibition of Both Histone Deacetylase and DNA Methyltransferase. *J. Org. Chem.* **2003**, *68*, 3866–3873. [CrossRef] [PubMed]

110. Park, Y.; Liu, Y.; Hong, J.; Lee, C.O.; Cho, H.; Kim, D.K.; Im, K.S.; Jung, J.H. New Bromotyrosine Derivatives from an Association of Two Sponges, Jaspis W Ondoensis and Poecillastra W Ondoensis. *J. Nat. Prod.* **2003**, *66*, 1495–1498. [CrossRef] [PubMed]

111. Yang, Q.; Liu, D.; Sun, D.; Yang, S.; Hu, G.; Wu, Z.; Zhao, L. Synthesis of the Marine Bromotyrosine Psammaplin F and Crystal Structure of a Psammaplin a Analogue. *Molecules* **2010**, *15*, 8784–8795. [CrossRef]

112. Mujumdar, P.; Teruya, K.; Tonissen, K.F.; Vullo, D.; Supuran, C.T.; Peat, T.S.; Poulsen, S.A. An Unusual Natural Product Primary Sulfonamide: Synthesis, Carbonic Anhydrase Inhibition, and Protein X-Ray Structures of Psammaplin C. *J. Med. Chem.* **2016**, *59*, 5462–5470. [CrossRef]

113. Kim, D.; Lee, I.S.; Jung, J.H.; Yang, S.I. Psammaplin a, a Natural Bromotyrosine Derivative from a Sponge, Possesses the Antibacterial Activity against Methicillin-Resistant *Staphylococcus aureus* and the DNA Gyrase-Inhibitory Activity. *Arch. Pharmacal Res.* **1999**, *22*, 25–29. [CrossRef]

114. TTabudravu, J.; Eijsink, V.; Gooday, G.; Jaspars, M.; Komander, D.; Legg, M.; Synstad, B.; van Aalten, D. Psammaplin a, a Chitinase Inhibitor Isolated from the Fijian Marine Sponge *Aplysinella rhax*. *Bioorganic Med. Chem.* **2002**, *10*, 1123–1128. [CrossRef]

115. Revelant, G.; Al-Lakkis-Wehbe, M.; Schmitt, M.; Alavi, S.; Schmitt, C.; Roux, L.; Al-Masri, M.; Schifano-Faux, N.; Maiereanu, C.; Tarnus, C.; et al. Exploring S1 Plasticity and Probing S1' Subsite of Mammalian Aminopeptidase N/Cd13 with Highly Potent and Selective Aminobenzosuberone Inhibitors. *Bioorganic Med. Chem.* **2015**, *23*, 3192–3207. [CrossRef]

116. Kim, T.H.; Kim, H.S.; Kang, Y.J.; Yoon, S.; Lee, J.; Choi, W.S.; Jung, J.H.; Kim, H.S. Psammaplin a Induces Sirtuin 1-Dependent Autophagic Cell Death in Doxorubicin-Resistant Mcf-7/Adr Human Breast Cancer Cells and Xenografts. *Biochim. Biophys. Acta (BBA)-Gen. Subj.* **2015**, *1850*, 401–410. [CrossRef]

117. Ratovitski, E.A. Tumor Protein (Tp)-P53 Members as Regulators of Autophagy in Tumor Cells Upon Marine Drug Exposure. *Mar. Drugs* **2016**, *14*, 154. [CrossRef] [PubMed]

118. Zhou, Y.-D.; Li, J.; Du, L.; Mahdi, F.; Le, T.P.; Chen, W.-L.; Swanson, S.M.; Watabe, K.; Nagle, D.G. Biochemical and Anti-Triple Negative Metastatic Breast Tumor Cell Properties of Psammaplins. *Mar. Drugs* **2018**, *16*, 442. [CrossRef] [PubMed]

119. Ahn, M.Y.; Jung, J.H.; Na, Y.J.; Kim, H.S. A Natural Histone Deacetylase Inhibitor, Psammaplin a, Induces Cell Cycle Arrest and Apoptosis in Human Endometrial Cancer Cells. *Gynecol. Oncol.* **2008**, *108*, 27–33. [CrossRef] [PubMed]

120. Kim, H.J.; Kim, J.H.; Chie, E.K.; Da Young, P.; Kim, I.A.; Kim, I.H. Dnmt (DNA Methyltransferase) Inhibitors Radiosensitize Human Cancer Cells by Suppressing DNA Repair Activity. *Radiat. Oncol.* **2012**, *7*, 1–10. [CrossRef]

121. Kim, D.H.; Shin, J.; Kwon, H.J. Psammaplin A Is a Natural Prodrug That Inhibits Class I Histone Deacetylase. *Exp. Mol. Med.* **2007**, *39*, 47–55. [CrossRef]

122. Jing, Q.; Hu, X.; Ma, Y.; Mu, J.; Liu, W.; Xu, F.; Li, Z.; Bai, J.; Hua, H.; Li, D. Marine-Derived Natural Lead Compound Disulfide-Linked Dimer Psammaplin A: Biological Activity and Structural Modification. *Mar. Drugs* **2019**, *17*, 384. [CrossRef] [PubMed]

123. Nicolaou, K.C.; Hughes, R.; Pfefferkorn, J.A.; Barluenga, S.; Roecker, A.J. Combinatorial Synthesis through Disulfide Exchange: Discovery of Potent Psammaplin a Type Antibacterial Agents Active against Methicillin-Resistant *Staphylococcus aureus* (MRSA). *Chem. –A Eur. J.* **2001**, *7*, 4280–4295. [CrossRef]

124. Nicolaou, K.C.; Hughes, R.; Pfefferkorn, J.A.; Barluenga, S. Optimization and Mechanistic Studies of Psammaplin a Type Antibacterial Agents Active against Methicillin-Resistant *Staphylococcus aureus* (MRSA). *Chem. –A Eur. J.* **2001**, *7*, 4296–4310. [CrossRef]

125. Alonso, I.P.; Sanchez, Y.M.A.; Ruiz, G.A.; González, M.L.R.; Hernández-Zanuy, A. Identificación De Actividad Inhibidora De Aminopeptidasa N Aislada De Riñón Porcino, En Invertebrados Marinos De La Plataforma Insular De La Habana/Identification of Porcine Kidney Aminopeptidase N Inhibitory Activity, in Marine Invertebrates from Havana Coastline. *Rev. Cuba. Cienc. Biológicas* **2016**, *5*, 15.

126. Alonso, I.P.; Pedroso, A.; Sánchez, Y.M.A.; Valdés-Tresanco, M.E.; Méndez, L.R.; Fortun, S. La Aminopeptidasa a De Mamíferos: Características Bioquímicas, Funciones Fisiológicas Y Su Implicación En Procesos Fisiopatológicos En Humanos/Aminopeptidase a from Mammals: Biochemical Characteristics, Physiological Roles and Implication in Physiopathological Processes in Humans. *Rev. Cuba. Cienc. Biológicas* **2018**, *6*, 20.

127. Göhring, B.; Holzhausen, H.; Meye, A.; Heynemann, H.; Rebmann, U.; Langner, J.; Riemann, D. Endopeptidase 24.11/Cd10 Is Down-Regulated in Renal Cell Cancer. *Int. J. Mol. Med.* **1998**, *2*, 409–423. [CrossRef] [PubMed]

128. Tonna, S.; Dandapani, S.V.; Uscinski, A.; Appel, G.B.; Schlöndorff, J.S.; Zhang, K.; Denker, B.M.; Pollak, M.R. Functional Genetic Variation in Aminopeptidase a (Enpep): Lack of Clear Association with Focal and Segmental Glomerulosclerosis (Fsgs). *Gene* **2008**, *410*, 44–52. [CrossRef]

129. del Carmen Puertas, M.; Martínez-Martos, J.M.; Cobo, M.; Lorite, P.; Sandalio, R.M.; Palomeque, T.; Torres, M.I.; Carrera-González, M.P.; Mayas, M.D.; Ramírez-Expósito, M.J. Plasma Renin–Angiotensin System-Regulating Aminopeptidase Activities Are Modified in Early Stage Alzheimer's Disease and Show Gender Differences but Are Not Related to Apolipoprotein E Genotype. *Exp. Gerontol.* **2013**, *48*, 557–564. [CrossRef] [PubMed]

130. Blanco, L.; Sanz, B.; Perez, I.; Sánchez, C.E.; Cándenas, M.L.; Pinto, F.M.; Gil, J.; Casis, L.; López, J.I.; Larrinaga, G. Altered Glutamyl-Aminopeptidase Activity and Expression in Renal Neoplasms. *BMC Cancer* **2014**, *14*, 386. [CrossRef]

131. Bodineau, L.; Frugiere, A.; Marc, Y.; Inguimbert, N.; Fassot, C.; Balavoine, F.; Roques, B.; Llorens-Cortes, C. Orally Active Aminopeptidase a Inhibitors Reduce Blood Pressure: A New Strategy for Treating Hypertension. *Hypertension* **2008**, *51*, 1318–1325. [CrossRef] [PubMed]

132. Matsui, M.; Fowler, J.H.; Walling, L.L. Leucine Aminopeptidases: Diversity in Structure and Function. *Biol. Chem.* **2006**, *387*, 1535–1544. [CrossRef] [PubMed]

133. Scranton, M.A.; Yee, A.; Park, S.-Y.; Walling, L.L. Plant Leucine Aminopeptidases Moonlight as Molecular Chaperones to Alleviate Stress-Induced Damage. *J. Biol. Chem.* **2012**, *287*, 18408–18417. [CrossRef]

134. Chao, W.S.; Gu, Y.-Q.; Pautot, V.; Bray, E.A.; Walling, L.L. Leucine Aminopeptidase Rnas, Proteins, and Activities Increase in Response to Water Deficit, Salinity, and the Wound Signals Systemin, Methyl Jasmonate, and Abscisic Acid. *Plant Physiol.* **1999**, *120*, 979–992. [CrossRef]

135. Alén, C.; Sherratt, D.J.; Colloms, S. Direct Interaction of Aminopeptidase a with Recombination Site DNA in Xer Site-Specific Recombination. *EMBO J.* **1997**, *16*, 5188–5197. [CrossRef]

136. Behari, J.; Stagon, L.; Calderwood, S.B. Pepa, a Gene Mediating Ph Regulation of Virulence Genes in *Vibrio cholerae*. *J. Bacteriol.* **2001**, *183*, 178–188. [CrossRef]

137. Aly, A.S.; Vaughan, A.M.; Kappe, S.H. Malaria Parasite Development in the Mosquito and Infection of the Mammalian Host. *Annu. Rev. Microbiol.* **2009**, *63*, 195–221. [CrossRef] [PubMed]

138. Goldberg, D.E. Complex Nature of Malaria Parasite Hemoglobin Degradation. *Proc. Natl. Acad. Sci. USA* **2013**, *110*, 5283–5284. [CrossRef] [PubMed]

139. Skinner-Adams, T.S.; Stack, C.M.; Trenholme, K.R.; Brown, C.L.; Grembecka, J.; Lowther, J.; Mucha, A.; Drag, M.; Kafarski, P.; McGowan, S.; et al. *Plasmodium falciparum* Neutral Aminopeptidases: New Targets for Anti-Malarials. *Trends Biochem. Sci.* **2010**, *35*, 53–61. [CrossRef] [PubMed]

140. Calic, P.P.; Vinh, N.B.; Webb, C.T.; Malcolm, T.R.; Ngo, A.; Lowes, K.; Drinkwater, N.; McGowan, S.; Scammells, P.J. Structure-Based Development of Potent Plasmodium Falciparum M1 and M17 Aminopeptidase Selective and Dual Inhibitors Via S1'-Region Optimisation. *Eur. J. Med. Chem.* **2023**, *248*, 115051. [CrossRef] [PubMed]

141. Drinkwater, N.; Vinh, N.B.; Mistry, S.N.; Bamert, R.S.; Ruggeri, C.; Holleran, J.P.; Loganathan, S.; Paiardini, A.; Charman, S.A.; Powell, A.K.; et al. Potent Dual Inhibitors of *Plasmodium falciparum* M1 and M17 Aminopeptidases through Optimization of S1 Pocket Interactions. *Eur. J. Med. Chem.* **2016**, *110*, 43–64. [CrossRef]

142. Bauvois, B.; Dauzonne, D. Aminopeptidase-N/Cd13 (Ec 3.4. 11.2) Inhibitors: Chemistry, Biological Evaluations, and Therapeutic Prospects. *Med. Res. Rev.* **2006**, *26*, 88–130. [CrossRef]

143. Kancharla, P.; Li, Y.; Yeluguri, M.; Dodean, R.A.; Reynolds, K.A.; Kelly, J.X. Total Synthesis and Antimalarial Activity of 2-(P-Hydroxybenzyl)-Prodigiosins, Isoheptylprodigiosin, and Geometric Isomers of Tambjamine Myp1 Isolated from Marine Bacteria. *J. Med. Chem.* **2021**, *64*, 8739–8754. [CrossRef]

144. Nweze, J.A.; Mbaoji, F.N.; Li, Y.-M.; Yang, L.-Y.; Huang, S.-S.; Chigor, V.N.; Eze, E.A.; Pan, L.-X.; Zhang, T.; Yang, D.-F. Potentials of Marine Natural Products against Malaria, Leishmaniasis, and Trypanosomiasis Parasites: A Review of Recent Articles. *Infect. Dis. Poverty* **2021**, *10*, 1–19. [CrossRef]

145. Zayed, A.; Negm, W.; Kabbash, A.; Ezzat, S.M. Marine-Derived Metabolites as Antimalarial Candidates Targeting Various Life Stages. *J. Adv. Med. Pharm. Res.* **2022**, *3*, 12–18. [CrossRef]

146. Singh, H.; Parida, A.; Debbarma, K.; Ray, D.P.; Banerjee, P. Common Marine Organisms: A Novel Source of Medicinal Compounds. *Int. J. Bioresour. Sci.* **2020**, *7*, 39–49. [CrossRef]
147. Zhang, M.; Tian, Z.; Wang, J.; Tian, X.; Wang, C.; Cui, J.; Huo, X.; Feng, L.; Yu, Z.; Ma, X. Visual Analysis and Inhibitor Screening of Leucine Aminopeptidase, a Key Virulence Factor for Pathogenic Bacteria-Associated Infection. *ACS Sens.* **2021**, *6*, 3604–3610. [CrossRef] [PubMed]
148. Fang, C.; Zhang, J.; Yang, H.; Peng, L.; Wang, K.; Wang, Y.; Zhao, X.; Liu, H.; Dou, C.; Shi, L.; et al. Leucine Aminopeptidase 3 Promotes Migration and Invasion of Breast Cancer Cells through Upregulation of Fascin and Matrix Metalloproteinases-2/9 Expression. *J. Cell. Biochem.* **2019**, *120*, 3611–3620. [CrossRef] [PubMed]
149. Yang, H.; Dai, G.; Wang, S.; Zhao, Y.; Wang, X.; Zhao, X.; Zhang, H.; Wei, L.; Zhang, L.; Guo, S.; et al. Inhibition of the Proliferation, Migration, and Invasion of Human Breast Cancer Cells by Leucine Aminopeptidase 3 Inhibitors Derived from Natural Marine Products. *Anti-Cancer Drugs* **2020**, *31*, 60–66. [CrossRef] [PubMed]

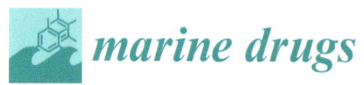

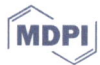

Article

Generation of Bioactive Peptides from *Porphyridium* sp. and Assessment of Their Potential for Use in the Prevention of Hypertension, Inflammation and Pain

Maria Hayes [1,*], Rotimi E. Aluko [2,3], Elena Aurino [1,4] and Leticia Mora [5]

1 Department of Food BioSciences, Teagasc Food Research Centre, Ashtown, D15 DY05 Dublin, Ireland; elena.aurino@teagasc.ie
2 Department of Food and Human Nutritional Sciences, University of Manitoba, Winnipeg, MB R3T 2N2, Canada; rotimi.aluko@umanitoba.ca
3 Richardson Centre for Food Technology and Research, University of Manitoba, Winnipeg, MB R3T 2N2, Canada
4 Department of Chemical, Materials and Industrial Production Engineering, University of Naples Federico II, 80126 Naples, Italy
5 Instituto de Agroquímica y Tecnología de Alimentos (CSIC), Avenue Agustín Escardino 7, Valencia, 46980 Paterna, Spain; lemoso@iata.csic.es
* Correspondence: maria.hayes@teagasc.ie; Tel.: +353-18059957

Citation: Hayes, M.; Aluko, R.E.; Aurino, E.; Mora, L. Generation of Bioactive Peptides from *Porphyridium* sp. and Assessment of Their Potential for Use in the Prevention of Hypertension, Inflammation and Pain. *Mar. Drugs* 2023, 21, 422. https://doi.org/10.3390/md21080422

Academic Editors: Francesc Xavier Avilés and Isel Pascual

Received: 25 June 2023
Revised: 21 July 2023
Accepted: 23 July 2023
Published: 25 July 2023

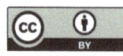

Abstract: Inflammation, hypertension, and negative heart health outcomes including cardiovascular disease are closely linked but the mechanisms by which inflammation can cause high blood pressure are not yet fully elucidated. Cyclooxygenase (COX) enzymes play a role in pain, inflammation, and hypertension development, and inhibition of these enzymes is currently of great interest to researchers and pharmaceutical companies. Non-steroidal anti-inflammatory drugs are the drug of choice in terms of COX inhibition but can have negative side effects for consumers. Functional food ingredients containing cyclooxygenase inhibitors offer a strategy to inhibit cyclooxygenases without negative side effects. Several COX inhibitors have been discovered, to date, from marine and other resources. We describe here, for the first time, the generation and characterization of a bioactive hydrolysate generated using Viscozyme® and Alcalase from the red microalga *Porphyridium* sp. The hydrolysate demonstrates in vitro COX-1 inhibitory activity and antihypertensive activity in vivo, assessed using spontaneously hypertensive rats (SHRs). Peptides were identified and sequenced using MS and assessed using an in silico computational approach for potential bioactivities. The peptides predicted to be bioactive, including GVDYVRFF, AIPAAPAAPAGPKLY, and LIHADPPGVGL were chemically synthesized and cyclooxygenase inhibition was confirmed. Peptides AIPAAPAAPAGPKLY and LIHADPPGVGL had COX-1 IC_{50} values of 0.2349 mg/mL (0.16 µM) and 0.2193 mg/mL (0.2 µM), respectively. The hydrolysate was included in a food carrier (jelly candies) and an antihypertensive effect was observed in SHRs.

Keywords: *Porphyridium* sp.; peptides; cyclooxygenase enzymes; hypertension; inflammation; animal health; spontaneously hypertensive rats; pain relief

1. Introduction

High blood pressure or hypertension and diseases associated with inflammation, including rheumatoid arthritis, asthma, mental illness such as depression, and gastrointestinal issues such as inflammatory bowel disease, are common conditions that may co-exist together, especially in elderly populations [1]. Inflammatory pain results in the mobilization of white blood cells and antibodies, leading to swelling and fluid accumulation. Inflammatory mediators sensitize noxious signals, pain fibers become active, and pain persists. Non-steroidal anti-inflammatory drugs (NSAIDs) such as aspirin, ibuprofen, and valdecoxib inhibit cyclooxygenase enzymes (COX-1 and COX-2 enzymes E.C.1.14.99.1) and find use in preventing inflammation and pain [2].

However, treatment with NSAIDS may have severe side effects, including ulcers, heartburn, diarrhea, and constipation. Gastrointestinal erosions and renal and hepatic insufficiency are mostly associated with COX-1 inhibitors [3]. Moreover, COX-2 inhibitors can increase blood pressure and increase the risk of atherothrombosis [4]. Natural cyclooxygenase inhibitors may provide pain relief without negative health effects. There is a need, therefore, to find new compounds to treat pain, inflammation, and hypertension without negative side effects [5].

The potential health benefits of algal oils, polysaccharides, and endogenous peptides derived from the red microalgae *Porphyridium* sp. are well known and several patents regarding their potential application as functional supplement ingredients, medicines, or topical applications exist in the literature [6–8]. *Porphyridium* species produce sulfated exopolysaccharides (EPSs) in a layer that surrounds the cytoplasmic membrane of the microalga and this mucilage is associated with antimicrobial, antiviral, antioxidant, and anti-inflammatory activities [9]. The protein and peptides derived from this alga also have interesting health beneficial activities. *Porphyridium* sp. are rich in proteins and make ideal candidates for generation of bioactive hydrolysates. Bioactive hydrolysates impart health benefits to the consumer that go beyond basic human nutrition based on peptides found within the hydrolysates and permeate fractions that can inhibit enzymes that play a role in human health. Peptides previously identified from protein hydrolysates can inhibit enzymes including Angiotensin-Converting Enzyme 1 (ACE-1), Renin, Dipeptidyl peptidase IV (DPP-IV), and cyclooxygenases, which play a part in the development of high blood pressure, type-2-diabetes (T2D), inflammation, and pain, respectively. Previously, the two dipeptides with amino acid single letter sequences HE and GP demonstrated anti-atherosclerotic effects on foam cell formation in the RAW264.7 cell line [10]. Peptide inhibitors of the enzyme ACE-1 are also important for the development of new alternatives to Captopril® for control of hypertension, and significant research has been carried out recently concerning the development of ACE-1 inhibitory hydrolysates from dairy, microalgae, meat, seaweed, and cereal proteins [11–16].

The aim of this work is to produce a bioactive protein hydrolysate from *Porphyridium* sp. using enzymatic hydrolysis and 3 kDa molecular weight cut off (MWCO) filtration. The enzymes Viscozyme® and Alcalase® were used to generate hydrolysates. An in vitro bioassay found that the 3 kDa MWCO permeate from the *Porphyridium* sp. hydrolysate significantly inhibited the COX-1 enzyme compared to the positive control Resveratrol®. Peptides were subsequently identified from the permeate fraction using mass spectrometry. In silico analysis of identified peptides in combination with chemical synthesis, and in vitro COX-1 and COX-2 inhibition assays, identified several bioactive peptides within the hydrolysate. Furthermore, an in vivo trial performed in spontaneously hypertensive rats (SHRs) using the *Porphyridium* sp. hydrolysate alone and the hydrolysate included in the carrier food jelly sweets determined antihypertensive effects of the hydrolysate and survival of this antihypertensive activity once formulated in a food carrier. Jellies and gummies are a popular class of confectionary and product launches making health, functionality, fortified, and sustainability claims have increased [17]. In vivo results were compared to the commercially available antihypertensive drug Captopril© (positive control) and a saline solution (negative control). Results demonstrate the antihypertensive and COX-1 inhibitory bioactivities associated with a *Porphyridium* sp. hydrolysate produced in a controlled manner. Bioactive peptides with COX-1 inhibitory activities (in vitro) were identified and their enzyme inhibitory IC_{50} values are comparable to previously reported COX-1 inhibitors derived from natural products. The developed jelly sweet products have potential for use as antihypertensive products to control blood pressure and may help to ameliorate pain and inflammation in consumers. However, further in vivo trials are required to validate results obtained in vitro.

2. Results

2.1. Proximate Compositional Analysis of Porphyridium sp. and Generated Hydrolysates

The protein, fat, moisture, and ash content of the whole *Porphyridium* sp. biomass was determined using AOAC methods as described in the Materials and Methods section. The protein content was 13.99% (dry weight basis), fat content was 4.82%, moisture was 9.68%, and ash content was 28.55%. A yield of 8.99% (dry weight) was obtained for the hydrolysate, which had a protein, fat, moisture, and ash content of 11.90%, 1.32%, 9.46%, and 28.96%, respectively.

2.2. In Vitro Screening for Cyclooxygenase 1 and 2 Inhibition

The *Porphyridium* sp. hydrolysate inhibited COX-1 by 92.14% ($\pm$3.16) when assayed at a concentration of 1 mg/mL (Figure 1). The microalgal hydrolysate inhibited COX-2 by 32.25% when assayed at a concentration of 1 mg/mL. All assays were carried out in triplicate ($n = 9$).

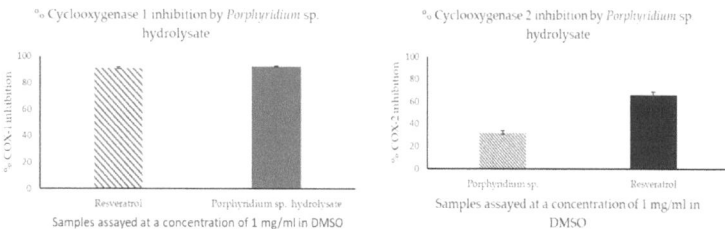

Figure 1. Cyclooxygenase (COX-1 and COX-2) inhibition by the *Porphyridium* sp. hydrolysate assayed at a concentration of 1 mg/mL in DMSO. Control used was Resveratrol, a known COX-1 inhibitor, assayed at 1 mg/mL concentration ($n = 9$).

Three peptides found in the *Porphyridium* sp. hydrolysate and identified using MS to have amino acid sequences GVDYVRFF, AIPAAPAAPAGPKLY, and LIHADPPGVGL with PeptideRanker scores of 0.857, 0.768, and 0.743, respectively, were assessed for their ability to inhibit COX-1 and COX-2 in vitro. The peptide GVDYDRFF inhibited COX-1 by 29.72% only. Peptides AIPAAPAAPAGPKLY and LIHAAPPGVG had COX-1 IC_{50} values of 0.2349 mg/mL (0.16 μM) and 0.2193 mg/mL (0.2 μM), respectively, based on assessment of five concentrations (1 mg/mL, 0.5 mg/mL, 0.25 mg/mL, 0.125 mg/mL, 0.0625 mg/mL) used to determine the standard curve and COX IC_{50} values ($n = 3$). However, none of the peptides inhibited COX-2 by greater than 30% when assayed at a concentration of 1 mg/mL.

2.3. Mass Spectrometry and In Silico Analysis of Peptides

2.3.1. Peptides Identified Using Mass Spectrometry

Following MS analysis, seventy-two peptides were identified in the *Porphyridium* sp. hydrolysate generated using Viscozyme® and Alcalase®. Only three peptide sequences were subsequently synthesized based on in silico analysis. These peptides were GVDYVRFF, corresponding to a peptide fragment found in the protein Phycoerythrin beta subunit (Accession number: tr|A0A5J4Z524|A0A5J4Z524_PORPP). The second peptide, with the amino acid sequence AIPAAPAAPAGPKLY, was derived from a putative transport protein found in *Porphyridium purpurem* (Accession number: tr|A0A5J4YZ45|A0A5J4YZ45_PORPP), and the third peptide LIHADPPGVGL corresponds with the amino acid sequence found in an uncharacterized protein found in *Porphyridium purpurem* (Accession number: tr|A0A5J4Z524|A0A5J4Z524_PORPP). These peptides were selected for synthesis based on their PeptideRanker scores but also based on the presence of amino acids such as Y, F, and L at the terminal end of the peptide.

2.3.2. Determination of the PeptideRanker Scores, Novelty, and Potential Bioactivities of Peptides

PeptideRanker (http://distilldeep.ucd.ie/PeptideRanker/, accessed on 7 January 2023) is an open source software resource, used to predict the potential bioactivity of peptides based on a novel N-to-1 neural network [18]. PeptideRanker ranks the probability that a peptide sequence will be bioactive. The peptides with amino acid sequences GVDYVRFF, AIPAAPAAPAGPKLY, and LIHADPPGVGL have PeptideRanker scores of 0.857, 0.768, and 0.743, respectively (the highest scores of all identified peptides). PeptideRanker scores indicate that these peptides are likely to have bioactivity. Acceptable probability values for bioactivity are between 0.5 and 1.0. PeptideRanker scores obtained for other peptides identified in this study are shown in Table 1. Values greater than 0.5 are reported.

A search of the BIOPEP-UWM database (https://biochemia.uwm.edu.pl/biopep-uwm/, accessed on 7 January 2023) [19], UniProt Peptide Search (WoS—https://www.uniprot.org/tool-dashboard, accessed on 21 July 2023), and PubMed-indexed papers determined the novelty of the seven peptides identified and shown in Table 1. Of the peptides analyzed and listed in Table 1, their amino acid sequences were not identified in previously published papers concerning seaweed proteins and bioactive peptides, and the peptides are novel to the best of our knowledge.

A simulated digestion of identified novel peptides was performed using Peptide Cutter software (http://web.expasy.org/peptide_cutter/, accessed on 7 January 2023) [20]. This was carried out to assess if bioactive peptides could potentially survive gastrointestinal (GI) digestion or whether they are pro-peptides. Peptides shown in Table 1 were digested using enzymes found in the GI tract, including pepsin (pH 1.3), trypsin, and chymotrypsin. All peptides were cleaved into shorter peptide fragments and, in some instances, digested peptides were identified as having additional bioactivities (Table 1). Simulated GI digestion of the seven peptides produced smaller peptides such as the active dipeptide VR derived from GVDYVRFF. VR has shown ACE-1 and DPP-IV inhibitory activities [19,21,22]. Simulated digestion of the peptide LIHADPPGVGL produced the previously identified DPP-IV and DPP-III inhibitory dipeptide IH [23,24], and the ACE-1 inhibitory tri-peptide GVG was previously identified in the antihypertensive peptide VAPGVG [25].

2.3.3. Chemical Synthesis of Selected Peptides

Peptides identified as having potential bioactivities with the amino acid sequences GVDYVRFF, AIPAAPAAPAGPKLY, and LIHADPPGVGL were chemically synthesized by GenScript Biotech (Leiden, The Netherlands). GenScript also verified the purity of the peptide by analytical RP-HPLC–MS. The primary structure and the theoretical values of the selected peptides were determined using PepDraw (https://www2.tulane.edu/~biochem/WW/PepDraw/, accessed on 16 June 2023) as shown in Figure 2.

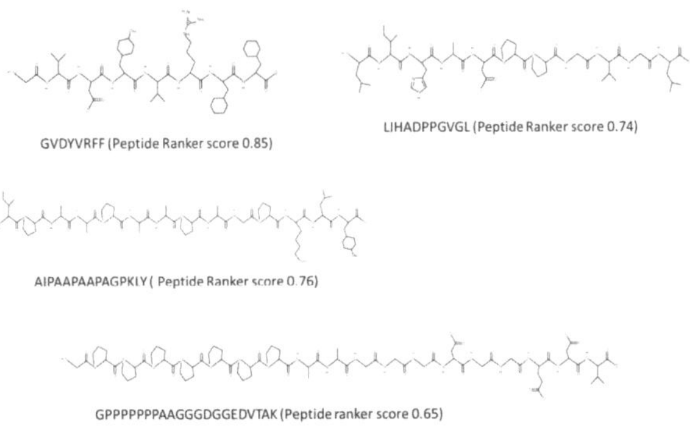

GVDYVRFF (Peptide Ranker score 0.85)

LIHADPPGVGL (Peptide Ranker score 0.74)

AIPAAPAAPAGPKLY (Peptide Ranker score 0.76)

GPPPPPPPAAGGGDGGEDVTAK (Peptide ranker score 0.65)

Figure 2. Chemical structure and characteristics of synthesized peptides derived from the *Porphyridium* sp. hydrolysate. Chemical structures were drawn using PepDraw (PepDraw (tulane.edu))–accessed on 16 June 2023.

Table 1. Peptide sequences identified from *Porphyridium* sp. hydrolysate permeate fraction generated using *Viscozyme*, Alcalase, and bioactivities of peptide fragments obtained after simulated gastrointestinal digestion.

Peptide Amino Acid Sequence (Single Letter Code)	Protein of Origin	Accession Code	Peptide Ranker Value *	PreAIP RF *† Combined Values	BIOPEP Search **	Expasy Peptide Cutter ***	Bioactivities Associated with Peptide Fragments	Peptide Charge
Porphyridium sp. Peptides Generated from Hydrolysis								
GVDYVRFF	Uncharacterized protein OS = *Porphyridium purpureum* OX = 35,688 GN = FVE85_6371 PE = 4 SV = 1	tr | A0A5J4Z524 | A0A5J4Z524_PORPP	0.857	0.374 Low confidence	Novel	GVD, Y, VR, E, F	GVD-alpha amylase inhibitor; VR-DPP-IV and ACE inhibitor peptide	0
AIPAAPAAPAGPKLY	Putative transporter YrhG OS = *Porphyridium purpureum* OX = 35,688 GN = FVE85_0107 PE = 4 SV = 1	tr | A0A5J4YZ45 | A0A5J4YZ45_PORPP	0.768	0.262 Negative AIP	Novel	AIPAAPAAPAGPK; L, Y	All novel but GPK occurs at the C-terminal end of antioxidative, antibacterial, osteoanabolic and calcium binding peptides found in BIOPEP	1
LIHADPPGVGL	Uncharacterized protein OS = *Porphyridium purpureum* OX = 35,688 GN = FVE85_6371 PE = 4 SV = 1	tr | A0A5J4Z524 | A0A5J4Z524_PORPP	0.743	0.390 Medium confidence AIP	Novel	L, IH, ADPPGVG, L	IH-DPP-IV inhibitor & DPP-III inhibitor; GVG occurs in alpha amylase and ACE-I inhibitors	−1
GLDAGLSHCGVVNVCIP	UDP-glucose/GDP-mannose dehydrogenase OS = *Ectocarpus siliculosus* OX = 2880 GN = Esi_0052_0113 PE = 4 SV = 1	tr | D8LPB4 | D8LPB4_ECTSI	0.729	0.500 High confidence AIP	Novel	G, L, DAG, L, SH, CGVVNVCIP	DAG-found in ACE-1 and antioxidative peptides; SH is a DPP-IV inhibitory peptide	−1
LIHADPPGVGLITGF	Uncharacterized protein OS = *Porphyridium purpureum* OX = 35,688 GN = FVE85_6371 PE = 4 SV = 1	tr | A0A5J4Z524 | A0A5J4Z524_PORPP	0.716	0.369 low confidence AIP	Novel	L, IH, ADPPGVG, L, TG, F	IH- DPP-IV inhibitor and DPP-III inhibitor, GVG occurs in alpha amylase and ACE-I inhibitor peptides, TG-DPP-IV inhibitor and ACE-1 inhibitor	−1

Table 1. Cont.

Peptide Amino Acid Sequence (Single Letter Code)	Protein of Origin	Accession Code	Peptide Ranker Value *	PreAIP RF *† Combined Values	BIOPEP Search **	Expasy Peptide Cutter ***	Bioactivities Associated with Peptide Fragments	Peptide Charge
AIPAAPAAPAGPK	Putative transporter YrhG OS = Porphyridium purpureum OX = 35,688 GN = FVE85_0107 PE = 4 SV = 1	tr | A0A5J4YZ45 | A0A5J4YZ45_PORPP	0.709		Novel	AIPAAPAAPAGPK	All novel but GPK occurs at the C-terminal end of antioxidative, antibacterial, osteoanabolic and calcium binding peptides found in BIOPEP	1
GPPPPPPAASGGDCGGEDVTAK	Adenylyl cyclase-associated protein 2 OS = Porphyridium purpureum OX = 35,688 GN = FVE85_5192 PE = 3 SV = 1	tr | A0A5J4Z4T9 | A0A5J4Z4T9_PORPP	0.659	0.469 High confidence AIP	Novel	Resistance to cleavage by Trypsin, Chymotrypsin and Pepsin	TAK found in the immunomodulator peptide RTAKV	−2
AAGGSLFEEYMR	Protein PYP1 OS = Porphyridium purpureum OX = 35,688 GN = FVE85_6364 PE = 4 SV = 1	tr | A0A5J4Z4701 A0A5J4Z470_PORPP	0.648	0.461 Medium confidence AIP	Novel	AAGGS, L, F, EE, Y, M, R	GGS found in the sequence of an ACE-1 inhibitory peptide YAGGS	−1
LFDGKVCTMLIIIT	NADH-ubiquinone oxidoreductase chain 5 OS = Rhodogorgon sp. OX = 2,485,824 GN = ND5 PE = 3 SV = 1	tr | A0A3G3MIM01 A0A3G3MIM0_9FLOR	0.641	0.545 High confidence AIP	Novel	L, F, DGK, VCTM, L, IIIT	all novel peptide fragments- no assigned bioactivities but IT is found in the ACE-1 inhibitory peptides ITT and ITK	0
LDSHLPINLPQGL	Ribulose bisphosphate carboxylase large chain (Fragment) OS = Porphyridium purpureum OX = 35,688 GN = rbcL PE = 3 SV = 1	tr | Q1WFR3 | Q1WFR3_PORPP	0.619	0.428 Medium confidence AIP	Novel	L, DSH, L, PINL, PQG, L	PQG occurs at the end of the PEP inhibitory peptide PPPPGCGPQPRP-PQG	−1

Porphyridium sp. Peptides Generated from Hydrolysis

* PeptideRanker http://bioware.ucd.ie/~compass/biowareweb/, accessed on 25 July 2022; PreAIP ** http://kurata14.bio.kyutech.ac.jp/PreAIP/, accessed on 19 July 2023; ** BIO-PEP-UWM https://biochemia.uwm.edu.pl/biopep-uwm/, accessed on 8 January 2023; *** PeptideCutter-SIB Swiss Institute of Bioinformatics Expasy, accessed on 7 January 2023.

43

2.4. Product Development–Production of Jelly Candies

For the development of the jelly candies containing the *Porphyridium* sp. hydrolysate, several tests were performed to determine effective combinations of different proportions of the hydrolysate, gelatin, and flavor ingredients until an appealing visual texture resulted.

2.5. In Vivo Antihypertensive Trial

The antihypertensive effect of the *Porphyridium* sp. hydrolysate and the jellies containing the *Porphyridium* sp. hydrolysate was evaluated. Jellies contained 3.36% (w/w) of the *Porphyridium* sp. hydrolysate. The antihypertensive effect is based on changes in hypertension physiological parameters including systolic blood pressure (SBP), diastolic blood pressure (DBP), mean arterial pressure (MAP), and heart rate (HR) after oral administration of SHRs. The *Porphyridium* sp. hydrolysate and jellies formulated with this hydrolysate reduced SBP by −1.54 mm Hg and −6.17 mm Hg, respectively, compared to Captopril®, which reduced SBP by −18.21 mmHg after 24 hrs. The maximal reduction of SBP observed for *Porphyridium* sp. hydrolysate was −11.67 mm Hg after 4 h and −18.97 mm Hg for *Porphyridium* sp. hydrolysate containing jellies after 2 h post oral gavage. Saline solution had no SBP-reducing effect when assessed (Figure 3a).

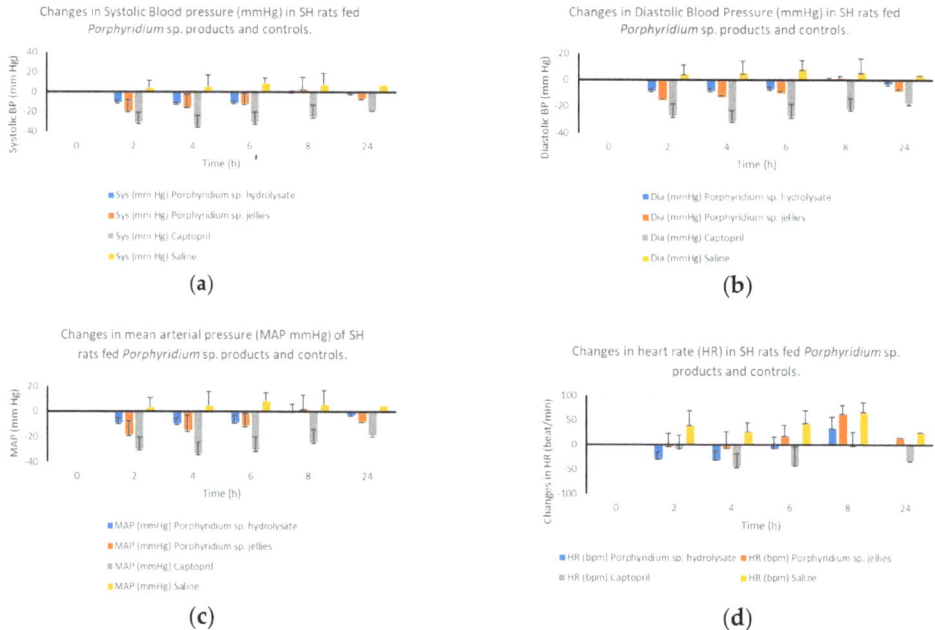

Figure 3. (**a**): The effect of the *Porphyridium* sp. hydrolysate and jellies containing 3.36% dry weight of hydrolysate on SBP compared to the positive control Captopril© and a saline solution (negative control). (**b**): The effect of the *Porphyridium* sp. hydrolysate and jellies containing 3.36% dry weight of hydrolysate on DBP compared to the positive control Captopril© and a saline solution (negative control). (**c**): Reductions in MAP (mm Hg) observed following oral gavage of *Porphyridium* sp. hydrolysate, jellies containing the hydrolysate, saline, and the positive control Captopril©. (**d**): Changes in HR following oral gavage of the *Porphyridium* sp. hydrolysate, jellies, and controls.

The *Porphyridium* sp. hydrolysate and jellies formulated with this hydrolysate reduced DBP by −2.99 mm Hg and −7.99 mm Hg, respectively, compared to Captopril®, which reduced DBP by −17.66 mmHg after 24 h. The maximal reduction of DBP observed for *Porphyridium* sp. hydrolysate was −7.46 mm Hg after 4 h and −15.43 mm Hg for *Porphyridium* sp. hydrolysate containing jellies after 2 h post oral gavage, compared to

−27.30 mmHg for Captopril©. Saline solution again had no DBP-reducing effect when assessed (Figure 3b).

MAP was reduced by −2.31 mmHg and −7.54 mm Hg after 24 h following oral gavage of the *Porphyridium* sp. hydrolysate and jellies, respectively. This was compared to a MAP reduction of −33.7 mmHg observed following oral gavage of SHRs with Captopril© (Figure 3c).

The decrease in HR also happened with a maximum reduction of 31 beats per min after 4 h following oral gavage of the *Porphyridium* sp. hydrolysate and a maximum reduction of 6 beats per min after 4 h following oral gavage of the *Porphyridium* sp. containing jellies and 45 beats per min after 4 h following oral gavage of Captopril©.

2.6. Statistical Analysis

All the experiments were performed in triplicate, and results are expressed as the mean ± standard deviation (SD) of the two replicates using EXCEL 2010. All measurements were carried out either in triplicate ($n = 3$) or ($n = 9$). Statistical analysis was performed using Excel 2010. one-way ANOVA and a post hoc Tukey's HSD test was applied. In all cases, the criterion for statistical significance was $p < 0.05$.

3. Discussion

Protein was extracted from *Porphyridium* sp. biomass using a combination of Viscozyme and Alcalase. This combination of enzymes was used previously to extract proteins from seaweed biomass including *Chondrus crispus* and, indeed, microalgae such as *Nannochloropsis gaditana* [26,27]. A yield of 11.90% protein (dry weight basis) resulted. Previous studies reported protein yields using Alcalase alone of 35.1% [28]. The enzymes Alcalase, Thermolysin, and Bromelain are the most commonly used enzymes to generate bioactive peptides from biomass including algae [28]. We employed the enzyme mixture Viscozyme in our work as the mixture contains enzymes with the potential to break down the cell wall polysaccharides composed of galactose, glucose, xylose, and glucuronic acid found in *Porphyridium* species. Viscozyme contains cellulases, hemicellulases, including xylanase, and endoglucanases. Alcalase was then applied to the mixture to generate bioactive peptides from the released protein. Alcalase is widely used for this purpose in the processing and manufacture of hydrolysates containing bioactive peptides from high-protein-containing foods [29] and was applied previously to algae for this purpose by our group [30,31] and by other researchers [32].

Bioactive peptides are less than 10 kDa in size. The generated hydrolysate was passed through a 10 kDa molecular weight cut off (MWCO) filter to enrich for a permeate rich in peptides. Following MS analysis, seventy-two peptides were identified in the permeate fraction and three peptides were selected for chemical synthesis based on their novelty and predicted bioactivities using PeptideRanker. The peptides selected for synthesis, namely GVDYVRFF, AIPAAPAAPAGALLY, and LIHADPPGVGL, were not found in the BIOPEP-UWM™ database of bioactive peptides (https://biochemia.uwm.edu.pl/biopep-uwm/, accessed on 8 January 2023) or in the PepBank database (http://pepbank.mgh.harvard.edu, accessed on 8 January 2023). Analysis of these peptide sequences using PeptideRanker (http://bioware.ucd.ie/~compass/biowareweb/, accessed on 25 July 2022) and PreAIP (accessed on 19 July 2023) found that they were very likely to be bioactive as they all had scores greater than 0.74 (PeptideRanker) and many peptides were identified as having potential to be anti-inflammatory by the PreAIP program. The AF scores obtained in PreAIP for the peptides compared favorably to the score obtained for the anti-inflammatory rice peptides identified previously by Qu [33]. PeptideRanker was trained at a threshold of 0.5, i.e., any peptide predicted to have a score greater than the 0.5 threshold is labeled as bioactive. The chosen peptides were also selected based on the presence of the amino acids phenylalanine (F), tyrosine (Y), and leucine (L). The side chains of phenylalanine and leucine are long carbon chains or rings, which makes them bulky. Branched chain amino acids are essential for the cellular signaling function and when found in peptides they

45

may be ideal for disease prevention [34]. The selected peptides have a bulky side chain aromatic amino acid at the C-terminal end of the peptide. In previously identified ACE-1 inhibitor peptides, tyrosine, phenylalanine, and tryptophan residues are often present at the C-terminus, particularly for the di-and tripeptide inhibitors [35,36]. Following simulated digestion using the Expasy peptide cutter, the peptide GVDYVRFF generated the dipeptide VR and the free amino acid F at the C-terminal end. VR was previously identified as an ACE-1 and DPP-IV inhibitory peptide [21,22]. The free amino acid phenylalanine (F) is found at the C-terminal end of previously identified ACE-I inhibitory peptides VVF, DF, and PDLVF [37,38]. AIPAAPAAPAGALLY was digested into the peptides AIPAAPAA and PAGPK and the free amino acids L and Y. GPK, found at the C-terminal end of PAGPK, occurs in eight known bioactive peptides listed in BIOPEP™ and has known antibacterial and antioxidant and calcium-binding properties [39,40]. The peptide LIHADPPGVGL resulted in peptides IH and ADPPGVP and the free amino acid L following simulated digestion. The dipeptide IH is a known dipeptidyl peptidase IV (DPP-IV) inhibitory peptide [23], which indicates that the hydrolysate may also have anti-type 2 diabetes (T2D) properties following ingestion by animals.

The rules concerning COX enzyme inhibition by bioactive peptides are not well deciphered to date. Several researchers have an interest in peptide inhibition of COX enzymes as existing COX inhibitors, such as the non-steroidal anti-inflammatory drugs (NSAIDs) rofecoxib and valdecoxib, which are known cardiovascular toxins and so have been withdrawn from the market [41]. Over 140 dipeptides were previously screened for their ability to inhibit COX-2 [42]. In this work, the *Porphyridium* sp. hydrolysate inhibited COX-1 by 92.14% ($\pm$3.16) and the chemically synthesized peptides AIPAAPAAPAGPKLY and LIHADPPGVGL had COX-1 IC$_{50}$ values of 0.2349 mg/mL (0.16 μM) and 0.2193 mg/mL (0.2 μM), respectively, when assayed at 1 mg/mL concentrations compared to the positive control Resveratrol®. The peptide GVDYVRFF did not inhibit COX-1 significantly. COX-2 was not significantly inhibited by the *Porphyridium* sp. hydrolysate or the synthesized peptides identified in the hydrolysate. Natural-product-based COX 1 inhibitors discovered to date seem better than NSAIDs in terms of side effects such as thrombotic cardiovascular events (COX-2 inhibitors) or gastrointestinal erosions, and renal and hepatic insufficiency (COX-1 inhibitors). Natural compound inhibitors of COX-1 and COX-2 are generally supposed to be devoid of severe side effects. The COX-1 IC$_{50}$ values obtained for AIPAAPAAPAGPKLY and LIHADPPGVGL compare favorably with COX IC$_{50}$ values previously determined for natural product COX-1 inhibitors. Previously, researchers identified a peptide named RQ-9 with the sequence RLARAGLAQ that was found to inhibit COX activity with a COX-1 IC$_{50}$ value of 0.31 μg/mL and a COX-2 IC$_{50}$ value of 4.77 μg/mL [43].

COX-1 inhibitors are associated with side effects including heart health issues. In this study, a *Porphyridium* sp. hydrolysate with COX-1 inhibitory activity was fed to SH rats and no adverse effects were observed. Antihypertensive activity resulted. The SH rat is a well-established model of human essential hypertension. Various studies to determine the antihypertensive effects of food-derived bioactive peptides have used spontaneous hypertensive animals as a model system [44,45]. A decrease in SBP and DBP as well as MAP resulted, following consumption of the hydrolysate and hydrolysate included at 3.36% (total weight) in jelly candies, up to 6 h post consumption and compared to the positive control Captopril©. This result compares favorably with results obtained concerning antihypertensive activity in SH rats observed following administration by the oral route of hydrolysates of royal jelly where blood pressure slowly decreased with time by about 15 mmHg from the previous level after 8 h in the control group [46]. The food carrier used in this study (jelly candies) proved effective at maintaining the bioactivity of the *Porphyridium* sp. hydrolysate and actually increased antihypertensive activity by ~20% compared to the hydrolysate alone in relation to SBP and DBP. This may be due to release of gelatin/collagen peptides following digestion in the SHR that could further enhance antihypertensive activity. However, we did not include hydrolyzed gelatin as a control. A study carried out recently by Cao and colleagues [47] identified that bovine-gelatin-derived peptides (BGPs) reduced blood pressure, triglyceride levels, and the low-density lipoprotein cholesterol/high-density lipoprotein cholesterol ratio in SHRs. This was achieved through downregulation of angiotensin converting enzyme (ACE-1), angiotensin II (Ang II), and Ang II type 1 receptor (AT1R) levels and upregulation of Ang II type 2 receptor (AT2R) levels. *Porphyridium* sp. were previously shown to lower plasma cholesterol levels in animals through different physiological mechanisms [33].

4. Materials and Methods

4.1. Porphyridium sp. Hydrolysate and Permeate Generation

Freeze-dried *Porphyridium* sp. biomass was cultivated and processed by Thomas More (Geel, Belgium) and VITO (Mol, Belgium). To freeze dry, *Porphyridium* sp. microalgae were suspended in ddH$_2$O (10%, w/v) and placed in a water bath (Grant JB Aqua 12 water bath, Grant instrument, England, UK) at 80 °C for 10 min to deactivate endogenous enzymes present in the biomass. The pH of the mixture was adjusted using 1M HCl and the enzyme Viscozyme was added to the sample (1% w/w). The mixture was incubated at 45 °C for 2 h with stirring at 220 rpm in a shaking incubator. Samples were removed from the incubator after 2 h and subsequently were heat-deactivated in a water bath at 80 °C × 10 min. The pH of the mixture was adjusted to 8–8.5 using 1M NaOH and the enzyme Alcalase was added to the mixture. The temperature was maintained at 55 °C and stirred at 220 rpm. To assess the efficiency of the enzymatic process, the permeate yield, protein recovery, and the degree of hydrolysis (DH) were calculated as follows:

$$\% \text{ permeate yield } [g/g] = \frac{\text{mass of permeate}}{\text{mass of whole biomass}} \times 100$$

$$\% \text{ protein recovery } [g/g] = \frac{\text{mass of protein in the permeate}}{\text{mass of protein in the whole biomass}} \times 100$$

The degree of hydrolysis (DH) was calculated at the end of each hydrolysis stage using the trichloroacetic acid (TCA) method described previously by Hoyle and colleagues [48]. A sample of 1 mL of the hydrolysate was collected after the deactivation step and added to 1 mL of 20% (w/v) TCA. The solutions were left to settle for 30 min and then centrifuged at 7800× g × 15 min. The percentage protein in the supernatant and the hydrolysate sample were assessed using the QuantiPro BCA Assay kit (Sigma, St. Louis, MO, USA) as per the manufacturer's instructions and DH was calculated as follows:

$$\text{DH}\% = \frac{\text{TCAsoluble N in the supernatant}}{\text{total N in the hydrolysate}} \times 100$$

The hydrolysate obtained was filtered using a 3 kDa molecular weight cut-off (MWCO) membrane filter (Millipore, Tullagreen, Carrigtwohill, Co. Cork, Ireland), and a permeate and a retentate fraction recovered.

Proximate compositional analysis was performed on the whole biomass and hydrolysates. The nitrogen percentage in the samples was determined using the LECO FP628 (LECO Corp., St Joseph, MI, USA) protein analyzer by applying the Dumas AOAC method 992.15 (1990) [49]. The protein content was obtained using a conversion factor of 6.25. The percentage lipid in each sample was assessed using the Oracle NMR Smart Trac rapid Fat analyzer (CEM Corporation, Matthews, NC, USA) using AOAC official methods 985.14. The ash and moisture content of the samples was determined as described previously [49].

4.2. In Vitro Bioactivities Assessment

4.2.1. In Vitro Screening for Cyclooxygenase (COX-1 and COX-2) Inhibitory Activities

In vitro assays to determine COX inhibition were performed using cell-free assays as described previously [30,50]. The hydrolysate or peptides were incubated independently with ovine recombinant COX-1 (Cayman Chemicals, Hamburg, Germany) or human recombinant COX-2 (Cayman Chemicals, Hamburg, Germany). Resveratrol (Merck, Dublin,

Ireland) was used as a positive control. The assay was performed in accordance with the manufacturers' instructions. Briefly, the assay measures the peroxidase components of COXs in the presence and absence of COX inhibitors or test components. Peroxidase activity is measured colorimetrically and the appearance of oxidized N, N, N', N'-tetramethyl-p-phenylenediamine (TMPD) is observed at 590 nm. The percentage of COX-1 or COX-2 inhibition is calculated based on the increase or decrease in absorbance observed at 590 nm in the presence or absence of the test component (control or test). The assay is carried out using a 96-well plate and includes a background well containing 160 μL of the assay buffer (0.1 M Tris-HCL, pH8) and 10 μL of Hemin. The 100% initial activity is observed in triplicate and wells contain 150 μL of the assay buffer, 10 μL of Hemin, and 10 μL of either COX-1 or COX-2 enzymes. Inhibitor wells contain 150 μL of assay buffer, 10 μL of Hemin, and 10 μL of enzyme, and 10 μL of the test inhibitor (algal extract) or the positive control (Resveratrol). Test compounds were dissolved in dimethyl sulfoxide (DMSO). Following addition of all elements to the wells, the plate is incubated at 25 °C for two minutes. A colorimetric substrate is added to all wells and immediately 20 μL of arachidonic acid is subsequently added. The absorbance of all wells is measured at 590 nm.

The average absorbance of all wells is calculated. The absorbance of the background wells is subtracted from all wells. The absorbance value for the test sample is subtracted from the initial activity absorbance value and subsequently this is divided by the 100% initial activity absorbance value. The percentage COX-1/COX-2 inhibition is calculated by multiplying this final value by 100. COX-1 and COX-2 IC_{50} values relate to the concentrations that give 50% inhibition.

4.2.2. Mass Spectrometry in Tandem and In Silico Analysis

The *Porphyridium* sp. 3 kDa MWCO permeate fraction was processed for mass spectrometry analysis using the Preomics Phoenix Clean-up Kit (96×), (Preomics, D-82152 Planegg/Martinsried, Germany) in accordance with the manufacturers' instructions and as described previously [30]. The sample was acidified and hydrophobic and hydrophilic contaminants removed using a series of wash steps and peptides eluted from the cartridge and prepared in loading buffer for LC-MS/MS analysis. Peptides were identified using a mass spectrometer nanoESI qQTOF (6600 plus TripleTOF, AB SCIEX, Framingham, MA, USA) using liquid chromatography and tandem mass spectrometry (LC–MS/MS). A total of 1 μL of microalgal permeate was loaded onto a trap column (3 μ C18-CL 120 Å, 350 μM × 0.5 mm; Eksigent, Redwood City, CA, USA) and desalted with 0.1% TFA (trifluoroacetic acid) at 5 μL/min for 5 min. The peptides were then loaded onto an analytical column (3 μ C18-CL 120 Å, 0.075 × 150 mm) equilibrated in 5% acetonitrile (ACN) 0.1% formic acid (FA). Elution was carried out with a linear gradient from 5 to 40% B in A for 20 min, where solvent A was 0.1% FA and solvent B was ACN with 0.1% FA) at a flow rate of 300 nL/min. The sample was ionized in an electrospray source of Optiflow < 1 μL Nano applying 3.0 kV to the spray emitter at 200 °C. Analysis was carried out in a data-dependent mode. Survey MS1 scans were acquired from 350 to 1400 m/z for 250 ms. The quadrupole resolution was set to 'LOW' for MS2 experiments, which were acquired from 100 to 1500 m/z for 25 ms in 'high sensitivity' mode. The following switch criteria were used: charge: 1+ to 4+; minimum intensity; 100 counts per second (cps). Up to 50 ions were selected for fragmentation after each survey scan. Dynamic exclusion was set to 15 s. The system sensitivity was controlled by analyzing 500 ng of K562 protein extract digest (SCIEX); in these conditions, 1819 proteins were identified (FDR < 1%) in a 20 min gradient. Protein Pilot v 5.0. (SCIEX Framingham, MA, USA) default parameters were used to generate the peak list directly from 6600 plus TripleTOF wiff files. The Paragon algorithm of ProteinPilot v 5.0 was used to search the SwisProt and Uniprot Prot-Algae database with the following parameters: no enzyme specificity, IAM cys-alkylation, no taxonomy restriction, and the search effort set to throughout. Peptides were identified with a confidence of ≥95%.

The potential of identified peptides to be bioactive was predicted using the PeptideRanker tool [18] (http://bioware.ucd.ie/~compass/biowareweb/, accessed on the

7 January 2023) and peptide scores were obtained. The novelty of identified peptides was determined by performing a literature and database search in BIOPEP-UWM (http://www.uwm.edu.pl/biochemia/index.php/en/biopep, accessed on 3 January 2023). In addition, peptide sequences were assessed using the anti-inflammatory peptide predictor PreAIP (http://kurata1.bio.kyutech.ac.jp/PreAIP/, accessed on 17 July 2023) [51].

4.3. Chemical Synthesis of Peptides

Bioactive peptides predicted to be bioactive using PeptideRanker and with the amino acid sequences GVDYVRFF, AIPAAPAAPAGPKLY, and LIHADPPGVGL were chemically synthesized by GenScript Biotech (Leiden, The Netherlands). GenScript also verified the purity of the peptide by analytical RP-HPLC–MS. The primary structure and the theoretical values of the selected peptides was determined using PepDraw (https://www2.tulane.edu/~biochem/WW/PepDraw/, accessed on 8 January 2023).

4.4. Product Formulation

Ingredients used for jelly candy production included: 0.5 g of the hydrolysate (3.36% of dry weight ingredients), 0.75 g agar (Merck, Dublin, Ireland), 0.75 g pectin (Merck, Dublin, Ireland), 0.75 g of guar gum (Sigma Aldrich, Dublin, Ireland), 0.2 mL of liquid sucrose (Dr Oetker, Dublin 12, Ireland), 0.5 mL of liquid food coloring (pink) (Dr Oetker, Dublin 12, Ireland), 0.5 mL orange extract (Dr Oetker, Dublin 12, Ireland), 3.5 sheets (approximately 12 g) of sheet bovine derived gelatin (Dr Oetker, Dublin 12, Ireland), 57 mL of ddH$_2$O. The jelly candies (jellies) were manufactured as described previously [17,52]. A cold-set approach was used. Once achieved, the mixture was poured into polyethylene molds (2 × 1.5 cm) and refrigerated for 24 h at between 2 and 8 °C. The formulation used for the jelly candies was as follows: 6 g of *Porphyridium* sp. hydrolysate, 570 mL of ddH$_2$O, 0.75 g agar, 0.75 g pectin, 0.75 g guar gum, 5 g liquid sucrose, 1 g ascorbic acid, 1 mL food coloring (red), 1 mL of lemon extract essence, and 12 g of bovine gelatin (~3.5 sheets). All the *Porphyridium* sp. jellies produced were removed from the molds and stored in a freezer at −80 °C until the time of further analysis. The bioactive hydrolysate was added at a concentration of 3.36% (w/v) to the formulation. Jellies were rolled in cornstarch to prevent sticking following removal from molds.

4.5. In Vivo Trial in SHRs

Animal model and experimental design: Spontaneously hypertensive rats (SHRs), implanted with Data Sciences International (DSI) HD-S10 telemetry transmitters (DSI, St. Paul, MN, USA), were purchased from Envigo RMS, LLC (Indianapolis, IN, USA) and used without further alteration. The rats were housed under a 12 h day and night cycle at 21 °C with regular chow feed and tap water provided ad libitum. Animal experiments were carried out following the Canadian Council on Animal Care Ethics guidelines with a protocol approved by the University of Manitoba Fort Garry Campus Animal Care Committee. For each experiment, there were four rats per group: phosphate buffered saline (PBS), Captopril (50 mg/kg body weight (wt) dissolved in PBS), and sample (100 mg/kg body wt dissolved in PBS). Each rat was orally gavaged with a 1 mL solution using a disposable plastic syringe; blood pressure was then recorded continuously in freely moving rats for 24 h by telemetry. Results are reported as changes in values of the SBP, DBP, MAP, and HR at different time points over a 24 h period minus their baseline measurements at time zero.

Telemetry recording and signal processing: Systolic and diastolic blood pressure (SBP and DBP) measurements were performed in a quiet room with each rat cage placed on top of one receiver (Model RPC-1, DSI instruments, St. Paul, MN, USA). Real time experimental data (including heart rates (HRs)) were recorded continuously using the Ponemah 6.1 data acquisition software (DSI instruments, MN, USA). The system was attached to an APR-1 atmospheric-pressure monitor (DSI instruments, MN, USA), which normalized the transmitted pressure values and ensured that the recorded blood pressure signals were not dependent on changes in atmospheric pressure. The zero time values for each measured parameter were then subtracted from the respective values obtained at 2, 4, 6, 8, and 24 h, where the most notable changes were observed. The rat experiments were performed in four replicates and standard deviations were calculated using Excel.

5. Conclusions

Bioactive peptides were successfully generated from the red microalga *Porphyridium* sp. and displayed ACE-1 and COX-1 inhibitory activities in vitro. In vivo studies in SHRs confirmed an antihypertensive effect of this hydrolysate and additionally, the antihypertensive effect of the hydrolysate was enhanced when included in a gelatin carrier at a concentration of 3.36%. Additional bioactivities were assigned to peptides found in the hydrolysate using in silico methods including PreAIP and Peptide Ranker. The hydrolysate ingredient and the gelatin confectionary hold potential for use in the prevention of high blood pressure and pain in humans and animals but further in vivo trials are required to validate these findings.

Author Contributions: Conceptualization, M.H.; methodology, M.H., E.A., L.M. and R.E.A.; software, M.H.; validation, M.H., R.E.A. and L.M.; formal analysis, M.H.; investigation, M.H.; resources, M.H.; data curation, M.H.; writing—original draft preparation, M.H.; writing—review and editing, M.H., L.M. and R.E.A.; visualization, M.H.; supervision, M.H.; project administration, M.H.; funding acquisition, M.H. All authors have read and agreed to the published version of the manuscript.

Funding: NORTH-WEST EUROPE INTERREG funded this research, grant number NWE 639, as part of the IDEA project (Implementation and development of economic viable algae-based value chains in Northwest Europe) 2017–2023. We thank VITO (Leen Bastiaens and Queenie Simons) for supply of microalgae and Thomas More University additionally.

Institutional Review Board Statement: The study was conducted in accordance with the Declaration of Helsinki, and approved by the University of Manitoba Fort Garry Campus Animal Care Committee (Ethics Committee) and in accordance with the guidelines of the Canadian Council on Animal Care Ethics guidelines.

Data Availability Statement: Further data is available from the corresponding author.

Conflicts of Interest: The authors declare no conflict of interest.

References

1. Chen, L.; Deng, H.; Cui, H.; Fang, J.; Zuo, Z.; Deng, J.; Li, Y.; Wang, X.; Zhao, L. Inflammatory responses and inflammation-associated diseases in organs. *Oncotarget* **2017**, *9*, 7204–7218. [CrossRef]
2. Parisien, M.; Lima, L.V.; Dagostino, C.; El-Hachem, N.; Drury, G.L.; Grant, A.V.; Huising, J.; Verma, V.; Meloto, C.B.; Silva, J.R.; et al. Acute inflammatory response via neutrophil activation protects against the development of chronic pain. *Sci. Transl. Med.* **2022**, *14*, eabj9954. [CrossRef] [PubMed]
3. Süleyman, H.; Demircan, B.; Karagöz, Y. Anti-inflammatory and side effects of cyclooxygenase inhibitors. *Pharmacol. Rep.* **2007**, *59*, 247–258. [PubMed]
4. Patrono, C. Cardiovascular effects of cyclooxygenase-2 inhibitors: A mechanistic and clinical perspective. *Br. J. Clin. Pharmacol.* **2016**, *82*, 957–964. [CrossRef]
5. Attiq, A.; Jalil, J.; Husain, K.; Ahmad, W. Raging the War Against Inflammation With Natural Products. *Front. Pharmacol.* **2018**, *9*, 976. [CrossRef] [PubMed]
6. Sun, L.; Wang, C.; Shi, Q.; Ma, C. Preparation of different molecular weight polysaccharides from *Porphyridium cruentum* and their antioxidant activities. *Int. J. Biol. Macromol.* **2009**, *45*, 42–47. [CrossRef]
7. Dillon, H.; Sumanchi, A.; Rao, K. US20070167398A1. In *Methods and Compositions for Reducing Inflammation and Preventing Oxidative Damage*; Current Holdrs TerraVia Holdings Inc.: Dallas, TX, USA, 2007.
8. Sekar, S.; Chandramohan, M. Phycobiliproteins as a commodity: Trends in applied research, patents and commercialization. *J. Appl. Phycol.* **2008**, *20*, 113–136. [CrossRef]
9. Risjani, Y.; Mutmainnah, N.; Manurung, P.; Wulan, S.N.; Yunianta. Exopolysaccharide from *Porphyridium cruentum* (*purpureum*) is Not Toxic and Stimulates Immune Response against Vibriosis: The Assessment Using Zebrafish and White Shrimp *Litopenaeus vannamei*. *Mar. Drugs.* **2021**, *19*, 133. [CrossRef]
10. Kavitha, M.D.; Gouda, K.G.M.; Aditya Rao, S.J.; Shilpa, T.S.; Shetty, N.P.; Sarada, R. Atheroprotective effect of novel peptides from Porphyridium purpureum in RAW 264.7 macrophage cell line and its molecular docking study. *Biotechnol. Lett.* **2019**, *41*, 91–106. [CrossRef]

11. Mora, L.; Gallego, M.; Toldrá, F. ACEI-Inhibitory Peptides Naturally Generated in Meat and Meat Products and Their Health Relevance. *Nutrients* **2018**, *10*, 1259. [CrossRef]
12. Di Bernardini, R.; Mullen, A.M.; Bolton, D.; Kerry, J.; O'Neill, E.; Hayes, M. Assessment of the angiotensin-I-converting enzyme (ACE-I) inhibitory and antioxidant activities of hydrolysates of bovine brisket sarcoplasmic proteins produced by papain and characterisation of associated bioactive peptidic fractions. *Meat Sci.* **2012**, *90*, 226–235. [CrossRef]
13. Hayes, M.; Mora, L.; Lucakova, S. Identification of Bioactive Peptides from *Nannochloropsis oculata* Using a Combination of Enzymatic Treatment, in Silico Analysis and Chemical Synthesis. *Biomolecules* **2022**, *12*, 1806. [CrossRef]
14. Bleakley, S.; Hayes, M.; O' Shea, N.; Gallagher, E.; Lafarga, T. Predicted Release and Analysis of Novel ACE-I, Renin, and DPP-IV Inhibitory Peptides from Common Oat (*Avena sativa*) Protein Hydrolysates Using in Silico Analysis. *Foods* **2017**, *6*, 108. [CrossRef] [PubMed]
15. Shannon, E.; Conlon, M.; Hayes, M. In vitro enzyme inhibitory effects of green and brown Australian seaweeds and potential impact on metabolic syndrome. *J. Appl. Phycol.* **2023**, *35*, 893–910. [CrossRef]
16. Hayes, M.; Stanton, C.; Slattery, H.; O'Sullivan, O.; Hill, C.; Fitzgerald, G.F.; Ross, R.P. Casein fermentate of Lactobacillus animalis DPC6134 contains a range of novel propeptide Angiotensin-Converting Enzyme inhibitors. *Appl. Environ. Microbiol.* **2007**, *73*, 14. [CrossRef] [PubMed]
17. Teixeira-Lemos, E.; Almeida, A.R.; Vouga, B.; Morais, C.; Correia, I.; Pereira, P.; Guiné, R.P. Development and characterization of healthy gummy jellies containing natural fruits. *Open Agric.* **2021**, *6*, 466–478. [CrossRef]
18. Mooney, C.; Haslam, N.; Pollastri, G.; Shields, D.C. Towards the improved discovery and design of functional peptides: Common features of diverse classes permit generalised prediction of bioactivity. *PLoS ONE* **2012**, *7*, e45012. [CrossRef]
19. Minkiewicz, P.; Iwaniak, A.; Darewicz, M. BIOPEP-UWM Database of Bioactive Peptides: Current Opportunities. *Int. J. Mol. Sci.* **2019**, *20*, 5978. [CrossRef]
20. Gasteiger, E.; Hoogland, C.; Gattiker, A.; Duvaud, S.; Wilkins, M.R.; Appel, R.D.; Bairoch, A. *Protein Identification and Analysis Tools on the Expasy Server*; Walker, J.M., Ed.; The Proteomics Protocols Handbook, Humana Press; Full text—Copyright Humana Press: Totowa, NJ, USA, 2005.
21. Gomez-Ruiz, J.A.; Ramos, M.; Recio, I. Identification of novel angiotensin-converting enzyme inhibitory peptides from ovine milk proteins by CE-MS and chromatographic techniques. *Electrophoresis* **2007**, *28*, 4202–4211. [CrossRef]
22. Nongonierma, A.B.; FitzGerald, R.J. Inhibition of dipeptidyl peptidase IV (DPP-IV) by proline containing casein derived peptides. *J. Funct. Foods* **2013**, *5*, 1909–1917. [CrossRef]
23. Lan, V.T.T.; Ito, K.; Ohno, M.; Motoyama, T.; Ito, S.; Kawarasaki, Y. Analyzing a dipeptide library to identify human dipeptidyl peptidase IV inhibitor. *Food Chem.* **2015**, *175*, 66–73. [CrossRef]
24. Dhanda, S.; Singh, H.; Singh, J. Hydrolysis of various bioactive peptides by goat brain dipeptidyl peptidase III. *Cell Biochem. Funct.* **2008**, *23*, 339–345. [CrossRef]
25. Hatakenaka, T.; Kato, T.; Okamoto, K. In Vitro and In Silico Studies on Angiotensin I-Converting Enzyme Inhibitory Peptides Found in Hydrophobic Domains of Porcine Elastin. *Molecules* **2023**, *28*, 3337. [CrossRef] [PubMed]
26. Naseri, A.; Jacobsen, C.; Sejberg, J.J.P.; Pedersen, T.E.; Larsen, J.; Hansen, K.M.; Holdt, S.L. Multi-Extraction and Quality of Protein and Carrageenan from Commercial Spinosum (*Eucheuma denticulatum*). *Foods* **2020**, *9*, 1072. [CrossRef]
27. Blanco-Llamero, C.; García-García, P.; Señoráns, F.J. Combination of Synergic Enzymes and Ultrasounds as an Effective Pretreat-ment Process to Break Microalgal Cell Wall and Enhance Algal Oil Extraction. *Foods* **2021**, *10*, 1928. [CrossRef] [PubMed]
28. Safi, C.; Rodriguez, L.C.; Mulder, W.; Engelen-Smit, N.; Spekking, W.; Broek, L.V.D.; Olivieri, G.; Sijtsma, L. Energy consumption and water-soluble protein release by cell wall disruption of *Nannochloropsis gaditana*. *Bioresour. Technol.* **2017**, *239*, 204–210. [CrossRef] [PubMed]
29. Toldrá, F.; Mora, L. Proteins and Bioactive Peptides in High Protein Content Foods. *Foods* **2021**, *10*, 1186. [CrossRef]
30. Purcell, D.; Packer, M.A.; Hayes, M. Angiotensin-I-Converting Enzyme Inhibitory Activity of Protein Hydrolysates Generated from the Macroalga *Laminaria digitata* (Hudson) JV Lamouroux 1813. *Foods* **2022**, *11*, 1792. [CrossRef] [PubMed]
31. Fitzgerald, C.; Mora-Soler, L.; Gallagher, E.; O' Connor, P.; Prieto, J.; Soler-Vila, A.; Hayes, M. Isolation and Characteri zation of Bioactive Pro-Peptides with in Vitro Renin Inhibitory Activities from the Macroalga *Palmaria palmata*. *J. Agric. Food Chem.* **2012**, *60*, 7421–7427. [CrossRef]
32. Admassu, H.; Abdalbasit, M.; Gasmalla, A.; Yang, R.; Zhao, W. Bioactive peptides derived from seaweed protein and their health benefits: Antihypertensive, antioxidant and antidiabetic properties. *J. Food Sci.* **2018**, *83*, 6–16. [CrossRef] [PubMed]
33. Qu, T.; He, S.; Ni, C.; Wu, Y.; Xu, Z.; Chen, M.L.; Li, H.; Cheng, Y.; Wen, L. In Vitro Anti-Inflammatory Activity of Three Peptides Derived from the Byproduct of Rice Processing. *Plant Foods Hum Nutr.* **2022**, *77*, 172–180. [CrossRef] [PubMed]
34. Dullius, A.; Fassina, P.; Giroldi, M.; Goettert, M.I.; Volken de Souza, C.F. A biotechnological approach for the production of branched chain amino acid containing bioactive peptides to improve human health: A review. *Food Res. Int.* **2020**, *131*, 109002. [CrossRef] [PubMed]
35. Manoharan, S.; Shuib, A.S.; Abdullah, N. Structural characteristics and antihypertensive effects of angiotensin-1-converting enzyme inhibitory peptides in the Renin-Angiotensin and Kallikrein Kinin systems. *Afr. J. Tradit. Complement. Altern. Med.* **2017**, *14*, 383–406. [CrossRef] [PubMed]
36. He, R.; Aluko, R.E.; Ju, X.-R. Evaluating Molecular Mechanism of Hypotensive Peptides Interactions with Renin and Angiotensin Converting Enzyme. *PLoS ONE* **2014**, *9*, e91051. [CrossRef]

37. Wu, J.; Aluko, R.E.; Nakai, S. Structural requirements of Angiotensin-I-converting enzyme inhibitory activity—Structure activity relationship study of di- and tripeptides. *J. Agric. Food Chem.* **2006**, *54*, 732–738. [CrossRef]
38. Torkova, A.; Kononikhin, A.; Bugrova, A.; Khotchenkov, V.; Tsentalovich, M.; Medvedeva, U. Effect of in vitro gastrointestinal digestion on bioactivity of poultry protein hydrolysate. *Curr. Res. Nutr. Food Sci.* **2016**, *4* (Suppl. S2), 77–78.
39. Chi, C.F.; Wang, B.; Wang, Y.M.; Zhang, B.; Deng, S.J. Isolation and characterization of three antioxidant peptides from protein hydrolysate of bluefin leatherjacket (*Navodon septentrionalis*) heads. *J. Funct. Foods* **2015**, *12*, 1–10. [CrossRef]
40. He, J.; Guo, H.; Zhang, M.; Wang, M.; Sun, L.; Zhuang, Y. Purification and characterization of a novel calcium-binding heptapeptide from the hydrolysate of tilapia bone with its osteogenic activity. *Foods* **2022**, *11*, 468. [CrossRef]
41. Dogne, J.M.; Supuran, C.T.; Pratico, D. Adverse cardiovascular effects of the coxibs. *J. Med. Chem.* **2005**, *48*, 2251–2257. [CrossRef]
42. Fosgerau, K.; Hoffmann, T. Peptide therapeutics: Current status and future directions. *Drug Discov. Today* **2015**, *20*, 122–128. [CrossRef]
43. Złotek, U.; Jakubczyk, A.; Rybczyńska-Tkaczyk, K.; Ćwiek, P.; Baraniak, B.; Lewicki, S. Characteristics of New Peptides GQL-GEHGGAGMG, GEHGGAGMGGGQFQPV, EQGFLPGPEESGR, RLARAGLAQ, YGNPVGGVGH, and GNPVGGVGHGTTGT as Inhibitors of Enzymes Involved in Metabolic Syndrome and Antimicrobial Potential. *Molecules* **2020**, *25*, 2492. [CrossRef] [PubMed]
44. Igarashi, K.; Yoshioka, K.; Mizutani, K.; Miyakoshi, M.; Murakami, T.; Akizawa, T. Blood pressure-depressing activity of a peptide derived from silkworm fibroin in spontaneously hypertensive rats. *Biosci. Biotechnol. Biochem.* **2006**, *70*, 517–520. [CrossRef] [PubMed]
45. Marczak, E.D.; Usui, H.; Fujita, H.; Yang, Y.; Yokoo, M.; Lipkowski, A.W.; Yoshikawa, M. New antihypertensive peptides isolated from rapeseed. *Peptides* **2003**, *24*, 791–798. [CrossRef] [PubMed]
46. Takaki-Doi, S.; Hashimoto, K.; Yamamura, M.; Kamei, C. Antihypertensive activities of royal jelly protein hydrolysate and its fractions in spontaneously hypertensive rats. *Acta Med. Okayama.* **2009**, *63*, 57–64. [CrossRef]
47. Cao, S.; Wang, Z.; Xing, L.; Zhou, L.; Zhang, W. Bovine Bone Gelatin-Derived Peptides: Food Processing Characteristics and Evaluation of Antihypertensive and Antihyperlipidemic Activities. *J. Agric. Food Chem.* **2022**, *70*, 9877–9887. [CrossRef]
48. Hoyle, N.T.; Merritt, J.H. Quality of fish protein hydrolysates from herring (*Clupea harengus*). *J. Food Sci.* **1994**, *59*, 76–79. [CrossRef]
49. Association of Official Analytical Chemists. *Official Methods of Analysis of AOAC International*; AOAC International: Rockville, MD, USA, 1998.
50. Willenberg, I.; Meschede, A.K.; Gueler, F.; Jang, M.-S.; Shushakova, N.; Schebb, N.H. Food Polyphenols Fail to Cause a Biologically Relevant Reduction of COX-2 Activity. *PLoS ONE* **2015**, *10*, e0139147. [CrossRef]
51. Khatun, M.S.; Hasan, M.M.; Kurata, H. PreAIP: Computational prediction of anti-inflammatory peptides by integrating multiple complementary features. *Front. Genet.* **2019**, *10*, 129. [CrossRef]
52. Purwaningtyas, H.P.; Suhartakik, N.; Mustofa, A. Formulation of jelly from candy Betel (*Piper betle* L.)—Suji (*Pleomele angustofolia*) leaf extract. *J. Teknol. Dan Ind. Pangan* **2017**, *2*, 25–30. (In Indonesian)

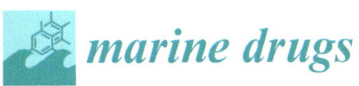

Review

Enzyme Inhibitors from Gorgonians and Soft Corals

Andrea Córdova-Isaza [1,2,†], Sofía Jiménez-Mármol [1,2,†], Yasel Guerra [1,2,*] and Emir Salas-Sarduy [3,4,*]

1 Ingeniería en Biotecnología, Facultad de Ingeniería y Ciencias Aplicadas, Universidad de Las Américas, Quito 170125, Ecuador
2 Grupo de Bio-Quimioinformática, Universidad de Las Américas, Quito 170125, Ecuador
3 Instituto de Investigaciones Biotecnológicas (IIB) "Dr. Rodolfo A. Ugalde", Consejo Nacional de Investigaciones Científicas y Técnicas (CONICET), Buenos Aires B1650HMP, Argentina
4 Escuela de Bio y Nanotecnología (EByN), Universidad de San Martín (UNSAM), Buenos Aires B1650HMP, Argentina
* Correspondence: yasel.guerra.borrego@udla.edu.ec (Y.G.); esalas@iib.unsam.edu.ar (E.S.-S.); Tel.: +593-2-3981000 (ext. 964) (Y.G.); +54-11-4006-1500 (ext. 2120) (E.S.-S.)
† These authors contributed equally to this work.

Abstract: For decades, gorgonians and soft corals have been considered promising sources of bioactive compounds, attracting the interest of scientists from different fields. As the most abundant bioactive compounds within these organisms, terpenoids, steroids, and alkaloids have received the highest coverage in the scientific literature. However, enzyme inhibitors, a functional class of bioactive compounds with high potential for industry and biomedicine, have received much less notoriety. Thus, we revised scientific literature (1974–2022) on the field of marine natural products searching for enzyme inhibitors isolated from these taxonomic groups. In this review, we present representative enzyme inhibitors from an enzymological perspective, highlighting, when available, data on specific targets, structures, potencies, mechanisms of inhibition, and physiological roles for these molecules. As most of the characterization studies for the new inhibitors remain incomplete, we also included a methodological section presenting a general strategy to face this goal by accomplishing STRENDA (Standards for Reporting Enzymology Data) project guidelines.

Keywords: enzyme inhibitors; natural products; gorgonian; soft coral; enzyme kinetics; inhibitor characterization; STRENDA guidelines

Citation: Córdova-Isaza, A.; Jiménez-Mármol, S.; Guerra, Y.; Salas-Sarduy, E. Enzyme Inhibitors from Gorgonians and Soft Corals. *Mar. Drugs* **2023**, *21*, 104. https://doi.org/10.3390/md21020104

Academic Editors: Francesc Xavier Avilés and Isel Pascual

Received: 23 December 2022
Revised: 28 January 2023
Accepted: 28 January 2023
Published: 31 January 2023

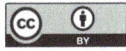

1. Introduction

Enzyme inhibitors are ubiquitous in nature and, as key regulators of enzyme activity, play pivotal roles in the physiology of all living forms. At a molecular level, endogenous inhibitors regulate enzymatic processes such as metabolism and nutrition, transport, signal transduction, DNA damage repair, apoptosis, cell differentiation, and cell cycle progression, among others. Therefore, many enzyme inhibitors are directly involved in critical events in the context of health and disease [1–8]. Natural enzyme inhibitors also target exogenous enzymes, such as those from invading or competing organisms. Pathogenic viruses, bacteria, fungi, and parasites usually depend on enzymes as virulence factors to guarantee successful colonization and survival. Additionally, digestive enzymes can be used as part of the offensive armamentarium of living organisms in highly crowded environments to avoid competition. Thus, endogenous enzyme inhibitors result in effective defensive immune or anti-predatory mechanisms against such molecular weapons [9,10]. Consequently, natural enzyme inhibitors have received notorious attention as a research subject and have found numerous biomedical [11,12], industrial [13], and environmental applications [14,15].

Marine environments house many different organisms which produce a huge diversity of bioactive molecules. In particular, they have proven to be a prolific source of novel enzyme inhibitors with unique functional features. Inhibitors for all major enzyme classes have been isolated and characterized from marine sources, including kinases [16–19], proteases [20], phospholipases [21], glucosidases [22], cholinesterases [23,24], topoisomerases [25], and DNA polymerases [26], among others. Accordingly, many of them have found interesting investigational, biomedical, and biotechnological applications [27–29]. The anthozoan sub-class Octocorallia, including over 3000 extant species of soft corals, gorgonian, and sea pens, has been considered a promising reservoir of unique natural products with unusual bioactivities [30]. Octocorals are widely distributed in all marine environments around the world and comprise three taxonomic orders: Helioporacea, Pennatulacea, and Alcyonaceae [30]. Although not strict in a taxonomic sense, the term "soft coral" is commonly applied to organisms in the Pennatulacea and Alcyonaceae orders with their polyps embedded within a fleshy mass of coenenchymal tissue [31]. Similarly, the term "gorgonian" is used to designate multiple species of the Alcyonaceae order producing a skeletal axis (or axial-like layer) composed of calcite and the proteinaceous material gorgonin [31]. Both soft corals and gorgonians have been found to be sources of numerous natural products with high structural diversity and interesting bioactivities, with terpenoids, steroids, and alkaloids as the most popular [4]. Although less represented in the scientific literature, several fascinating enzyme inhibitors have been also reported from these sources [32].

Due to their great diversity and potential, there is a sustained interest in identifying new enzyme inhibitors from these marine organisms. In the past decade, we worked actively on the prospection and characterization of protease inhibitory activities in the aqueous extracts of invertebrates from the Caribbean Sea [33–36]. Our interest focused on tight-binding protease inhibitors from the gorgonian *Plexaura homomalla*, and by transference, in related taxonomic classes such as soft corals. Thus, in this work, we decided to review recent progress in the identification and enzymological characterization of enzyme inhibitors from these marine organisms. From this literature analysis, protein-tyrosine phosphatase 1B (PTP1B) and the ubiquitin-proteasome system emerged as the enzymes most frequently targeted by novel inhibitors, while terpenes and terpenoids predominated among inhibitors. We also observed that, in contrast with the detailed structural studies present in almost all the studies, the enzymological characterization was insufficient or absent for many of the newly reported inhibitors. Critical aspects of inhibition, such as reversibility, time dependency, inhibition type, and the value for the inhibition thermodynamic constant K_i [37], must be properly determined so that these bioactive molecules find applications according to their potential. Considering that most novel inhibitors are indeed identified in laboratories not specialized in enzymology, we also included in this review a final section with strategic recommendations on how to conduct such kind of characterization, using STRENDA (Standards for Reporting Enzymology Data) guidelines as a methodological framework [37–39].

2. Enzyme Inhibitors Isolated from Gorgonians and Soft Corals

Figure 1 graphically resumes relevant statistics on the collected information describing enzyme inhibitors from soft corals and gorgonians. We found and processed over 50 scientific reports, published between 1974 and 2022, which contained 127 inhibitor molecules (Supplementary Tables S1 to S3). Concerning their origin, soft corals were the preferred source for the prospection of new inhibitors in this period (Figure 1A), accounting for about 64% of the reviewed papers. This tendency was confirmed in the last 5 years when the proportion increased to 81% (Figure 1B). Considering that 206 original papers from this field (i.e., search terms: "natural product" AND "soft coral" OR "gorgonian" NOT "Review") were deposited in PUBMED in the period 1974–2022, the class of enzyme inhibitors seemed to be a predominant one, representing nearly 25% of the total scientific production.

For classification purposes, the target enzymes for the reported inhibitors were grouped into four major classes (i.e., hydrolases, oxidoreductases, transferases, and translocases) according to the reaction type they catalyze. Hydrolases and transferases were, by far, the most abundant among them (Figure 1C and Table 1).

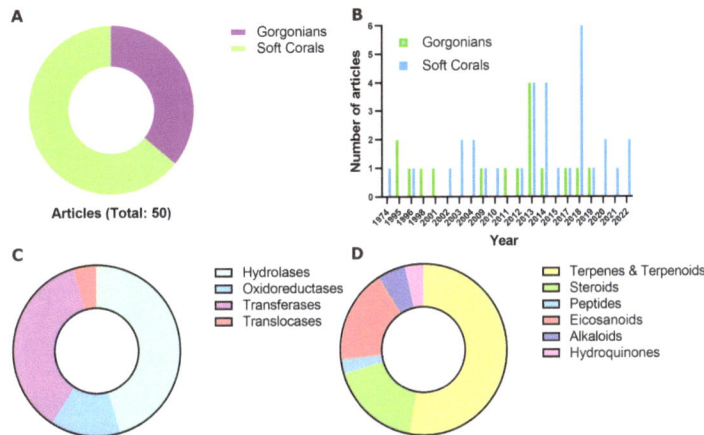

Figure 1. Distribution of the reviewed enzyme inhibitors isolated from soft corals and gorgonians. Inhibitors were classified according to their organism of origin (**A**), publication date (**B**), principal classes of targeted enzymes (**C**), and molecular structure (**D**).

Table 1. List of enzymes targeted by the inhibitors isolated from soft corals and gorgonians. Associated diseases and/or processes are also indicated.

Enzyme	EC Number	Class	Disease/Process
Protein tyrosine phosphatase 1B	3.1.3.48	Hydrolase	Cancer
Acetylcholinesterase	3.1.1.7	Hydrolase	Alzheimer's disease
HIV-1 protease	3.4.23.16	Hydrolase	HIV-AIDS
Elastase	3.4.21.11	Hydrolase	Immune response/inflammation
3CLpro Enzyme	3.4.22.69	Hydrolase	COVID-19
Ubiquitin-proteasome system	3.4.25.1	Hydrolase	Neurodegenerative/ immune-related/cancer
Phosphodiesterase-4	3.1.4.53	Hydrolase	Inflammatory/asthma/chronic obstructive pulmonary diseases
α-glucosidase	3.2.1.207	Hydrolase	Type II diabetes
Histone deacetylase 6	3.5.1.98	Hydrolase	Immunoregulation
Phospholipase A2	3.1.1.4	Hydrolase	Cancer/inflammation/atherosclerosis
5α-Reductase	1.3.1.22	Oxidoreductase	Benign hyperplasia/ male pattern baldness
Cytochrome P450 1A	1.14.14.1	Oxidoreductase	Cancer
Tyrosinase	1.14.18.1	Oxidoreductase	Development of skin-whitening agents
Tyrosine kinase p56[lck]	2.7.10.2	Transferase	Inflammatory/ autoimmune disorders
IKKbeta kinase	2.7.11.10	Transferase	Inflammatory diseases
Epidermal growth factor receptor kinase	2.7.10.1	Transferase	Cancer
Protein kinase C	2.7.11.13	Transferase	Cancer/neurological/ cardiovascular disorders
Human tumor-related protein kinases	-	Transferase	Cancer
Casitas B-lineage lymphoma proto-oncogene B	2.3.2.27	Transferase	Cancer
Farnesyl protein transferase	2.5.1.58	Transferase	Cancer
Glutathione S-transferase	2.5.1.18	Transferase	Cancer
H (+)-pyrophosphatase	7.1.3.1	Translocase	-

Lastly, we grouped inhibitors by targets and tabulated their structures, potencies (predominantly as half-maximal inhibitory concentrations or IC_{50} values), and source organism. Inhibitors were classified into six major classes (i.e., terpenes and terpenoids, steroids, peptides, eicosanoids, alkaloids, and hydroquinones), and showed relatively low structural diversity. As expected, more than half of the inhibitory molecules identified in this period from soft corals and gorgonians were terpenes and terpenoids (Figure 1D), two classes that have historically dominated the literature on coral-derived natural products. Surprisingly, the functional characterization of novel enzyme inhibitors was biased toward cellular toxicity studies and not toward the in-depth understanding of their inhibitory activity. In the few cases where further enzymological information was available (e.g., inhibition mechanism, the value for the thermodynamic constant K_i, or target specificity), we included it within the text.

2.1. Hydrolases

2.1.1. Protein Tyrosine Phosphatase 1B (PTP1B) (EC 3.1.3.48)

The enzyme PTP1B is known as a target in the search for new drugs in the treatment of type 2 diabetes, obesity, and breast cancer [40–42]. This enzyme is one of the most used targets in the evaluation of marine compounds as enzyme inhibitors from soft corals. Twenty-eight molecules from seven soft coral and gorgonian species have been reported as PTP1B inhibitors (Table 2 and Figure 2). Most of these compounds are diterpenes or diterpenoids, with a few cases of steroids. The soft coral *Sarcophyton trocheliophorum Marenzeller* is the source of the highest number of isolated PTP1B inhibitors, such as the capnosane-type diterpenes Sarsolides A (**1**) and B (**2**) [43], the cembrane diterpenoids sarcophytonolide N (**3**), sarcrassin E (**4**), cembrene C (**5**), 4Z,12Z,14E-sarcophytolide (**6**), ketoemblide (**7**) [44], and the diterpenoid Methyl sarcotroate B (**8**) (Table 2 and Figure 2) [45]. The inhibitory results from capnosane-type diterpenes suggest that the presence of an exomethylene $\Delta 10$ (17) of the capnosane skeleton may play an important role in inhibitory activity [43]. In a similar way, some preliminary structure–function relationships could be proposed for the cembrane diterpenoids. The most potent molecules, sarcophytonolide N and sarcrassin E, have a dienoate moiety at C-1 through C-18, while the presence of an α-β-unsaturated lactone in sarcrassin E seems to be not essential for the inhibition. On the other hand, the presence of the methyl ester group at C-18 in sarcophytonolide N and sarcrassin E increases the inhibitory activity. The lack of cytotoxicity against human cell lines A-549 and HL-60 makes these compounds promising hits for the development of a new class of PTP1B inhibitors [43]. Methyl sarcotroates B is the only PTP1B inhibitor isolated from a marine organism containing a hydroperoxide group [43].

Table 2. PTP1B inhibitors isolated from soft corals and gorgonians.

Compound	IC_{50} (µM)	Source	Classification	Reference
Sarsolides A (**1**)	6.8			[43]
Sarsolides B (**2**)	27.1			
Sarcophytonolide N (**3**)	5.95	*Sarcophyton trocheliophorum Marenzeller*	Soft coral	
Sarcrassin E (**4**)	6.33			[44]
Cembrene C (**5**)	26.6			
4Z,12Z,14E-sarcophytolide (**6**)	15.4			
Ketoemblide (**7**)	27.2			
Methyl sarcotroates B (**8**)	6.97			[45]

Table 2. *Cont.*

Compound	IC$_{50}$ (μM)	Source	Classification	Reference
Sinulin D (**9**)	47,500	*Sinularia* sp.	Soft coral	[46]
(1*R*,3*S*,4*S*,7*E*,11*E*)-3,4-epoxycembra-7,11,15-triene (**10**)	12,500			
15-hydroxy-α-cadinol (**11**)	22,100			
Sinupol (**12**)	63.9	*Sinularia polydactyla*	Soft coral	[47]
(1*R*,4*aR*,6*S*,8*aS*)-6-((2*E*,4*E*)-6-hydroxy-6-methylhepta-2,4-dien-2-yl)-4,8*a*-dimethyl-1,2,4*a*,5,6,7,8,8*a*-octahyronaphthalen-1-ol (**13**)	75.5			
Sinulacetate (**14**)	51.8			
Linardosinene I (**15**)	10.67 [1]	*Litophyton nigrum*	Soft coral	[48]
Molestins C (**16**)	218	*Sinularia* cf. *molesta*	Soft coral	[49]
Molestins D (**17**)	344			
(5′*Z*)-5-(2′,6′-Dimethylocta-5′,7′-dienyl)-furan-3-carboxylic acid (**18**)	1.24			
(3β,4α,5α,8β)-4-methylergost-24(28)-ene-8-ol-3-monoacetate (**19**)	22.7	*Sinularia depressa*	Soft coral	[50]
(3β, 4α, 5α)-4-methylergost-24(28)-ene-3-ol (**20**)	19.5			
Ergost-4,24(28)-diene-3-one (**21**)	15.3			
7α-hydroxy-crassarosterol A (**22**)	33.05	*Sinularia flexibilis*	Soft coral	[51]
Lipidyl pseudopterane A (**23**)	71 [1]	*Pseudopterogorgia acerosa*	Gorgonian	[52]
Lipidyl pseudopterane B (**24**)	ND			
Lipidyl pseudopterane C (**25**)	ND			
Lipidyl pseudopterane D (**26**)	ND			
Lipidyl pseudopterane E (**27**)	ND			
Lipidyl pseudopterane F (**28**)	ND			

[1] μg/mL, ND—not determined.

PTP1B inhibitors have also been isolated from several species of the soft coral genus *Sinularia*. The cembranoids sinulin D (**9**) and (1*R*,3*S*,4*S*,7*E*,11*E*)-3,4-epoxycembra-7,11, 15-triene (**10**), together with the sesquiterpenoid 15-hydroxy-α-cadinol (**11**), were isolated from *Sinularia* sp. [46]. These three terpenoids showed IC$_{50}$ values in the millimolar range, which can be considered a weak inhibitory activity [46]. The prenyleudesmane-type diterpene sinupol (**12**), and (1*R*,4*aR*,6*S*,8*aS*)-6-((2*E*,4*E*)-6-hydroxy-6-methylhepta-2,4-dien-2-yl)-4,8*a*-dimethyl-1,2,4*a*,5,6,7,8,8*a*-octahyronaphthalen-1-ol (**13**) have been isolated from the soft coral *Sinularia polydactyla* [47]. Furthermore, the capnosane-type diterpenoid sinulacetate (**14**) and the nardosinane-type sesquiterpenoid linardosinene I (**15**) were found in *Sinularia polydactyla* and *Litophyton nigrum* [48], respectively. Additionally, the guaiane-type sesquiterpenes Molestins C (**16**) and D (**17**), together with the furanosesquiterpene (5′*Z*)-5-(2′,6′-Dimethylocta-5′,7′-dienyl)-furan-3-carboxylic acid (**18**), were isolated from *Sinularia* cf. *molesta* [49]. On the other hand, the steroids (3β,4α,5α,8β)-4-methylergost-24(28)-ene-8-ol-3-monoacetate (**19**), (3β,4α,5α)-4-methylergost-24(28)-ene-3-ol, ergost-4,24(28)-diene-3-one (**20**), and ergost-4,24(28)-diene-3-one (**21**) were isolated from *Sinularia depressa* [50], while the polyhydroxylated steroid 7α-hydroxy-crassarosterol A (**22**) was found in *Sinularia flexibilis* [51]. A potential role of substitution of hydroxyl groups in positions 3 and 8 is proposed, based on the results obtained from steroids with the same scaffold isolated from *Sinularia depressa*.

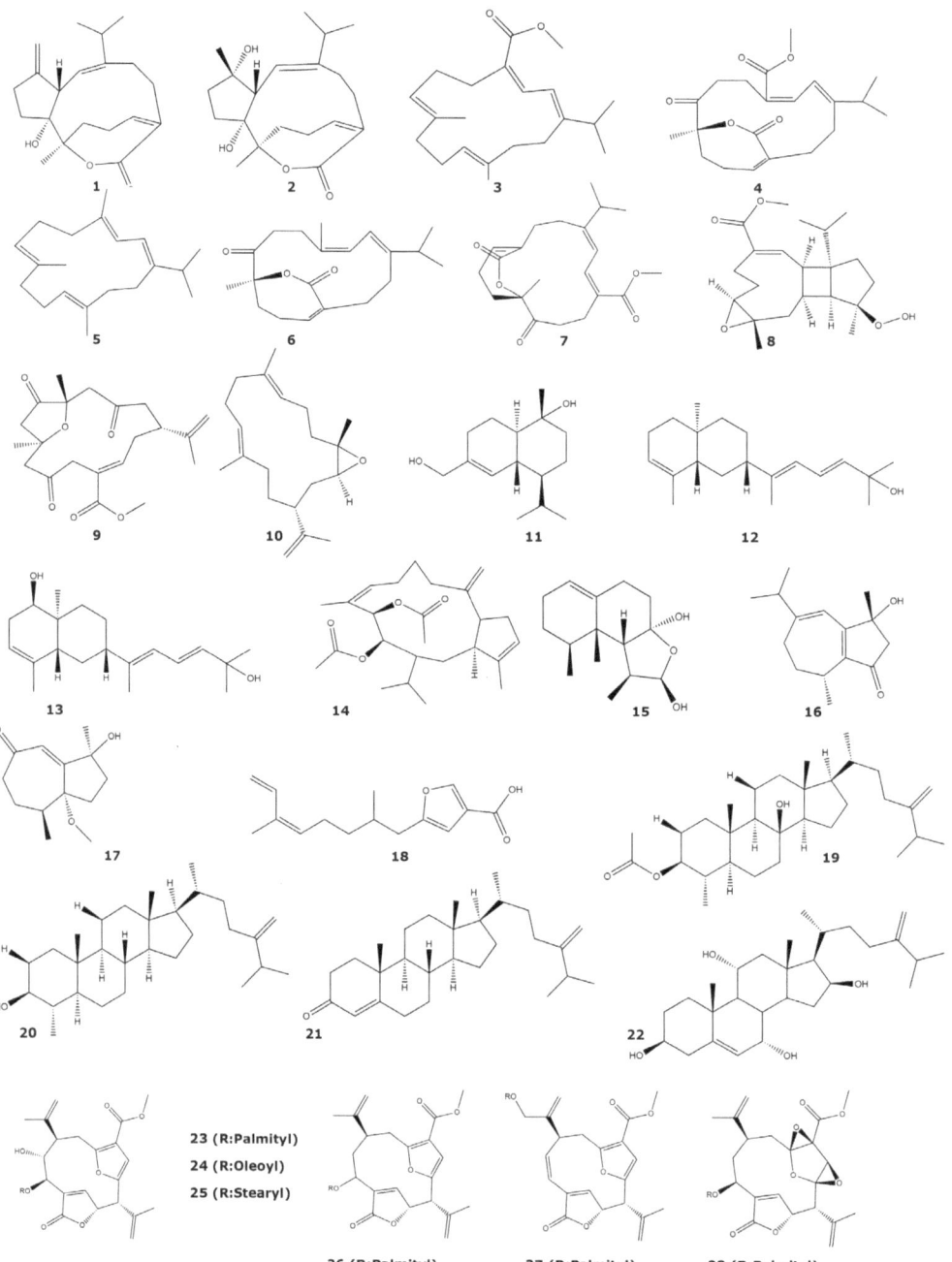

Figure 2. PTP1B inhibitors isolated from soft corals and gorgonians (compounds **1–28**).

Several new lipidyl pseudopteranes (**23–28**) with inhibitory activity towards PTP1B were found in the gorgonian *Pseudopterogorgia acerosa* [52]. These compounds were reported as the first pseudopterane diterpenes with a fatty acid moiety and, based on the enzymatic assays performed with several enzymes of the protein tyrosine phosphatase family, they have been described as selective inhibitors of PTP1B.

2.1.2. Acetylcholinesterase (EC 3.1.1.7)

The enzyme acetylcholinesterase is a validated drug target for the treatment of Alzheimer´s disease [53], with several inhibitors approved by the FDA for its clinical use [54]. All the acetylcholinesterase inhibitors described from soft coral and gorgonians are diterpenes or sesquiterpenes, with little or no quantitative data about their inhibition. The most potent and best-characterized inhibitors are the cembranes asperdiol (**29**) and 14-acetoxycrassine (**32**), isolated from the soft coral *Eunicea knighti* and the gorgonian *Pseudoplexaura porosa*, respectively (Table 3 and Figure 3) [55]. Other cembranes, with acetylcholinesterase inhibitory activity, were found in *Eunicea knighti* and *Pseudoplexaura flagellosa*; but no further kinetic characterization was performed [55]. Additionally, the diterpene sarcophine (**33**), produced by *Sarcophyton glaucum*, was described as a competitive inhibitor of acetylcholinesterase, although no IC$_{50}$ or K$_i$ value was reported [56]. In the same study, it was suggested that sarcophine (**33**) inhibits acetylcholinesterase through the formation of an adduct with the free cysteines of the enzyme. Other compounds, that have been classified as weak acetylcholinesterase inhibitors are the sesquiterpenoid sinuketal (**34**) and the cembranoid crassumolide E (**35**), which were isolated from *Sinularia* sp. and *Lobophytum* sp., respectively [46,57]. It should be noted that crassumolide E (**35**) was considered a weak inhibitor in comparison with galanthamine, although the minimal concentration of crassumolide E needed to inhibit the enzyme was in the nanomolar range.

Table 3. Inhibitors of the hydrolases acetylcholinesterase, HIV-1 protease, elastase, and 3CLpro isolated from soft corals and gorgonians.

Compound	IC$_{50}$ (μM)	Source	Classification	Reference
Acetylcholinesterase				
Asperdiol (**29**)	0.358			
Asperdiol diacetate (**30**)	ND	*Eunicea knighti*	Soft coral	[55]
8*R*-dihydroplexaurolone (**31**)	ND			
14-acetoxycrassine (**32**)	1.40	*Pseudoplexaura porosa*	Gorgonian	
Sarcophine (**33**)	ND	*Sarcophyton glaucum*	Soft coral	[56]
Sinuketal (**34**)	ND	*Sinularia* sp.	Soft coral	[46]
Crassumolide E (**35**)	ND	*Lobophytum* sp.	Soft coral	[57]
HIV-1 protease				
Alismol (**36**)	7.20			
7β-acetoxy-24-methylcholesta-5-24(28)-diene-3,19-diol (**37**)	4.85			
erythro-N-dodecanoyl-docosasphinga-(4*E*,8*E*)-dienine (**38**)	4.80	*Litophyton arboreum*	Soft coral	[58]
Sarcophytol M (**39**)	15.7			
Chimyl alcohol (**40**)	26.6			
Elastase				
PcKuz1	ND			
PcKuz2	ND	*Palythoa caribaeorum*	Soft coral	[59]
PcKuz3	ND			
(15R)-PGE2 (**41**)	ND			
(15R)-PGA2 (**42**)	ND	*Plexaura homomalla*	Gorgonian	[60]
(15*R*)-*O*Ac-PGA2 (**43**)	ND			
3CLpro				
Tuaimenal A (**44**)	21	*Duva florida*	Soft coral	[61]

ND—not determined.

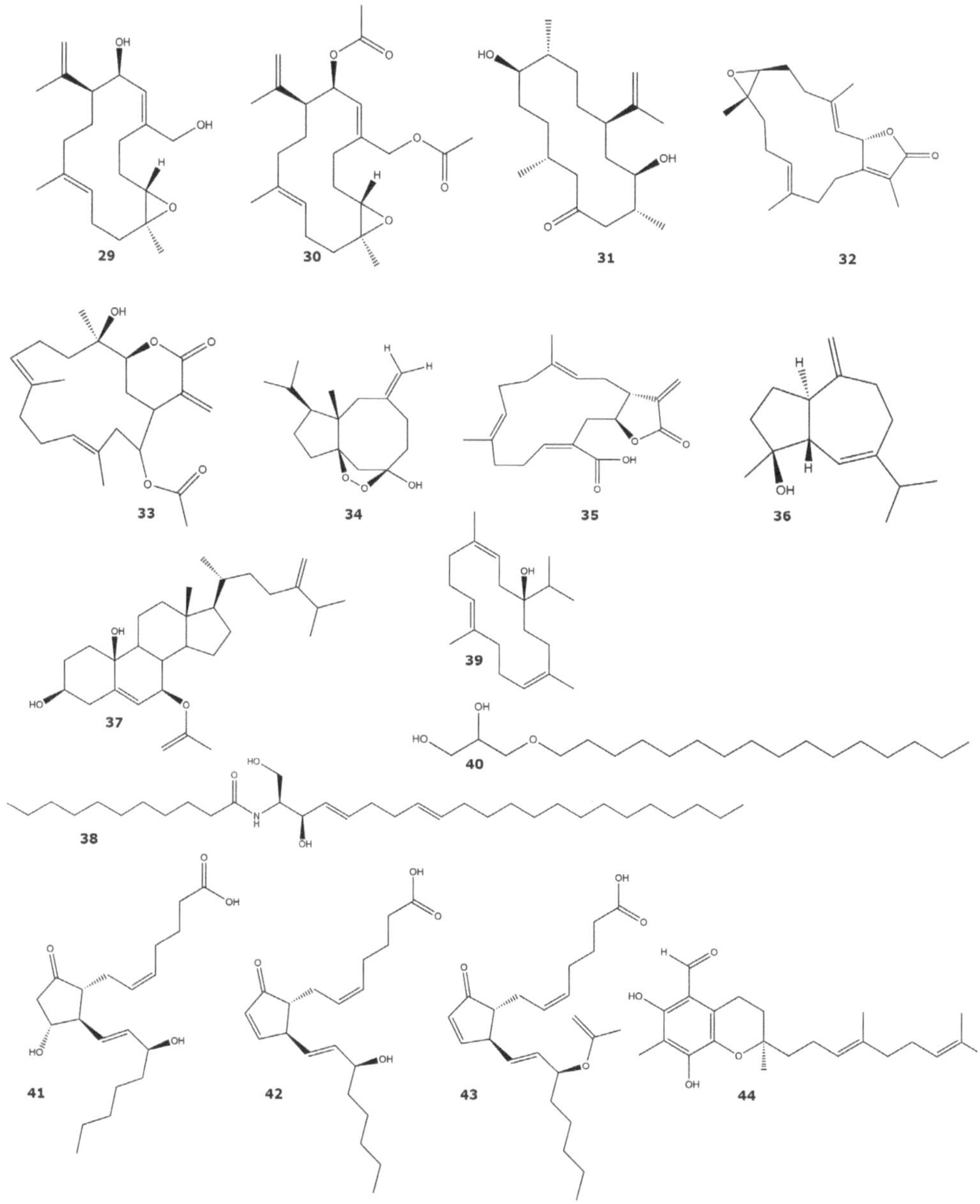

Figure 3. Hydrolase inhibitors isolated from soft corals and gorgonians (compounds **29–44**). Structures include inhibitors of acetylcholinesterase, HIV-1 protease, Elastase, and 3CLpro.

2.1.3. HIV-1 Protease (EC 3.4.23.16)

HIV-1 protease is a well-established drug target for the treatment of HIV-AIDS [62,63]. In fact, several inhibitors of this enzyme are used in highly active antiretroviral therapy used for the treatment of this disease [64]. Several molecules with inhibitory activity against the protease of HIV-1 have been identified from the soft coral *Litophyton arboreum* (Table 3 and Figure 3). The structural diversity among the compounds alismol (**36**), 7β-acetoxy-24-methylcholesta-5-24(28)-diene-3,19-diol (**37**), erythro-N-dodecanoyl-docosasphinga-(4*E*,8*E*)-dienine (**38**), sarcophytol M (**39**), and chimyl alcohol (**40**) is signifi-cant, with the presence of sesquiterpenes, diterpenes, glyceryl ethers, and steroids [58]. The most potent compounds are 7β-acetoxy-24-methylcholesta-5-24(28)-diene-3,19-diol (**37**) and erythro-N-dodecanoyl-docosasphinga-(4*E*,8*E*)-dienine (**38**) with remarkably similar potency against the HIV-1 protease.

2.1.4. Elastase (EC 3.4.21.11)

Elastases are serine proteases belonging to the chymotrypsin-like family. Human neutrophil elastase (HNE) is one of the best-characterized elastases, as it plays important roles in inflammation, the elimination and degradation of extracellular pathogens, and the activation of other proteases [65]. As a key inflammation mediator, the discovery and development of new HNE inhibitors have received significant interest [66].

Kunitz-like peptides 1–3 (PcKuz 1–3), isolated from *Palythoa caribaeorum*, are a few of the peptide-nature molecules described as enzyme inhibitors from soft corals [59]. However, the weak inhibitory activity against the serine proteases trypsin and elastase, and the results of toxicity tests with zebrafish larvae, lead the authors of this study to suggest that these peptides should be considered Kunitz-type neurotoxins rather than protease inhibitors.

Three prostaglandins (**41**–**43**) with inhibitory activity against elastase were isolated from the gorgonian *Plexaura homomalla* (Table 3 and Figure 3) [60]. These compounds showed similar potency, in terms of inhibition, in the kinetic assays performed in this study, but no IC_{50} or K_i values were reported. Based on the results of the kinetics assays, it seems that the presence of the carboxyl group is essential for elastase inhibition, since the molecules with an acetyl ester in this position showed no inhibition on the enzyme [60].

2.1.5. 3CLpro Enzyme (EC 3.4.22.69)

The main protease of severe acute respiratory syndrome coronavirus is critical for the replication cycle of these viruses [67]. The main protease of SARS-CoV-2 is a 3CLpro cysteine protease that performs the cleavage of 12 nonstructural proteins of the virus. Inhibitors of this protease have proved to be effective in the inhibition of viral replication in cell-based assays [68]. An inhibitor of the SARS-CoV-2 3CLpro protease, described as a cyclized merosesquiterpenoid with a new carbon scaffold and composed by a highly substituted chromene core, was found in *Duva florida* (Table 3 and Figure 3) [61]. This compound, named Tuaimenal A (**44**), showed no inhibitory activity against other cysteine proteases (*Fasciola hepatica* cathepsin L1 and L3, and human cathepsin L) or serine proteases (trypsin, chymotrypsin, and thrombin), suggesting a particular specificity towards 3CLpro protease. Cell-based studies have shown that Tuaimenal A (**44**) has low toxicity in cells that are sensitive to other protease inhibitors, highlighting the potential of this molecule as a hit in the development of new anti-coronavirus drugs.

2.1.6. Ubiquitin-Proteasome System (EC 3.4.25.1)

The ubiquitin–proteasome system plays a critical role in the maintenance of proteome homeostasis. Therefore, proteasome is considered an important target for the development of drugs for the treatment of diseases such as neurodegenerative disease, immune-related disease, and cancer [69]. Several inhibitors of the ubiquitin–proteasome system have been identified using a cell-based, high-content assay based on the measurement of aggregations of ubiquitinated proteins. Among these inhibitors are the cembrane-based molecules Sarcophytonin A (**45**) and Laevigatol A (**46**), which were isolated from the soft coral *Sarcophyton trocheliophorum*; as well as Sarcophytoxide (**47**) and Sarcophine (**33**), isolated from *Sarcophyton ehrenbergi* (Table 4 and Figure 4) [70]. Sarcophytonin A (**45**) and Sarcophine (**33**) seem to target the 19S proteasome, based on the results obtained by comparison to the mechanistic action of known proteasome inhibitors. All four compounds showed negligible cytotoxicity (ED_{50} > 25 μg/mL) to human HEK293T cells. In addition, the dolabellane-based compounds clavinflol C (**48**), stolonidiol (**49**), stolonidiol-17-acetate (**50**), and clavinflol B (**51**), and the secosteroid-based molecules 3β,11-dihydroxy-24-methyl-9,11-

secocholest-5-en-9,23-dione (**52**), and 3β,11-dihydroxy-24-methylene-9,11-secocholest-5-en-9,23-dione (**53**) were purified from *Clavularia flava* [71]. These six molecules have shown less cytotoxicity than the known proteasome inhibitors bortezimid and MG132.

Table 4. Inhibitors of the hydrolases ubiquitin–proteasome system and phosphodiesterase-4, isolated from soft corals and gorgonians.

Compound	IC$_{50}$ (µM)	Source	Classification	Reference
Ubiquitin–Proteasome system				
Sarcophytonin A (**45**)	ND	*Sarcophyton trocheliophorum*	Soft coral	[70]
Laevigatol A (**46**)	ND			
Sarcophytoxide (**47**)	ND	*Sarcophyton ehrenbergi*	Soft coral	
Sarcophine (**33**)	ND			
Clavinflol C (**48**)	ND	*Clavularia flava*	Soft coral	[71]
Stolonidiol (**49**)	ND			
Stolonidiol-17-acetate (**50**)	ND			
Clavinflol B (**51**)	ND			
3β,11-dihydroxy-24-methyl-9,11-secocholest-5-en-9,23-dione (**52**)	ND			
3β,11-dihydroxy-24-methylene-9,11-secocholest-5-en-9,23-dione (**53**)	ND			
Methyl (2R,3S,8S,9R,E)-8-hydroxy-15-methoxy-5-oxo-2,9-di(prop-1-en-2-yl)-4,14-dioxatricyclo [9.2.1.1^{3,6}] pentadeca-1(13),6,11-triene-12-carboxylate (**54**)	9.77	*Pseudopterogorgia acerosa*	Gorgonian	[72]
PNG 2 (**55**)	ND	*Telesto riisei*	Soft coral	[73]
PNG 3 (**56**)	ND			
PNG 4 (**57**)	ND			
Z-PNG 4 (**58**)	ND			
PNG 6 (**59**)	ND			
Phosphodiesterase-4				
Sarcoehrendin B (**60**)	3.7	*Sarcophyton ehrenbergi*	Soft coral	[74]
Sarcoehrendin D (**61**)	10.6			
Sarcoehrendin F (**62**)	12.1			
Sarcoehrendin H (**63**)	16.9			
Sarcoehrendin J (**64**)	7.2			
9α,15α-diacetoxy-11α-hydroxy-5Z,13E-prostadienoic acid methyl ester (**65**)	4.7			
(5Z,9α,11α,13E,15S)-11,15-bis(acetoxy)-9-hydroxyprosta-5,13-dien-1-oic acid methyl ester (**66**)	5.5			
9,11,15-triacetoxy PGF2α methyl ester (**67**)	1.4			
Malonganenone L (**68**)	8.5	*Echinogorgia pseudossapo*	Gorgonian	[75]
Malonganenone M (**69**)	ND			
Malonganenone N (**70**)	ND			
Malonganenone O (**71**)	ND			
Malonganenone P (**72**)	ND			
Malonganenone Q (**73**)	20.3			

ND—not determined.

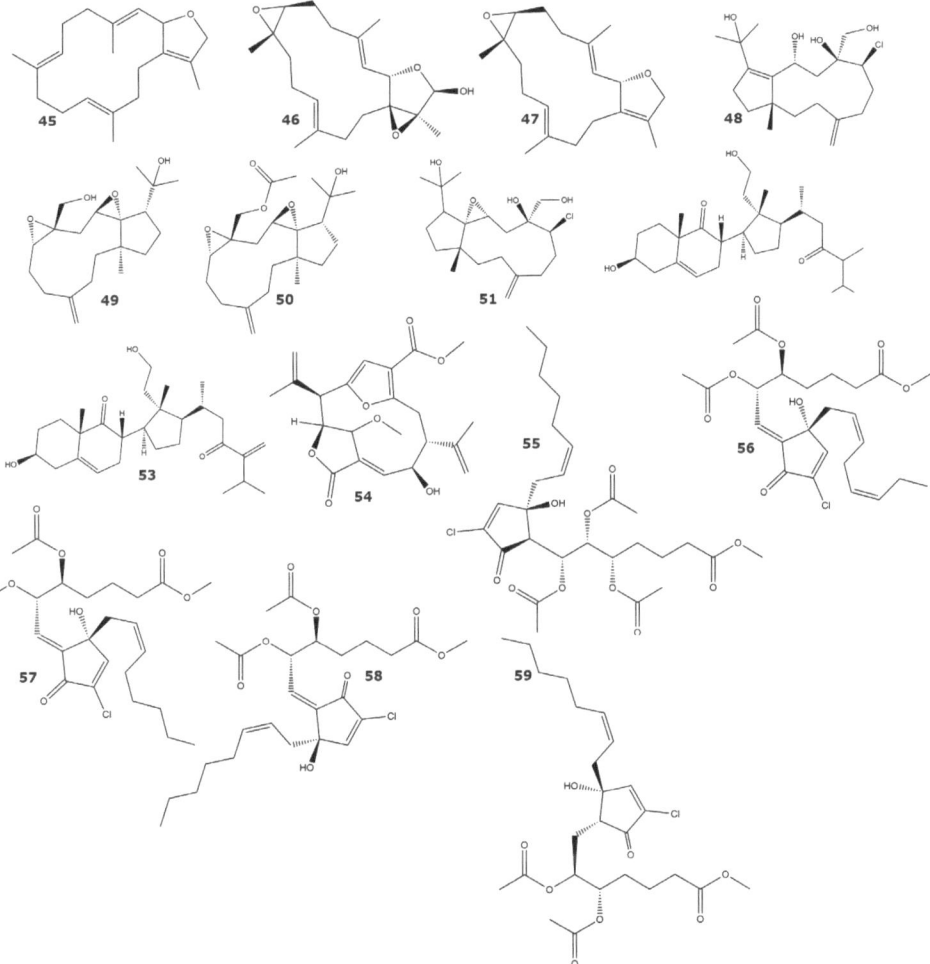

Figure 4. Inhibitors of the ubiquitin–proteasome system isolated from soft corals and gorgonians (compounds **45–59**).

A diterpenoid (**54**) found in the gorgonian *Pseudopterogorgia acerosa* inhibits the chymotrypsin-like activity of the ubiquitin–proteasome system, with no inhibition of its caspase-like activity [72].

Punaglandins are highly functional cyclopentadienone and cyclopentenone prostaglandins, chlorinated at the endocyclic R-carbon position. A group of these molecules, isolated from the soft coral *Telesto riisei*, were used to investigate the inhibition mechanism previously proposed for dienone prostaglandins [76]. In this study, the punaglandins PNG 2 (**55**), PNG 3 (**56**), PNG 4 (**57**), Z-PNG 4 (**58**), and PNG 6 (**59**) showed inhibitory activity against the ubiquitin isopeptidase using in vitro and in vivo assays (Table 4 and Figure 4) [73]. The use of these punaglandins demonstrates that the presence of chloride in endocyclic carbon increases the inhibitory activity in comparison to unchlorinated prostaglandins. Additionally, the results obtained suggest that the inhibitory activity of the prostaglandins is related to the olefin-ketone conjugation and the reactivity of the endocyclic carbon [73].

2.1.7. Phosphodiesterase-4 (EC 3.1.4.53)

The phosphodiesterases belong to a family of enzymes that catalyze the hydrolysis of the second messengers cyclic adenosine monophosphate (cAMP) and guanosine monophosphate (cGMP) [77]. Particularly, phosphodiesterase-4 is a promising drug target for diverse diseases including inflammatory, asthma, and chronic obstructive pulmonary disease [78]. Several prostaglandins showing inhibitory activity against phosphodiesterase-4 were isolated from the soft coral *Sarcophyton ehrenbergi*. A number of them were novel, such as compounds sarcoehrendin B (**60**), D (**61**), F (**62**), H (**63**), and J (**64**), while others, including 9α,15α-diacetoxy-11α-hydroxy-5Z,13E-prostadienoic acid methyl ester (**65**), (5Z,9α,11α,13E,15S)-11,15-bis(acetoxy)-9-hydroxyprosta-5,13-dien-1-oic acid methyl ester (**66**), and 9,11,15-triacetoxy PGF2α methyl ester (**67**), were already known molecules (Table 4 and Figure 5) [74]. Of these compounds, 5 showed IC_{50} values lower than 10 µM, while the inhibitory potency for 9,11,15-triacetoxy PGF2α methyl ester (**67**) was comparable to that of the positive control (rolipram). Based on the results obtained in this study, several structure–function relationships were proposed. For instance, the esterification at the OH-15 seems to be essential for a strong inhibitory activity, while the acetylation of OH-9 or OH-11 produces only a minor increase in activity [74].

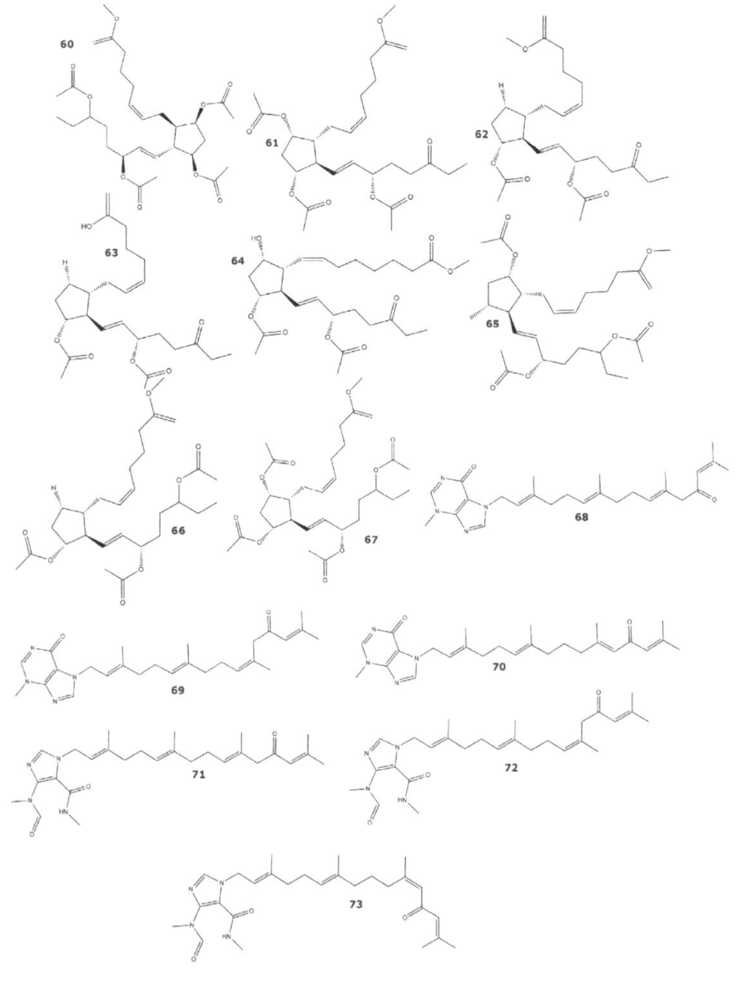

Figure 5. Phosphodiesterase-4 inhibitors isolated from soft corals and gorgonians (compounds **60–73**).

Moreover, six tetraprenylated alkaloids found in the gorgonian *Echinogorgia pseudossapo* showed inhibitory activity towards phosphodiesterase-4 [75]. These compounds are the melonganenones L–Q (**68–73**), with melonganenones L (**68**) and Q (**73**) exhibiting IC_{50} values of 8.5 and 20.3 µM, respectively (Table 4 and Figure 5). All six tetraprenylated alkaloids also showed inhibition against the phosphodiesterases PDE5A and PDE9A, but with weaker potency than towards PDE4 [75].

2.1.8. α-Glucosidase (EC 3.2.1.207)

α-Glucosidase is a key enzyme in carbohydrate metabolism, which regulates blood glucose. Through controlling postprandial glucose levels, this enzyme is a validated target for the treatment of type 2 diabetes, with several available inhibitors in the market [79,80]. Two cembranoid compounds with inhibitory activity towards α-glucosidase, sinulacrassin B (**74**) and S-(+)-cembrane A (**75**), were isolated from the soft coral *Sinularia crassa* (Table 5 and Figure 6) [81]. Both compounds showed higher inhibitory activity than 1-deoxynojirimycin, the positive control used in the enzymatic assay. In addition, these cembranoids were nontoxic towards human normal hepatocytes (LO2), with IC_{50} higher than 100 µM, providing a new scaffold for the development of anti-diabetes drugs.

Table 5. Inhibitors of hydrolases α-glucosidase, histone deacetylase 6, and phospholipase A2, isolated from soft corals and gorgonians.

Compound	IC_{50} (µM)	Source	Classification	Reference
α-glucosidase				
Sinulacrassin B (**74**)	10.65	*Sinularia crassa*	Soft coral	[81]
S-(+)-cembrane A (**75**)	30.31			
Histone deacetylase 6				
Methyl (1*S*, 4*S*, 5*R*, 9*S*9-4-((*Z*)-4-(3,3-dimethyloxiran-2-yl-)-1-hydrioxybut-2-en-2-yl)-1-methyl-6-methylene-10-oxabicyclo[7.1.0]decane-5-carboxylate (**76**)	80	*Xenia elongata*	Soft coral	[82]
Phospholipase A2				
Euplexide A (**77**)	ND	*Euplexaura anastomosans*	Gorgonian	[83]
Euplexide B (**78**)	ND			
Euplexide F (**79**)	ND			[84]
Euplexide G (**80**)	ND			
7α,8α-epoxy-3β,5α,6α-trihydroxycholestane (**81**)	ND	*Acabaria undulata*	Gorgonian	[85]
24-methyl-7α,8α-epoxy-3β,5α,6α-trihydroxycholest-22-ene (**82**)	ND			

ND—not determined.

2.1.9. Histone Deacetylase 6 (HDAC6) (EC3.5.1.98)

Histone deacetylases are enzymes that remove acetyl groups from histone and non-histone proteins, altering their stability and activity. Histone deacetylase 6 is a member of the Class IIb subfamily that participates in several biological processes including cell motility [86], cell survival [87], protein degradation [88], and immunoregulation [89]. A new diterpene, named methyl (1*S*, 4*S*, 5*R*, 9*S*9-4-((*Z*)-4-(3,3-dimethyloxiran-2-yl-)-1-hydrioxybut-2-en-2-yl)-1-methyl-6-methylene-10-oxabicyclo[7.1.0]decane-5-carboxylate (**76**), was found in the soft coral *Xenia elongata* (Table 5 and Figure 6) [82]. This molecule selectively inhibits histone deacetylase 6, with no detectable inhibitory activity against deacetylases from class I (HDAC1, HDAC2, HDAC3, and HDAC8) and IIA (HDAC4, HDAC5, HDAC7, and HDAC9).

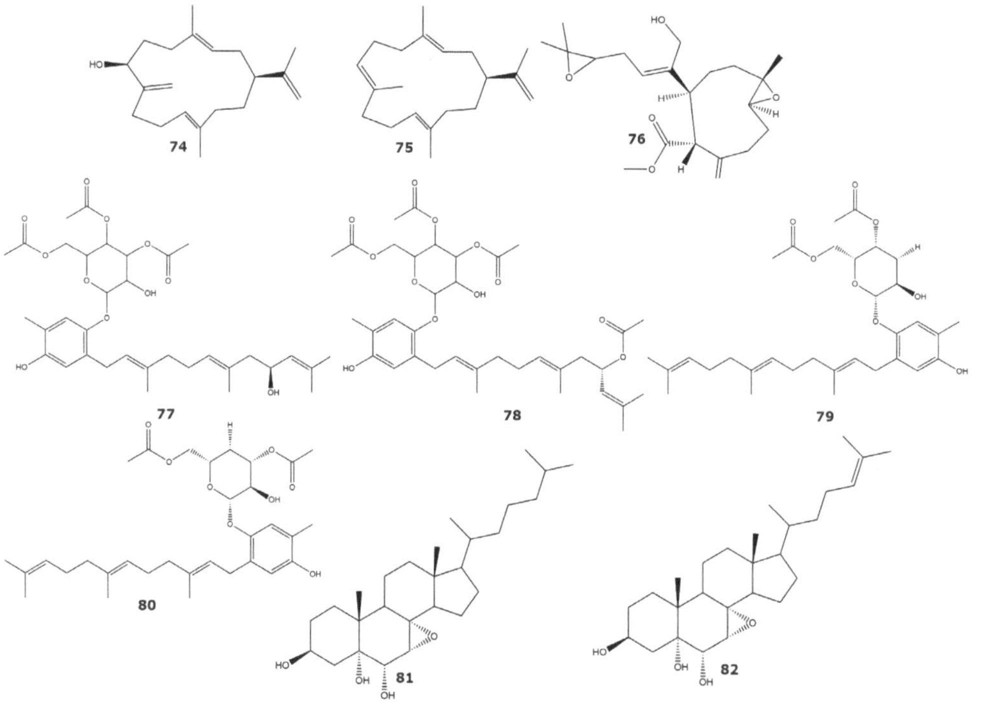

Figure 6. Hydrolase inhibitors isolated from soft corals and gorgonians (compounds **74–82**). Structures include inhibitors of α-glucosidase, Histone deacetylase 6 and Phospholipase A2.

2.1.10. Phospholipase A2 (PLA2) (EC 3.1.1.4)

Phospholipases A2 are esterases that cleave phospholipids and release fatty acids and lysophospholipids. These enzymes are considered as promising targets in the treatment of cancer, inflammation, and atherosclerosis, among other diseases [90–92]. Several PLA2 inhibitors have been found in the gorgonian *Euplexaura anastomosans*. These molecules, described as farnesylhydroquinone glycosides, were named Euplexides [83,84]. The euplexides A (**77**), B (**78**), F (**79**), and G (**80**) exhibited inhibitory activities against PLA2 ranging from 47 to 71% at 50 μg/mL, but no further kinetic characterization has been performed. Additionally, the steroids 7α,8α-epoxy-3β,5α,6α-trihydroxycholestane (**81**) and 24-methyl-7α,8α-epoxy-3β,5α,6α-trihydroxycholest-22-ene (**82**) have been isolated from the gorgonian *Acabaria undulata*, both with inhibitory activity towards PLA2 (Table 5 and Figure 6) [85].

2.2. Oxidoreductases

2.2.1. 5α-Reductase (EC 1.3.1.22)

The enzyme 5α-Reductase converts testosterone into the more potent androgen dihydrotestosterone. Inhibition of 5α-Reductase is a promising strategy in the treatment of benign hyperplasia and male pattern baldness [93,94]. Several soft steroidal molecules with inhibitory activity towards 5α-Reductase have been isolated from soft corals of the Adaman and Nicobar Islands. Some of these compounds were isolated from more than one species, such as the steroids 24-methylenecholest-5-ene-3β,7β, 16β-triol-3-O-α-l-fucopyranoside (**83**), that was found in three soft corals: *Sinularia crassa Tixier–Durivaul, Sinularia gravis Tixier–Durivault, Sinularia* sp., and 24-methylenecholest-5-ene-3β,7β, 16β-diol-3-O-α-l-fucopyranoside (**84**), isolated from *Sinularia* sp. and *Cladiella* sp. [95]. On the other hand, the molecules (24S)-24-methylcholestane-3β,5α,6β,7β-tetrol (**85**), and (24S)-24-methylcholestane-3β,5α,6β,25-tetrol (**86**) were isolated from *Lobophytum crassum* and

Lobophytum sp., respectively [95]. In a different study, the diterpenoid lemnabourside (**87**) was identified in the soft coral *Nephthea chabroli* [96], displaying weak inhibitory activity against 5α-Reductase (Table 6 and Figure 7) [96].

Table 6. Inhibitors of oxidoreductases isolated from soft corals and gorgonians.

Compound	IC$_{50}$ (µM)	Source	Classification	Reference
5α-Reductase				
24-methylenecholest-5-ene-3β,7β,16β-triol-3-O-α-l-fucopyranoside (**83**)	ND	*Sinularia crassa* Tixier–Durivaul	Soft coral	
		Sinularia gravis Tixier–Durivault	Soft coral	
		Sinularia sp.	Soft coral	[95]
24-methylenecholest-5-ene-3β,7β,16β-diol-3-O-α-l-fucopyranoside (**84**)	ND	*Sinularia* sp. *Cladiella* sp.	Soft coral Soft coral	
(24S)-24-methylcholestane-3β,5α,6β,7β-tetrol (**85**)	ND	*Lobophytum crassum*	Soft coral	
(24S)-24-methylcholestane-3β,5α,6β,25-tetrol (**86**)	ND	*Lobophytum* sp.	Soft coral	
Lemnabourside (**87**)	250	*Nephthea chabroli*	Soft coral	[96]
Cytochrome P450 1A				
12(S)-hydroperoxylsarcoph-10-ene, 8-epi-sarcophinone (**88**)	2.7			
8-epi-sarcophinone (**89**)	3.7	*Sarcophyton glaucum*	Soft coral	[97]
Ent-sarcophine (**90**)	3.4			
Tyrosinase				
4-(phenylsulfanyl)butan-2-one (**91**)	34.5 *	*Cladiella australis*	Soft coral	[98]

* K$_i$., ND—not determined.

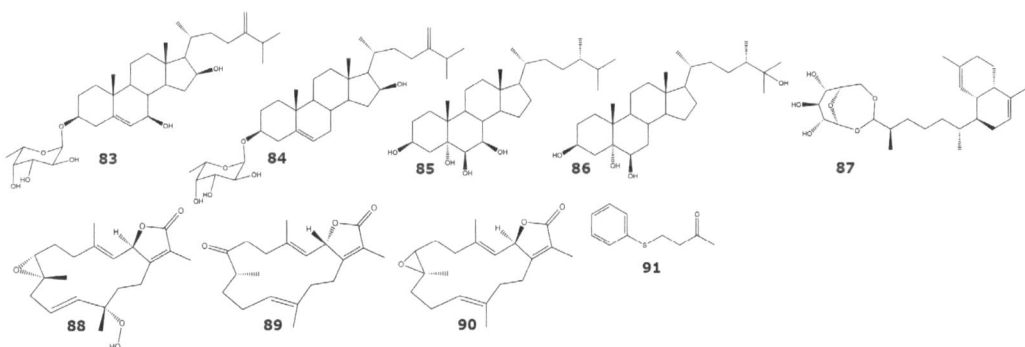

Figure 7. Oxidoreductase inhibitors isolated from soft corals and gorgonians (compounds **83–91**). Structures include inhibitors of 5α-Reductase, Cytochrome P450 1A, and Tyrosinase.

2.2.2. Cytochrome P450 1A (EC 1.14.14.1)

Cytochrome P450 enzymes are a superfamily with high versatility in drug metabolism, detoxification of xenobiotics, and biosynthesis of endogenous compounds [99]. Particularly, cytochrome P4501A is one of the most important enzymes involved in the tumorigenesis induced by environmental pollution [100]. Therefore, this enzyme has been considered as an attractive target for the development of anti-cancer drugs [99]. The cembranoids 12(S)-hydroperoxylsarcoph-10-ene (**88**), 8-epi-sarcophinone (**89**), and ent-sarcophine (**90**) were isolated from the Red Sea soft coral *Sarcophyton glaucum* (Table 6 and Figure 7) [97]. The results of the inhibition assays with these compounds revealed some interesting structure–

function relationships. For instance, the differences obtained for the inhibitory potency for ent-sarcophine (**90**) and sarcophine (**33**) suggest that the configurations of atoms C1 and C6 are essential for the inhibition of the cytochrome P450 1A [97].

2.2.3. Tyrosinase (EC 1.14.18.1)

Tyrosinase is a key enzyme which catalyzes a rate-limiting step in melanin synthesis, and the downregulation of its activity constitutes the most prominent approach for the development of melanogenesis inhibitors [101]. Thus, tyrosinase inhibitors are considered as promising candidates for the development of skin whitening agents [101]. The tyrosinase inhibitor 4-(phenylsulfanyl)butan-2-one (**91**) is isolated from the Formosan soft coral *Cladiella australis* (Table 6 and Figure 7). The kinetic characterization of this compound showed that it acts as a noncompetitive inhibitor of the mushroom tyrosinase, with a K_i value of 3.45×10^{-5} M. Additionally, in vitro cell-based assays revealed that 4-(phenylsulfanyl)butan-2-one (**91**) has low cytotoxicity towards several human cell lines [98].

2.3. Transferases

2.3.1. Tyrosine Kinase p56^{lck} (TK) (EC 2.7.10.2)

The tyrosine kinase p56^{lck} is a lymphocyte-specific protein tyrosine kinase that is a member of the Src family of non-receptor protein kinases [102]. This kinase is involved in the phosphorylation of several intracellular signaling proteins such as protein kinase C, phosphoinositide 3-kinase, and Zeta-chain-associated protein kinase 70 [103].

Since Tyrosine kinase p56^{lck} participates in T cell proliferation and differentiation, its inhibitors could be used in the treatment of several inflammatory and autoimmune disorders [103]. Two sterols, with inhibitory activity towards tyrosine kinase p56lck were isolated from the soft coral *Capnella lacertiliensis*: 12β-acetoxyergost-5-ene-3β,11β,16-triol (**92**), and 11β-acetoxyergost-5-ene-3β,12β,16-triol (93) (Table 7 and Figure 8) [104].

Table 7. Inhibitors of the transferases tyrosine kinase p56^{lck}, IKKbeta kinase, EGFR kinase, and protein kinase C, isolated from soft corals and gorgonians.

Compound	IC$_{50}$ (μM)	Source	Classification	Reference
Tyrosine kinase p56^{lck}				
12β-acetoxyergost-5-ene-3β,11β,16-triol (**92**)	ND	*Capnella lacertiliensis*	Soft coral	[104]
11β-acetoxyergost-5-ene-3β,12β,16-triol (**93**)	ND			
IKKbeta kinase				
3,4-epoxy,13-oxo,7E,11Z,15-cembratriene (**94**)	ND	*Sarcophyton* sp.	Soft coral	[105]
3,4-epoxy,13-oxo,7E,11E,15-cembratriene (**95**)	ND			
Astaxanthin (**96**)	ND	*Subergorgia* sp.	Gorgonian	
EGFR kinase				
Pachycladin A (**97**)	ND	*Cladiella pachyclados*	Soft coral	[106]
Protein kinase C (PKC)				
2S,4aS,5S,6S,8aS)-6-hydroxy-2-((1S,2R,3R)-3-((2R,E)-5-hydroxy-4,5,6-trimethylhept-3-en-2-yl)-2-(2-hydroxyethyl)-2-methylcyclopentyl)-5,8a-dimethyloctahydronaphthalen-1(2H)-one (**98**)	NA	*Pseudopterogorgia* sp.	Gorgonian	[107]
(2S,4aS,5S,6S,8aS)-6-hydroxy-2-((1S,2R,3R)-2-(2-hydroxyethyl)-2-methyl-3-((2R,5R,E)-4,5,6-trimethylhept-3-en-2-yl)cyclopentyl)-5,8a-dimethyloctahydronaphthalen-1(2H)-one (**99**)	NA			
3β, 11, 24-trihidroxy, 9,11-secogorgos-5-en-9-one (**100**)	NA			

ND—not determined, NA—not available.

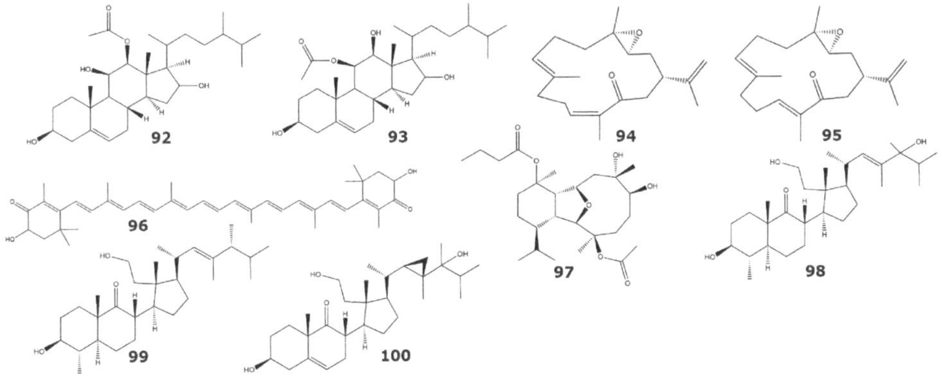

Figure 8. Transferase inhibitors isolated from soft corals and gorgonians (compounds **92–100**). Structures include inhibitors of Tyrosine kinase p56[lck], IKKbeta kinase, EGFR kinase, and protein kinase C.

2.3.2. IKKbeta Kinase (EC 2.7.11.10)

IKKbeta is one of the two catalytic units that compose the kinase complex IkB [108]. IKKbeta is involved in nuclear factor-KB signaling, and hence in the pathogenesis and progression of inflammatory diseases [109]. The cembranoids 3,4-epoxy,13-oxo,7E,11Z,15-cembratriene (**94**), and 3,4-epoxy,13-oxo,7E,11E,15-cembratriene (**95**) were isolated from the soft coral *Sarcophyton* sp. and both showed inhibitory activity against the IKKbeta kinase (Table 7 and Figure 8) [105]. In the same study, the carotenoid astaxanthin (**96**) was isolated from the gorgonian *Subergorgia* sp., and it showed inhibitory activity towards the IKKbeta kinase [105]. However, it is likely that astaxanthin is not produced by *Subergorgia* sp., but instead acquired from a marine bacteria or algae [110].

2.3.3. Epidermal Growth Factor Receptor Kinase (EGFR) (EC 2.7.10.1)

EGFR is a member of the epidermal growth factor receptor family. It was the first member of this family with supporting evidence linking its overexpression with cancer [111]. This relationship has been established for several types of cancer, including laryngeal [112], esophageal [113], and non-small cell lung cancer [114], among others. Thus, EGFR inhibitors are considered as attractive candidates for developing anticancer drugs. The pachycladin A (**97**) is a diterpenoid isolated from the soft coral *Cladiella pachyclados* and was able to inhibit the kinase enzymatic activity of the EGFR kinase 8 (Table 7 and Figure 8) [106]. The inhibition of pachycladin A (**97**) seems to be selective towards EGFR kinase since no inhibition was detected against the two other kinases from the EGFR family (HER2 and HER4).

2.3.4. Protein Kinase C (PKC) (EC 2.7.11.13)

Protein kinase C is a family of enzymes involved in cell signaling pathways that mediates critical events like cellular proliferation and gene expression regulation [115]. For these reasons, PKC is considered a key target for the treatment of various diseases, including cancer, and neurological and cardiovascular disorders [116–118]. Three new secosterols (**98–100**) showing PKC inhibitory activity in the micromolar range were isolated from the gorgonian *Pseudopterogorgia* sp. [107]. In this work, IC_{50} values ranged from 12 to 50 μM, but no individual values were reported for these compounds (Table 7 and Figure 8). Considering the role of PKC in inflammatory and proliferative processes, all these three molecules were evaluated in cell cultures and showed antiproliferative properties. For the compound (2S,4aS,5S,6S,8aS)-6-hydroxy-2-((1S,2R,3R)-2-(2-hydroxyethyl)-2-methyl-3-((2R,5R,E)-4,5,6-trimethylhept-3-en-2-yl)cyclopentyl)-5,8a-dimethyloctahydronaphthalen-1 (2H)-one (**99**), anti-inflammatory properties were also confirmed.

2.3.5. Human Tumor-Related Protein Kinases

Several 9,10 secosteroids were isolated from the gorgonian *Astrogorgia* sp. and assessed against 16 different human tumor-related protein kinases [119]. The kinases tested were AKT1 (RAC-alpha serine/threonine-protein kinase), ALK (Anaplastic lymphoma kinase), ARK5 (AMPK-related protein kinase 5), Aurora-B, AXL (AXL receptor tyrosine kinase), FAK (Focal adhesion kinase), IGF-1R (Insulin-like growth factor 1 receptor tyrosine kinase), MEK1wt (MAP kinase 1), METwt (MET receptor Tyrosine Kinase), NEK2 (NIMA-related Kinase 2), NEK6 (NIMA-related Kinase 6), PIM1 (Serine/threonine-protein kinase PIM-1), PLK1 (Serine/threonine-protein kinase PLK1), PRK1 (Serine/threonine-protein kinase N1), SRC (Proto-oncogene tyrosine-protein kinase Src), and VEGF-R2 (VEGFR2 receptor tyrosine kinase). The compounds calicoferols A (**101**) and E (**102**), and 24-exomethylenecalicoferol E (**103**), 9β-hydroxy-9,10-secosteroid astrogorgol F (**104**), and 9α-hydroxy-9,10-secosteroid astrogorgiadiol (**105**) showed significant inhibition against kinases LK, AXL, FAK, IGF1-R, MET wt, SRC, and VEGF-R2 (Table 8 and Figure 9) [119]. On the other hand, 9,16 di-oxygenated molecules, such as calicoferols I and B, showed weak inhibition ($IC_{50} > 100 \ \mu M$) against these kinases, pointing to the oxygenation at the C-16 as the cause for decreased inhibitory activity. The authors of this work concluded that the 9-oxygenated 9,10-secosterol nucleus is the basis of the inhibitory activity of these compounds towards the tested kinases. Additionally, the tetraprenylated alkaloid malonganenone D (**106**), isolated from the gorgonian *Euplexaura robusta*, has shown inhibitory activity against the MET Receptor Tyrosine Kinase, or c-Met [120]. This compound had been also previously isolated from the gorgonian *Euplexaura nuttingi* [121].

Table 8. Inhibitors of the transferases human tumor-related protein kinases, casitas B-lineage lymphoma proto-oncogene B (Cbl-b), farnesyl protein transferase, and glutathione S-transferase, isolated from soft corals and gorgonians.

Compound	IC$_{50}$ (µM)	Source	Classification	Reference
Human tumor-related protein kinases				
Calicoferol A (**101**)	9.33 (ALK), 38.1 (Aurora-B), 21.9 (AXL), 16.9 (FAK), 3.16 (IGF-1R), 34.0 (MET wt), 2.40 (SRC), 4.95 (VEGF-R2)			
Calicoferol E (**102**)	4.14 (ALK), 14.7 (AXL), 9.92 (FAK), 2.42 (IGF-1R), 47.7 (MET wt), 2.24 (SRC), 4.60 (VEGF-R2)			
24-exomethylenecalicoferol E (**103**)	4.36 (ALK), 20.2 (AXL), 10.7 (FAK), 2.30 (IGF-1R), 27.5 (MET wt), 1.48 (SRC), 4.85 (VEGF-R2)	*Astrogorgia* sp.	Gorgonian	[119]
9β-hydroxy-9,10-secosteroid astrogorgol F (**104**)	4.73 (ALK), 32.6 (AXL), 9.63 (FAK), 2.46 (IGF-1R), 71.5 (MET wt), 2.17 (SRC), 6.01 (VEGF-R2)			
9α-hydroxy-9,10-secosteroid astrogorgiadiol (**105**)	7.55 (ALK), 25.1 (Aurora-B), 16.9 (AXL), 13.2 (FAK), 2.77 (IGF-1R), 48.9 (MEK1 wt), 78.0 (MET wt), 1.91 (SRC), 4.35 (VEGF-R2)			
Malonganenone D (**106**)	ND	*Euplexaura robusta*	Gorgonian	[120]
Casitas B-lineage lymphoma proto-oncogene B (Cbl-b)				
Sinularamide A (**107**)	ND			
Sinularamide B (**108**)	ND			
Sinularamide C (**109**)	6.5	*Sinularia* sp.	Soft coral	[122]
Sinularamide D (**110**)	ND			
Sinularamide F (**111**)	ND			
Sinularamide G (**112**)	ND			
Farnesyl Protein Transferase				
1aR,4E,8E,11S,11aR,14aS,14bS)-1a,5,9,14a-tetramethyl-12-methylene-13-oxo-1a,2,3,6,7,10,11,11a,12,13,14a,14b-dodecahydrooxireno[2′,3′:13,14]cyclotetradeca[1,2-b]furan-11-yl acetate (**113**)	0.15	*Lobophytum cristagalli*	Soft coral	[123]
Glutathione S-transferase				
15(S)-PGA2 (**114**)	75.4			
15(R)-15-methyl PGA2 (**115**)	136.7			
15(S)-PGE2 (**116**)	312.2	*Plexaura homomalla* [1]	Gorgonian	[124]
15(R)-PGE2 (**117**)	ND			
15(S)-PGF2a (**118**)	334.6			

[1] Commercial compounds that represent the major classes of prostaglandins present in *P. homomalla*. ND—not determined.

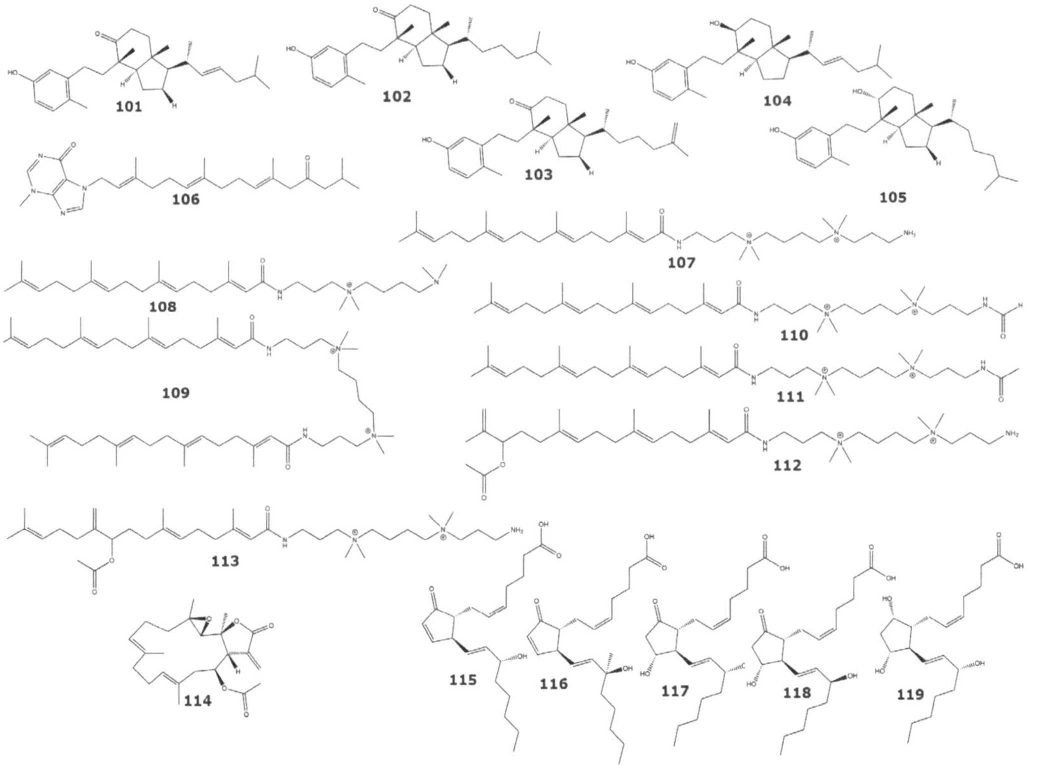

Figure 9. Transferase inhibitors isolated from soft corals and gorgonians (compounds (**101–119**). Structures include inhibitors of human tumor-related protein kinases, Casitas B-lineage lymphoma proto-oncogene B, Farnesyl Protein Transferase, and Glutathione S-transferase.

2.3.6. Casitas B-Lineage Lymphoma Proto-Oncogene B (Cbl-b) (E3-Ubiquitin Ligase) (EC 2.3.2.27)

Casitas B-lineage lymphoma proto-oncogene B (Cbl-b) is an E3 ubiquitin ligase that acts as an important regulator of the immune response [125]. Targeting this enzyme is a promising approach for the treatment of autoimmune diseases and cancer [126,127]. The Sinularamides A−G (**107−113**), isolated from the soft coral *Sinularia* sp., are a group of diterpenoids that inhibits Cbl-b enzyme [122]. The most potent of these compounds was the sinularamide C (**109**), displaying an IC_{50} value in the low micromolar range (Table 8 and Figure 9).

2.3.7. Farnesyl Protein Transferase (EC 2.5.1.58)

The farnesyl protein transferase is an enzyme that adds a 15-carbon isoprenoid to a cysteine amino acid of Ras protein [128]. Oncogenic mutations of Ras protein are quite common in cancer, making the protein that is involved in its post-transcriptional modification a promising way to block Ras signal transduction [129,130]. The molecule 1aR,4E,8E,11S,11aR,14aS,14bS)-1a,5,9,14a-tetramethyl-12-methylene-13-oxo-1a,2,3,6,7,10, 11, 11a,12,13,14a,14b-dodecahydrooxireno[2′,3′:13,14]cyclotetradeca[1,2-b]furan-11-yl acetate (**114**), with inhibitory activity towards recombinant human farnesyl protein transferase, was isolated from the soft coral *Lobophytum cristagalli* [123]. Kinetic assays suggest that this inhibitor competes with the Ras protein, substrate of the farnesyl protein transferase. The apparent K_i value determined in this kinetic characterization was 0.17 µM. However, the same inhibitor is noncompetitive with respect to the farnesyl pyrophosphate substrate. In the same study, this compound also inhibited the enzyme geranyl protein transferase-1, closely related to the farnesyl protein transferase, but with lower potency (IC$_{50}$: 5.3 μM) [123].

2.3.8. Glutathione S-Transferase (EC 2.5.1.18)

Glutathione S-transferases (GST) are a family of enzymes that catalyze the conjugation of glutathione to a wide number of xenobiotics, making them more hydrophilic and facilitating their elimination [131]. Although GST protects the cell from toxic products, it also reduces the effectiveness of certain anticancer drugs [132]. The use of inhibitors of GST could, therefore, increase the sensitivity of tumor cells to anticancer drugs [133].

Crude and aqueous extracts of the gorgonian *Plexaura homomalla* have shown inhibitory activity towards the GST enzyme from the gastropod *Cyphoma gibbosum*. The structural analysis of these extracts revealed the presence of several series of prostaglandins (**115-119**). The use of commercially available prostaglandins that represents the diversity of classes found in *P. homomalla* confirmed the capacity of the molecules 15(*S*)-PGA2 (**115**), 15(*R*)-15-methyl PGA2 (**116**), 15(*S*)-PGE2 (**117**), 15(*R*)-PGE2 (**118**), and 15(*S*)-PGF2a (**119**) to inhibit GST (Table 8 and Figure 9). The results of the enzymatic assays revealed that compounds with the cyclopentenone ring showed the highest inhibitory activity [124].

2.4. Translocases

H (+)-Pyrophosphatase (EC 7.1.3.1)

Vacuolar H(+)-pyrophosphatase is an electronic proton pump present in most land plants and in other organisms such as algae, bacteria, protozoa, and archaebacteria [134]. In plants, this enzyme participates in the cytosolic hydrolysis of PPi and in vacuole acidification [135]. Specific inhibitors of the enzyme would be useful for investigating its physiological role and its biochemical characteristics. Acylspermidines A (**120**), B (**121**), C (**122**), D (**123**), and E (**124**) (Figure 10) from the soft coral *Sinularia* sp. inhibit plant vacuolar H(+)-pyrophosphatase from *Vigna radiata cv. Wilczek* [136]. These acylspermidine derivates showed a noncompetitive inhibition toward the vacuolar H(+)-pyrophosphatase. However, these compounds did not inhibit the vacuolar H+-ATPase, plasma membrane H+-ATPase, mitochondrial ATPase, or cytosolic PPase, suggesting a specific inhibitory activity against the vacuolar H(+)-pyrophosphatase.

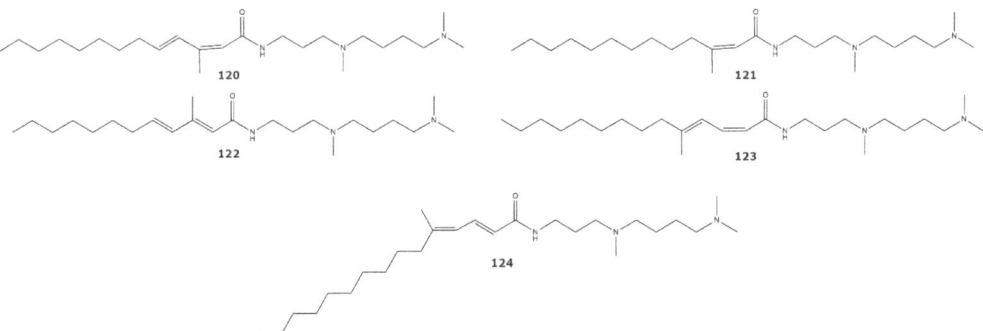

Figure 10. H(+)-pyrophosphatase inhibitors isolated from soft corals and gorgonians (compounds **120–124**).

3. Walking the Whole Path to Describe an Enzyme Inhibitory Activity: What Next, after Screening and Structure Elucidation?

Previous sections reveal that, despite the number of enzyme inhibitors identified in the last five decades from gorgonians and soft corals, none of them, to date, possess a complete enzymological characterization. Remarkably, in many of these works, not even an IC$_{50}$ value is calculated, but only an inhibition percentage at a fixed inhibitor concentration. This trend, which is extendable to other natural sources, reflects both (i) the lack of a uniform procedure for the enzymological characterization of inhibitors from marine organisms and (ii) the challenge that this goal represents for users unfamiliar with enzymology.

The STRENDA project provides guides for the minimal information set required for reporting enzymological data [38,39,137]. For inhibitors, report requirements include reversibility and time-dependency, inhibition type, Ki value, and the method used for its estimation [37]. Using these parameters as a reference, many reports of enzyme inhibitors, and particularly those from marine sources, appear noticeably incomplete. Although several factors might be involved, we believe that the scarcity of fully characterized inhibitors might be due to the lack of expertise of many laboratories in studying this bioactivity. Therefore, we believe that a brief description of critical steps might encourage the study of a higher number of novel enzyme inhibitors from this prominent source.

Figure 11 presents a general strategy for characterizing new enzyme inhibitors independent of their nature and origin, adapted from the one proposed by Copeland [138]. Although it admits some flexibility in the order of steps, the selected approach is, in our opinion, intuitive and the most convenient to implement in unexperienced laboratories. In brief, the strategy consists of five steps: (1) obtaining a preliminary assessment of inhibitory potency (i.e., the range of molar concentrations in which it effectively inhibits the target enzyme) by determining half-maximal inhibitory concentration (IC_{50}); (2) determining inhibition reversibility and temporal dependency; (3) elucidation of inhibition type; (4) estimation of K_i value; and (5) a specificity validation step.

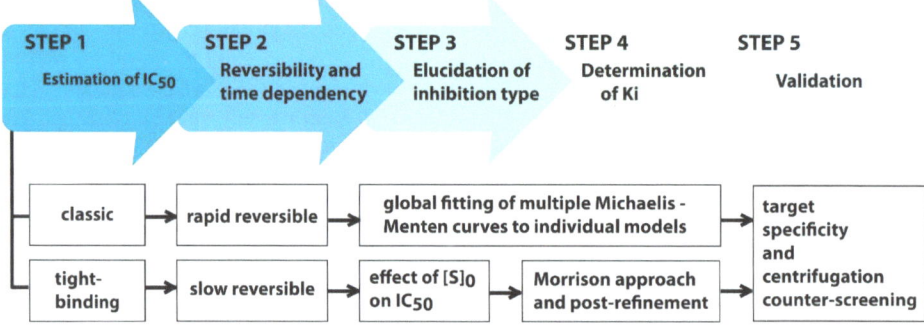

Figure 11. Proposed strategy for the characterization of reversible enzyme inhibitors from marine organisms according to STRENDA guidelines. The strategy is presented as a flowchart with five sequential steps. As alternative approaches or methodologies are possible in each step, two specific sequences are proposed according to the properties of the inhibitor (e.g., classic, rapid reversible inhibitor vs. tight-binding, slow reversible inhibitor).

Determining a preliminary estimate of inhibitor potency (Step 1) is critical, as this determines the most appropriate approach for further characterization steps (Figure 11). After estimating the IC_{50} value by quantifying the inhibition percentage at different inhibitor concentrations, the assessed inhibitors can be classified as classic (i.e., $IC_{50} \gg [E]_0$) or tight binding (i.e., $IC_{50} \approx [E]_0$). Importantly, caution is recommended when comparing IC_{50} values, as they reflect not only the potency of the inhibitor but also the experimental conditions used for its estimation [139].

Step 2 consists of assessing the reversibility of the enzyme–inhibitor interaction. This property can be determined by the jump dilution assay [138–140] or alternative interaction-based techniques [35,36,141,142]. Although irreversible and pseudo-irreversible inhibitors exist in nature [143–146], most of the enzyme inhibitors described so far from marine organisms belong to the reversible class. Other relevant aspects of inhibition, such as association (i.e., time-dependent inhibition) and dissociation kinetics, are also investigated at this stage.

Elucidation of inhibition type (Step 3) and the estimation of Ki value (Step 4) are typically performed simultaneously by measuring enzyme velocity while varying substrate and inhibitor concentrations. The potency of competitive, noncompetitive, and uncompetitive inhibitors variate distinctively as substrate concentration increases [139], a fact exploited to identify their inhibition mode [138,140]. Once the inhibition modality has been elucidated, diverse mathematical approaches are available to estimate the Ki value for classical inhibitors [147–149]. On the other hand, determining Ki values for tight-binding inhibitors requires a specific methodology [150,151], as many of the assumptions applied to derive the equations for classic inhibitors are no longer valid in such systems.

The strategy is completed with a specificity validation step (Step 5) to discard unspecific actuators or PAINS (pan-assay interference compounds), which can act over many different proteins or interfere with bioassays through diverse mechanisms [152,153]. As these compounds can occur in nature [154], the specificity of novel inhibitors should be assessed against related and unrelated off-target reporters [155]. Additionally, experimental conditions can be conveniently manipulated (e.g., by adding to the reaction mix appropriate amounts of detergents such as Triton X-100) to minimize the occurrence of aggregators, the most common cause of artificial enzyme inhibition during screenings [155–159].

4. Concluding Remarks and Future Perspectives

During the last five decades, gorgonians and soft corals remained as an important source of new enzyme inhibitors, producing more than 50 reports and 127 new inhibitory molecules. Mainly, these inhibitors remain uncharacterized from an enzymological point of view; therefore, little speculation is possible regarding their potencies and inhibition mechanisms. As expected, low affinity inhibitors with IC_{50} values in the high micromolar range predominated (putatively) among them. Of note, the Acetylcholinesterase inhibitors Asperdiol (**29**) and 14-acetoxycrassine (**32**) [55], the PTP1B inhibitor (5′Z)-5-(2′,6′-Dimethylocta-5′,7′-dienyl)-furan-3-carboxylic acid (**18**) [49], the Phosphodiesterase-4 inhibitor 9,11,15-triacetoxy PGF2α methyl ester (**67**) [74], and the farnesyl protein transferase inhibitor 1aR,4E,8E,11S,11aR,14aS,14bS)-1a,5,9,14a-tetramethyl-12-methylene-13-oxo-1a,2,3,6,7,10, 11,11a,12,13,14a,14b-dodecahydrooxireno[2′,3′:13,14]cyclotetradeca[1,2-*b*]furan-11-yl acetate (**114**) [123], displaying preliminary potency estimates or Ki values in the sub- or low-micromolar range, stand outs as the most promising and clearly merit in-depth characterization studies. Interestingly, human target enzymes involved in complex pathways for chronic disorders such as PTP1B (type 2 diabetes and obesity) or the Ubiquitin–Proteasome system (neurodegenerative disorders, cancer, etc.) clearly captured the attention of researchers in the field during the period analyzed, with 38 inhibitors combined. Other enzymes, such as the HIV-1 protease or human Phosphodiesterase-4, also received special attention.

Due to the limited scope of this issue and for the sake of space, the presented strategy is not an exhaustive guide for the functional characterization of new inhibitors. In contrast, it aims to summarize relevant concepts and set a framework to address this goal, in practice burdensome enough to cause a halt in the study of potentially interesting enzyme inhibitors. The infrastructure required for performing most enzymatic reactions is readily available in many academic institutions. Numerous substrate and enzyme preparations are commercially available at affordable prices and basic enzymology is part of almost every formation program in biological sciences. In addition, many enzymes are considered important biomolecules for industrial, biomedical, and environmental applications, making their activity modulation by specific inhibitors a topic of particular interest. Paradoxically, in-depth enzymological characterization of inhibitors seems to be the prerogative of only a few laboratories, resulting in the accumulation of reports describing bioactivity prospection in natural extracts with no follow-up. This is particularly true for, but not exclusive to, organisms of marine origin, which have constituted an abundant source of enzyme inhibitors with unique properties.

Therefore, we hope this effort can contribute to democratizing and popularizing the procedures required in enzymological practice to minimally characterize, according to STRENDA suggestions, new enzyme inhibitors from marine organisms. In addition, this work might also help to propagate the message of the STRENDA project, focusing on the uniformity, quality, and completeness of experimental data, and hence reproducibility, in enzymological practice. Adherence to these standards should significantly facilitate relaunching of high-quality enzymological research in the context of marine organisms.

Supplementary Materials: The following are available online at https://www.mdpi.com/article/10 .3390/md21020104/s1, Table S1: Complete dataset of enzyme inhibitors included in the manuscript., Table S2: Dataset of enzyme inhibitors isolated from soft corals, Table S3: Dataset of enzyme inhibitors isolated from gorgonians. For convenience, the three tables were included as separate sheets in a single excel file.

Author Contributions: Conceptualization, Y.G. and E.S.-S.; literature investigation, A.C.-I. and S.J.-M.; data curation, A.C.-I., S.J.-M., Y.G. and E.S.-S.; writing—original draft preparation, Y.G. and E.S.-S.; writing—review and editing, Y.G. and E.S.-S.; visualization, Y.G.; supervision, Y.G. and E.S.-S.; All authors have read and agreed to the published version of the manuscript.

Funding: This research was funded by Universidad de las Américas, Research Grant BIO.YGB.22.01 (Y.G.)

Institutional Review Board Statement: Not applicable.

Data Availability Statement: Not applicable.

Acknowledgments: This work is a posthumous tribute to the memory of María de Los Ángeles Chávez Planes (La Habana, 1941-La Habana, 2021), who dedicated most of her life to the identification and characterization of tight-binding protease inhibitors from marine invertebrates, the formation of new generations of scientists and spreading biochemistry knowledge through the teaching of Enzymology.

Conflicts of Interest: The authors declare no conflict of interest.

References

1. Zakiyanov, O.; Kalousová, M.; Zima, T.; Tesař, V. Matrix Metalloproteinases and Tissue Inhibitors of Matrix Metalloproteinases in Kidney Disease. *Adv. Clin. Chem.* **2021**, *105*, 141–212. [CrossRef] [PubMed]
2. Amin, F.; Khan, M.S.; Bano, B. Mammalian Cystatin and Protagonists in Brain Diseases. *J. Biomol. Struct. Dyn.* **2020**, *38*, 2171–2196. [CrossRef] [PubMed]
3. Spinale, F.G.; Villarreal, F. Targeting Matrix Metalloproteinases in Heart Disease: Lessons from Endogenous Inhibitors. *Biochem. Pharmacol.* **2014**, *90*, 7–15. [CrossRef] [PubMed]
4. Małgorzewicz, S.; Skrzypczak-Jankun, E.; Jankun, J. Plasminogen Activator Inhibitor-1 in Kidney Pathology (Review). *Int. J. Mol. Med.* **2013**, *31*, 503–510. [CrossRef] [PubMed]
5. Pini, L.; Giordani, J.; Ciarfaglia, M.; Pini, A.; Arici, M.; Tantucci, C. Alpha1-Antitrypsin Deficiency and Cardiovascular Disease: Questions and Issues of a Debated Relation. *J. Cardiovasc. Med. Hagerstown Md.* **2022**, *23*, 637–645. [CrossRef]
6. Zarkadoulas, N.; Pergialiotis, V.; Dimitroulis, D.; Stefanidis, K.; Verikokos, C.; Perrea, D.N.; Kontzoglou, K. A Potential Role of Cyclin-Dependent Kinase Inhibitor 1 (P21/WAF1) in the Pathogenesis of Endometriosis: Directions for Future Research. *Med. Hypotheses* **2019**, *133*, 109414. [CrossRef]
7. Grey, W.; Izatt, L.; Sahraoui, W.; Ng, Y.-M.; Ogilvie, C.; Hulse, A.; Tse, E.; Holic, R.; Yu, V. Deficiency of the Cyclin-Dependent Kinase Inhibitor, CDKN1B, Results in Overgrowth and Neurodevelopmental Delay. *Hum. Mutat.* **2013**, *34*, 864–868. [CrossRef]
8. Sviderskaya, E.V.; Gray-Schopfer, V.C.; Hill, S.P.; Smit, N.P.; Evans-Whipp, T.J.; Bond, J.; Hill, L.; Bataille, V.; Peters, G.; Kipling, D.; et al. P16/Cyclin-Dependent Kinase Inhibitor 2A Deficiency in Human Melanocyte Senescence, Apoptosis, and Immortalization: Possible Implications for Melanoma Progression. *J. Natl. Cancer Inst.* **2003**, *95*, 723–732. [CrossRef]
9. Shakeel, M.; Xu, X.; De Mandal, S.; Jin, F. Role of Serine Protease Inhibitors in Insect-Host-Pathogen Interactions. *Arch. Insect Biochem. Physiol.* **2019**, *102*, e21556. [CrossRef]
10. Bao, J.; Liu, L.; An, Y.; Ran, M.; Ni, W.; Chen, J.; Wei, J.; Li, T.; Pan, G.; Zhou, Z. Nosema Bombycis Suppresses Host Hemolymph Melanization through Secreted Serpin 6 Inhibiting the Prophenoloxidase Activation Cascade. *J. Invertebr. Pathol.* **2019**, *168*, 107260. [CrossRef]
11. Uemura, D.; Kawazoe, Y.; Inuzuka, T.; Itakura, Y.; Kawamata, C.; Abe, T. Drug Leads Derived from Japanese Marine Organisms. *Curr. Med. Chem.* **2021**, *28*, 196–210. [CrossRef]

12. Luesch, H.; MacMillan, J.B. Targeting and Extending the Eukaryotic Druggable Genome with Natural Products. *Nat. Prod. Rep.* **2020**, *37*, 744–746. [CrossRef]
13. Parvez, S.; Kang, M.; Chung, H.-S.; Bae, H. Naturally Occurring Tyrosinase Inhibitors: Mechanism and Applications in Skin Health, Cosmetics and Agriculture Industries. *Phytother. Res. PTR* **2007**, *21*, 805–816. [CrossRef]
14. Mathialagan, R.; Mansor, N.; Al-Khateeb, B.; Mohamad, M.H.; Shamsuddin, M.R. Evaluation of Allicin as Soil Urease Inhibitor. *Procedia Eng.* **2017**, *184*, 449–459. [CrossRef]
15. Matczuk, D.; Siczek, A. Effectiveness of the Use of Urease Inhibitors in Agriculture: A Review. *Int. Agrophys.* **2021**, *35*, 197–208. [CrossRef]
16. Qiao, G.; Bi, K.; Liu, J.; Cao, S.; Liu, M.; Pešić, M.; Lin, X. Protein Kinases as Targets for Developing Anticancer Agents from Marine Organisms. *Biochim. Biophys. Acta Gen. Subj.* **2021**, *1865*, 129759. [CrossRef]
17. Ning, C.; Wang, H.-M.D.; Gao, R.; Chang, Y.-C.; Hu, F.; Meng, X.; Huang, S.-Y. Marine-Derived Protein Kinase Inhibitors for Neuroinflammatory Diseases. *Biomed. Eng. Online* **2018**, *17*, 46. [CrossRef]
18. Ruocco, N.; Costantini, S.; Palumbo, F.; Costantini, M. Marine Sponges and Bacteria as Challenging Sources of Enzyme Inhibitors for Pharmacological Applications. *Mar. Drugs* **2017**, *15*, 173. [CrossRef]
19. Li, T.; Wang, N.; Zhang, T.; Zhang, B.; Sajeevan, T.P.; Joseph, V.; Armstrong, L.; He, S.; Yan, X.; Naman, C.B. A Systematic Review of Recently Reported Marine Derived Natural Product Kinase Inhibitors. *Mar. Drugs* **2019**, *17*, 493. [CrossRef]
20. Rauf, A.; Khalil, A.A.; Olatunde, A.; Khan, M.; Anwar, S.; Alafnan, A.; Rengasamy, K.R. Diversity, Molecular Mechanisms and Structure-Activity Relationships of Marine Protease Inhibitors—A Review. *Pharmacol. Res.* **2021**, *166*, 105521. [CrossRef]
21. Folmer, F.; Jaspars, M.; Schumacher, M.; Dicato, M.; Diederich, M. Marine Natural Products Targeting Phospholipases A2. *Biochem. Pharmacol.* **2010**, *80*, 1793–1800. [CrossRef] [PubMed]
22. Trang, N.T.H.; Tang, D.Y.Y.; Chew, K.W.; Linh, N.T.; Hoang, L.T.; Cuong, N.T.; Yen, H.T.; Thao, N.T.; Trung, N.T.; Show, P.L.; et al. Discovery of α-Glucosidase Inhibitors from Marine Microorganisms: Optimization of Culture Conditions and Medium Composition. *Mol. Biotechnol.* **2021**, *63*, 1004–1015. [CrossRef] [PubMed]
23. Lins Alves, L.K.; Cechinel Filho, V.; de Souza, R.L.R.; Furtado-Alle, L. BChE Inhibitors from Marine Organisms—A Review. *Chem. Biol. Interact.* **2022**, *367*, 110136. [CrossRef] [PubMed]
24. Prasasty, V.; Radifar, M.; Istyastono, E. Natural Peptides in Drug Discovery Targeting Acetylcholinesterase. *Molecules* **2018**, *23*, 2344. [CrossRef]
25. Dassonneville, L.; Wattez, N.; Baldeyrou, B.; Mahieu, C.; Lansiaux, A.; Banaigs, B.; Bonnard, I.; Bailly, C. Inhibition of Topoisomerase II by the Marine Alkaloid Ascididemin and Induction of Apoptosis in Leukemia Cells. *Biochem. Pharmacol.* **2000**, *60*, 527–537. [CrossRef]
26. Myobatake, Y.; Takeuchi, T.; Kuramochi, K.; Kuriyama, I.; Ishido, T.; Hirano, K.; Sugawara, F.; Yoshida, H.; Mizushina, Y. Pinophilins A and B, Inhibitors of Mammalian A-, B-, and Y-Family DNA Polymerases and Human Cancer Cell Proliferation. *J. Nat. Prod.* **2012**, *75*, 135–141. [CrossRef]
27. Moreno, R.I.; Zambelli, V.O.; Picolo, G.; Cury, Y.; Morandini, A.C.; Marques, A.C.; Sciani, J.M. Caspase-1 and Cathepsin B Inhibitors from Marine Invertebrates, Aiming at a Reduction in Neuroinflammation. *Mar. Drugs* **2022**, *20*, 614. [CrossRef]
28. Della Sala, G.; Agriesti, F.; Mazzoccoli, C.; Tataranni, T.; Costantino, V.; Piccoli, C. Clogging the Ubiquitin-Proteasome Machinery with Marine Natural Products: Last Decade Update. *Mar. Drugs* **2018**, *16*, 467. [CrossRef]
29. Tischler, D. A Perspective on Enzyme Inhibitors from Marine Organisms. *Mar. Drugs* **2020**, *18*, 431. [CrossRef]
30. Raimundo, I.; Silva, S.G.; Costa, R.; Keller-Costa, T. Bioactive Secondary Metabolites from Octocoral-Associated Microbes-New Chances for Blue Growth. *Mar. Drugs* **2018**, *16*, 485. [CrossRef]
31. McFadden, C.S.; Sánchez, J.A.; France, S.C. Molecular Phylogenetic Insights into the Evolution of *Octocorallia*: A Review. *Integr. Comp. Biol.* **2010**, *50*, 389–410. [CrossRef]
32. Ezzat, S.M.; Bishbishy, M.H.E.; Habtemariam, S.; Salehi, B.; Sharifi-Rad, M.; Martins, N.; Sharifi-Rad, J. Looking at Marine-Derived Bioactive Molecules as Upcoming Anti-Diabetic Agents: A Special Emphasis on PTP1B Inhibitors. *Molecules* **2018**, *23*, 3334. [CrossRef]
33. Ramírez, A.R.; Guerra, Y.; Otero, A.; García, B.; Berry, C.; Mendiola, J.; Hernández-Zanui, A.; de Los A Chávez, M. Generation of an Affinity Matrix Useful in the Purification of Natural Inhibitors of Plasmepsin II, an Antimalarial-Drug Target. *Biotechnol. Appl. Biochem.* **2009**, *52*, 149–157. [CrossRef]
34. Salas-Sarduy, E.; Cabrera-Muñoz, A.; Cauerhff, A.; González-González, Y.; Trejo, S.A.; Chidichimo, A.; de Los Angeles Chávez-Planes, M.; Cazzulo, J.J. Antiparasitic Effect of a Fraction Enriched in Tight-Binding Protease Inhibitors Isolated from the Caribbean Coral *Plexaura homomalla*. *Exp. Parasitol.* **2013**, *135*, 611–622. [CrossRef]
35. Salas-Sarduy, E.; Guerra, Y.; Covaleda Cortés, G.; Avilés, F.X.; Chávez Planes, M.A. Identification of Tight-Binding Plasmepsin II and Falcipain 2 Inhibitors in Aqueous Extracts of Marine Invertebrates by the Combination of Enzymatic and Interaction-Based Assays. *Mar. Drugs* **2017**, *15*, 123. [CrossRef]
36. Covaleda, G.; Trejo, S.A.; Salas-Sarduy, E.; Del Rivero, M.A.; Chavez, M.A.; Aviles, F.X. Intensity Fading MALDI-TOF Mass Spectrometry and Functional Proteomics Assignments to Identify Protease Inhibitors in Marine Invertebrates. *J. Proteom.* **2017**, *165*, 75–92. [CrossRef]
37. STRENDA Guidelines. Available online: https://www.beilstein-institut.de/en/projects/strenda/ (accessed on 22 December 2022).

38. Tipton, K.F.; Armstrong, R.N.; Bakker, B.M.; Bairoch, A.; Cornish-Bowden, A.; Halling, P.J.; Hofmeyr, J.-H.; Leyh, T.S.; Kettner, C.; Raushel, F.M.; et al. Standards for Reporting Enzyme Data: The STRENDA Consortium: What It Aims to Do and Why It Should Be Helpful. *Perspect. Sci.* **2014**, *1*, 131–137. [CrossRef]

39. Swainston, N.; Baici, A.; Bakker, B.M.; Cornish-Bowden, A.; Fitzpatrick, P.F.; Halling, P.; Leyh, T.S.; O'Donovan, C.; Raushel, F.M.; Reschel, U.; et al. STRENDA DB: Enabling the Validation and Sharing of Enzyme Kinetics Data. *FEBS J.* **2018**, *285*, 2193–2204. [CrossRef]

40. Villamar-Cruz, O.; Loza-Mejía, M.A.; Arias-Romero, L.E.; Camacho-Arroyo, I. Recent Advances in PTP1B Signaling in Metabolism and Cancer. *Biosci. Rep.* **2021**, *41*, BSR20211994. [CrossRef]

41. Combs, A.P. Recent Advances in the Discovery of Competitive Protein Tyrosine Phosphatase 1B Inhibitors for the Treatment of Diabetes, Obesity, and Cancer. *J. Med. Chem.* **2010**, *53*, 2333–2344. [CrossRef]

42. He, R.; Yu, Z.; Zhang, R.; Zhang, Z. Protein Tyrosine Phosphatases as Potential Therapeutic Targets. *Acta Pharmacol. Sin.* **2014**, *35*, 1227–1246. [CrossRef] [PubMed]

43. Liang, L.F.; Kurtán, T.; Mándi, A.; Gao, L.X.; Li, J.; Zhang, W.; Guo, Y.W. Sarsolenane and Capnosane Diterpenes from the Hainan Soft Coral *Sarcophyton trocheliophorum Marenzeller* as PTP1B Inhibitors. *Eur. J. Org. Chem.* **2014**, *2014*, 1841–1847. [CrossRef]

44. Liang, L.-F.; Gao, L.-X.; Li, J.; Taglialatela-Scafati, O.; Guo, Y.-W. Cembrane Diterpenoids from the Soft Coral *Sarcophyton trocheliophorum Marenzeller* as a New Class of PTP1B Inhibitors. *Bioorg. Med. Chem.* **2013**, *21*, 5076–5080. [CrossRef] [PubMed]

45. Liang, L.-F.; Kurtán, T.; Mándi, A.; Yao, L.-G.; Li, J.; Zhang, W.; Guo, Y.-W. Unprecedented Diterpenoids as a PTP1B Inhibitor from the Hainan Soft Coral *Sarcophyton trocheliophorum Marenzeller*. *Org. Lett.* **2013**, *15*, 274–277. [CrossRef] [PubMed]

46. Qin, G.-F.; Tang, X.-L.; Sun, Y.-T.; Luo, X.-C.; Zhang, J.; Van Ofwegen, L.; Sung, P.-J.; Li, P.-L.; Li, G.-Q. Terpenoids from the Soft Coral *Sinularia* sp. Collected in Yongxing Island. *Mar. Drugs* **2018**, *16*, 127. [CrossRef]

47. Ye, F.; Zhu, Z.-D.; Gu, Y.-C.; Li, J.; Zhu, W.-L.; Guo, Y.-W. Further New Diterpenoids as PTP1B Inhibitors from the Xisha Soft Coral *Sinularia polydactyla*. *Mar. Drugs* **2018**, *16*, 103. [CrossRef]

48. Yang, F.; Hua, Q.; Yao, L.-G.; Liang, L.-F.; Lou, Y.-X.; Lu, Y.-H.; An, F.-L.; Guo, Y.-W. One Uncommon Bis-Sesquiterpenoid from Xisha Soft Coral *Litophyton nigrum*. *Tetrahedron Lett.* **2022**, *88*, 153571. [CrossRef]

49. Chu, M.-J.; Tang, X.-L.; Han, X.; Li, T.; Luo, X.-C.; Jiang, M.-M.; van Ofwegen, L.; Luo, L.-Z.; Zhang, G.; Li, P.-L.; et al. Metabolites from the Paracel Islands Soft Coral *Sinularia* Cf. molesta. *Mar. Drugs* **2018**, *16*, 517. [CrossRef]

50. Liang, L.-F.; Wang, X.-J.; Zhang, H.-Y.; Liu, H.-L.; Li, J.; Lan, L.-F.; Zhang, W.; Guo, Y.-W. Bioactive Polyhydroxylated Steroids from the Hainan Soft Coral *Sinularia depressa Tixier-Durivault*. *Bioorg. Med. Chem. Lett.* **2013**, *23*, 1334–1337. [CrossRef]

51. Chen, W.-T.; Liu, H.-L.; Yao, L.-G.; Guo, Y.-W. 9,11-Secosteroids and Polyhydroxylated Steroids from Two South China Sea Soft Corals *Sarcophyton trocheliophorum* and *Sinularia flexibilis*. *Steroids* **2014**, *92*, 56–61. [CrossRef]

52. Kate, A.S.; Aubry, I.; Tremblay, M.L.; Kerr, R.G. Lipidyl Pseudopteranes A-F: Isolation, Biomimetic Synthesis, and PTP1B Inhibitory Activity of a New Class of Pseudopteranoids from the Gorgonian *Pseudopterogorgia acerosa*. *J. Nat. Prod.* **2008**, *71*, 1977–1982. [CrossRef]

53. Dos Santos, T.C.; Gomes, T.M.; Pinto, B.A.S.; Camara, A.L.; de Andrade Paes, A.M. Naturally Occurring Acetylcholinesterase Inhibitors and Their Potential Use for Alzheimer's Disease Therapy. *Front. Pharmacol.* **2018**, *9*, 1192. [CrossRef]

54. Haake, A.; Nguyen, K.; Friedman, L.; Chakkamparambil, B.; Grossberg, G.T. An Update on the Utility and Safety of Cholinesterase Inhibitors for the Treatment of Alzheimer's Disease. *Expert Opin. Drug Saf.* **2020**, *19*, 147–157. [CrossRef]

55. Castellanos, F.; Amaya-García, F.; Tello, E.; Ramos, F.A.; Umaña, A.; Puyana, M.; Resende, J.A.L.C.; Castellanos, L. Screening of Acetylcholinesterase Inhibitors in Marine Organisms from the Caribbean Sea. *Nat. Prod. Res.* **2019**, *33*, 3533–3540. [CrossRef]

56. Ne'eman, I.; Fishelson, L.; Kashman, Y. Sarcophine—A New Toxin from the Soft Coral *Sarcophyton glaucum* (Alcyonaria). *Toxicon* **1974**, *12*, 593–594. [CrossRef]

57. Bonnard, I.; Jhaumeer-Laulloo, S.B.; Bontemps, N.; Banaigs, B.; Aknin, M. New Lobane and Cembrane Diterpenes from Two Comorian Soft Corals. *Mar. Drugs* **2010**, *8*, 359–372. [CrossRef]

58. Ellithey, M.S.; Lall, N.; Hussein, A.A.; Meyer, D. Cytotoxic, Cytostatic and HIV-1 PR Inhibitory Activities of the Soft Coral *Litophyton arboreum*. *Mar. Drugs* **2013**, *11*, 4917–4936. [CrossRef]

59. Liao, Q.; Li, S.; Siu, S.W.I.; Yang, B.; Huang, C.; Chan, J.Y.-W.; Morlighem, J.-É.R.L.; Wong, C.T.T.; Rádis-Baptista, G.; Lee, S.M.-Y. Novel Kunitz-like Peptides Discovered in the Zoanthid *Palythoa caribaeorum* through Transcriptome Sequencing. *J. Proteome Res.* **2018**, *17*, 891–902. [CrossRef]

60. Reina, F.A.; Ramos, F.A.; Castellanos, L.; Aragón, M.; Ospina, L.F. Anti-Inflammatory R-Prostaglandins from Caribbean Colombian Soft Coral *Plexaura homomalla*. *J. Pharm. Pharmacol.* **2013**, *65*, 1643–1652. [CrossRef]

61. Avalon, N.E.; Nafie, J.; De Marco Verissimo, C.; Warrensford, L.C.; Dietrick, S.G.; Pittman, A.R.; Young, R.M.; Kearns, F.L.; Smalley, T.; Binning, J.M.; et al. Tuaimenal A, a Meroterpene from the Irish Deep-Sea Soft Coral *Duva florida*, Displays Inhibition of the SARS-CoV-2 3CLpro Enzyme. *J. Nat. Prod.* **2022**, *85*, 1315–1323. [CrossRef]

62. Erickson, J.W. The Not-so-Great Escape. *Nat. Struct. Biol.* **1995**, *2*, 523–529. [CrossRef] [PubMed]

63. Ghosh, A.K.; Osswald, H.L.; Prato, G. Recent Progress in the Development of HIV-1 Protease Inhibitors for the Treatment of HIV/AIDS. *J. Med. Chem.* **2016**, *59*, 5172–5208. [CrossRef] [PubMed]

64. Mocroft, A.; Lundgren, J.D. Starting Highly Active Antiretroviral Therapy: Why, When and Response to HAART. *J. Antimicrob. Chemother.* **2004**, *54*, 10–13. [CrossRef]

65. Bardoel, B.W.; Kenny, E.F.; Sollberger, G.; Zychlinsky, A. The Balancing Act of Neutrophils. *Cell Host Microbe* **2014**, *15*, 526–536. [CrossRef] [PubMed]
66. Crocetti, L.; Quinn, M.T.; Schepetkin, I.A.; Giovannoni, M.P. A Patenting Perspective on Human Neutrophil Elastase (HNE) Inhibitors (2014–2018) and Their Therapeutic Applications. *Expert Opin. Ther. Pat.* **2019**, *29*, 555–578. [CrossRef]
67. Luan, B.; Huynh, T.; Cheng, X.; Lan, G.; Wang, H.-R. Targeting Proteases for Treating COVID-19. *J. Proteome Res.* **2020**, *19*, 4316–4326. [CrossRef]
68. Hoffman, R.L.; Kania, R.S.; Brothers, M.A.; Davies, J.F.; Ferre, R.A.; Gajiwala, K.S.; He, M.; Hogan, R.J.; Kozminski, K.; Li, L.Y.; et al. Discovery of Ketone-Based Covalent Inhibitors of Coronavirus 3CL Proteases for the Potential Therapeutic Treatment of COVID-19. *J. Med. Chem.* **2020**, *63*, 12725–12747. [CrossRef]
69. Tundo, G.R.; Sbardella, D.; Santoro, A.M.; Coletta, A.; Oddone, F.; Grasso, G.; Milardi, D.; Lacal, P.M.; Marini, S.; Purrello, R.; et al. The Proteasome as a Druggable Target with Multiple Therapeutic Potentialities: Cutting and Non-Cutting Edges. *Pharmacol. Ther.* **2020**, *213*, 107579. [CrossRef]
70. Ling, X.-H.; Wang, S.-K.; Huang, Y.-H.; Huang, M.-J.; Duh, C.-Y. A High-Content Screening Assay for the Discovery of Novel Proteasome Inhibitors from Formosan Soft Corals. *Mar. Drugs* **2018**, *16*, 395. [CrossRef]
71. Chiu, C.-Y.; Ling, X.-H.; Wang, S.-K.; Duh, C.-Y. Ubiquitin-Proteasome Modulating Dolabellanes and Secosteroids from Soft Coral *Clavularia flava*. *Mar. Drugs* **2020**, *18*, 39. [CrossRef]
72. González, Y.; Doens, D.; Cruz, H.; Santamaría, R.; Gutiérrez, M.; Llanes, A.; Fernández, P.L. A Marine Diterpenoid Modulates the Proteasome Activity in Murine Macrophages Stimulated with LPS. *Biomolecules* **2018**, *8*, 109. [CrossRef]
73. Verbitski, S.M.; Mullally, J.E.; Fitzpatrick, F.A.; Ireland, C.M. Punaglandins, Chlorinated Prostaglandins, Function as Potent Michael Receptors to Inhibit Ubiquitin Isopeptidase Activity. *J. Med. Chem.* **2004**, *47*, 2062–2070. [CrossRef]
74. Cheng, Z.-B.; Deng, Y.-L.; Fan, C.-Q.; Han, Q.-H.; Lin, S.-L.; Tang, G.-H.; Luo, H.-B.; Yin, S. Prostaglandin Derivatives: Nonaromatic Phosphodiesterase-4 Inhibitors from the Soft Coral *Sarcophyton ehrenbergi*. *J. Nat. Prod.* **2014**, *77*, 1928–1936. [CrossRef]
75. Sun, Z.-H.; Cai, Y.-H.; Fan, C.-Q.; Tang, G.-H.; Luo, H.-B.; Yin, S. Six New Tetraprenylated Alkaloids from the South China Sea Gorgonian *Echinogorgia pseudossapo*. *Mar. Drugs* **2014**, *12*, 672–681. [CrossRef]
76. Mullally, J.E.; Moos, P.J.; Edes, K.; Fitzpatrick, F.A. Cyclopentenone Prostaglandins of the J Series Inhibit the Ubiquitin Isopeptidase Activity of the Proteasome Pathway. *J. Biol. Chem.* **2001**, *276*, 30366–30373. [CrossRef]
77. Liu, S.; Mansour, M.N.; Dillman, K.S.; Perez, J.R.; Danley, D.E.; Aeed, P.A.; Simons, S.P.; Lemotte, P.K.; Menniti, F.S. Structural Basis for the Catalytic Mechanism of Human Phosphodiesterase 9. *Proc. Natl. Acad. Sci. USA* **2008**, *105*, 13309–13314. [CrossRef]
78. Burgin, A.B.; Magnusson, O.T.; Singh, J.; Witte, P.; Staker, B.L.; Bjornsson, J.M.; Thorsteinsdottir, M.; Hrafnsdottir, S.; Hagen, T.; Kiselyov, A.S.; et al. Design of Phosphodiesterase 4D (PDE4D) Allosteric Modulators for Enhancing Cognition with Improved Safety. *Nat. Biotechnol.* **2010**, *28*, 63–70. [CrossRef]
79. Liu, Z.; Ma, S. Recent Advances in Synthetic α-Glucosidase Inhibitors. *ChemMedChem* **2017**, *12*, 819–829. [CrossRef]
80. Asano, N. Glycosidase Inhibitors: Update and Perspectives on Practical Use. *Glycobiology* **2003**, *13*, 93R–104R. [CrossRef]
81. Wu, M.-J.; Wang, H.; Jiang, C.-S.; Guo, Y.-W. New Cembrane-Type Diterpenoids from the South China Sea Soft Coral *Sinularia crassa* and Their α-Glucosidase Inhibitory Activity. *Bioorg. Chem.* **2020**, *104*, 104281. [CrossRef]
82. Andrianasolo, E.H.; Haramaty, L.; White, E.; Lutz, R.; Falkowski, P. Mode of Action of Diterpene and Characterization of Related Metabolites from the Soft Coral, *Xenia elongata*. *Mar. Drugs* **2014**, *12*, 1102–1115. [CrossRef] [PubMed]
83. Shin, J.; Seo, Y.; Cho, K.W.; Moon, S.-S.; Cho, Y.J. Euplexides A–E: Novel Farnesylhydroquinone Glycosides from the Gorgonian *Euplexaura anastomosans*. *J. Org. Chem.* **1999**, *64*, 1853–1858. [CrossRef] [PubMed]
84. Seo, Y.; Rho, J.R.; Cho, K.W.; Shin, J. New Farnesylhydroquinone Glycosides from the Gorgonian *Euplexaura anastomosans*. *Nat. Prod. Lett.* **2001**, *15*, 81–87. [CrossRef] [PubMed]
85. Shin, J.; Seo, Y.; Rho, J.-R.; Cho, K.W. Isolation of Polyhydroxysteroids from the Gorgonian *Acabaria undulata*. *J. Nat. Prod.* **1996**, *59*, 679–682. [CrossRef]
86. Zhang, X.; Yuan, Z.; Zhang, Y.; Yong, S.; Salas-Burgos, A.; Koomen, J.; Olashaw, N.; Parsons, J.T.; Yang, X.-J.; Dent, S.R.; et al. HDAC6 Modulates Cell Motility by Altering the Acetylation Level of Cortactin. *Mol. Cell* **2007**, *27*, 197–213. [CrossRef]
87. Lienlaf, M.; Perez-Villarroel, P.; Knox, T.; Pabon, M.; Sahakian, E.; Powers, J.; Woan, K.V.; Lee, C.; Cheng, F.; Deng, S.; et al. Essential Role of HDAC6 in the Regulation of PD-L1 in Melanoma. *Mol. Oncol.* **2016**, *10*, 735–750. [CrossRef]
88. Kawaguchi, Y.; Kovacs, J.J.; McLaurin, A.; Vance, J.M.; Ito, A.; Yao, T.P. The Deacetylase HDAC6 Regulates Aggresome Formation and Cell Viability in Response to Misfolded Protein Stress. *Cell* **2003**, *115*, 727–738. [CrossRef]
89. Keremu, A.; Aimaiti, A.; Liang, Z.; Zou, X. Role of the HDAC6/STAT3 Pathway in Regulating PD-L1 Expression in Osteosarcoma Cell Lines. *Cancer Chemother. Pharmacol.* **2019**, *83*, 255–264. [CrossRef]
90. Cummings, B.S. Phospholipase A2 as Targets for Anti-Cancer Drugs. *Biochem. Pharmacol.* **2007**, *74*, 949–959. [CrossRef]
91. Singh, N.; Jabeen, T.; Somvanshi, R.K.; Sharma, S.; Dey, S.; Singh, T.P. Phospholipase A2 as a Target Protein for Nonsteroidal Anti-Inflammatory Drugs (NSAIDS): Crystal Structure of the Complex Formed between Phospholipase A2 and Oxyphenbutazone at 1.6 A Resolution. *Biochemistry* **2004**, *43*, 14577–14583. [CrossRef]
92. Suckling, K. Phospholipase A2s: Developing Drug Targets for Atherosclerosis. *Atherosclerosis* **2010**, *212*, 357–366. [CrossRef]
93. Said, M.A.; Mehta, A. The Impact of 5α-Reductase Inhibitor Use for Male Pattern Hair Loss on Men's Health. *Curr. Urol. Rep.* **2018**, *19*, 65. [CrossRef]

94. Occhiato, E.G.; Guarna, A.; Danza, G.; Serio, M. Selective Non-Steroidal Inhibitors of 5 Alpha-Reductase Type 1. *J. Steroid Biochem. Mol. Biol.* **2004**, *88*, 1–16. [CrossRef]

95. Radhika, P.; Cabeza, M.; Bratoeff, E.; García, G. 5Alpha-Reductase Inhibition Activity of Steroids Isolated from Marine Soft Corals. *Steroids* **2004**, *69*, 439–444. [CrossRef]

96. Liu, W.K.; Wong, N.L.Y.; Huang, H.M.; Ho, J.K.C.; Zhang, W.H.; Che, C.T. Growth Inhibitory Activity of Lemnabourside on Human Prostate Cancer Cells. *Life Sci.* **2002**, *70*, 843–853. [CrossRef]

97. Hegazy, M.-E.F.; Eldeen, A.M.G.; Shahat, A.A.; Abdel-Latif, F.F.; Mohamed, T.A.; Whittlesey, B.R.; Paré, P.W. Bioactive Hydroperoxyl Cembranoids from the Red Sea Soft Coral *Sarcophyton glaucum*. *Mar. Drugs* **2012**, *10*, 209–222. [CrossRef]

98. Wu, S.-Y.S.; Wang, H.-M.D.; Wen, Y.-S.; Liu, W.; Li, P.-H.; Chiu, C.-C.; Chen, P.-C.; Huang, C.-Y.; Sheu, J.-H.; Wen, Z.-H. 4-(Phenylsulfanyl)Butan-2-One Suppresses Melanin Synthesis and Melanosome Maturation In Vitro and In Vivo. *Int. J. Mol. Sci.* **2015**, *16*, 20240–20257. [CrossRef]

99. Liu, J.; Sridhar, J.; Foroozesh, M. Cytochrome P450 Family 1 Inhibitors and Structure-Activity Relationships. *Molecules* **2013**, *18*, 14470–14495. [CrossRef]

100. Androutsopoulos, V.P.; Tsatsakis, A.M.; Spandidos, D.A. Cytochrome P450 CYP1A1: Wider Roles in Cancer Progression and Prevention. *BMC Cancer* **2009**, *9*, 187. [CrossRef]

101. Pillaiyar, T.; Manickam, M.; Namasivayam, V. Skin Whitening Agents: Medicinal Chemistry Perspective of Tyrosinase Inhibitors. *J. Enzyme Inhib. Med. Chem.* **2017**, *32*, 403–425. [CrossRef]

102. Marth, J.D.; Peet, R.; Krebs, E.G.; Perlmutter, R.M. A Lymphocyte-Specific Protein-Tyrosine Kinase Gene Is Rearranged and Overexpressed in the Murine T Cell Lymphoma LSTRA. *Cell* **1985**, *43*, 393–404. [CrossRef] [PubMed]

103. Kumar Singh, P.; Kashyap, A.; Silakari, O. Exploration of the Therapeutic Aspects of Lck: A Kinase Target in Inflammatory Mediated Pathological Conditions. *Biomed. Pharmacother. Biomed. Pharmacother.* **2018**, *108*, 1565–1571. [CrossRef] [PubMed]

104. Wright, A.D.; Goclik, E.; König, G.M. Oxygenated Analogues of Gorgosterol and Ergosterol from the Soft Coral *Capnella lacertiliensis*. *J. Nat. Prod.* **2003**, *66*, 157–160. [CrossRef] [PubMed]

105. Folmer, F.; Jaspars, M.; Solano, G.; Cristofanon, S.; Henry, E.; Tabudravu, J.; Black, K.; Green, D.H.; Küpper, F.C.; Aalbersberg, W.; et al. The Inhibition of TNF-Alpha-Induced NF-KappaB Activation by Marine Natural Products. *Biochem. Pharmacol.* **2009**, *78*, 592–606. [CrossRef]

106. Mohyeldin, M.M.; Akl, M.R.; Siddique, A.B.; Hassan, H.M.; El Sayed, K.A. The Marine-Derived Pachycladin Diterpenoids as Novel Inhibitors of Wild-Type and Mutant EGFR. *Biochem. Pharmacol.* **2017**, *126*, 51–68. [CrossRef]

107. He, H.; Kulanthaivel, P.; Baker, B.J.; Kalter, K.; Darges, J.; Cofield, D.; Wolff, L.; Adams, L. New Antiproliferative and Antiinflammatory 9,11-Secosterols from the Gorgonian *Pseudopterogorgia* sp. *Tetrahedron* **1995**, *51*, 51–58. [CrossRef]

108. Zandi, E.; Rothwarf, D.M.; Delhase, M.; Hayakawa, M.; Karin, M. The IκB Kinase Complex (IKK) Contains Two Kinase Subunits, IKKα and IKKβ, Necessary for IκB Phosphorylation and NF-KB Activation. *Cell* **1997**, *91*, 243–252. [CrossRef]

109. Senegas, A.; Gautheron, J.; Maurin, A.G.D.; Courtois, G. IKK-Related Genetic Diseases: Probing NF-KB Functions in Humans and Other Matters. *Cell. Mol. Life Sci. CMLS* **2015**, *72*, 1275–1287. [CrossRef]

110. Andersson, M.; Nieuwerburgh, L.V.; Snoeijs, P. Pigment Transfer from Phytoplankton to Zooplankton with Emphasis on Astaxanthin Production in the Baltic Sea Food Web. *Mar. Ecol. Prog. Ser.* **2003**, *254*, 213–224. [CrossRef]

111. Thompson, D.M.; Gill, G.N. The EGF Receptor: Structure, Regulation and Potential Role in Malignancy. *Cancer Surv.* **1985**, *4*, 767–788.

112. Wei, Q.; Sheng, L.; Shui, Y.; Hu, Q.; Nordgren, H.; Carlsson, J. EGFR, HER2, and HER3 Expression in Laryngeal Primary Tumors and Corresponding Metastases. *Ann. Surg. Oncol.* **2008**, *15*, 1193–1201. [CrossRef]

113. Wei, Q.; Chen, L.; Sheng, L.; Nordgren, H.; Wester, K.; Carlsson, J. EGFR, HER2 and HER3 Expression in Esophageal Primary Tumours and Corresponding Metastases. *Int. J. Oncol.* **2007**, *31*, 493–499. [CrossRef]

114. Riely, G.J.; Politi, K.A.; Miller, V.A.; Pao, W. Update on Epidermal Growth Factor Receptor Mutations in Non-Small Cell Lung Cancer. *Clin. Cancer Res. Off. J. Am. Assoc. Cancer Res.* **2006**, *12*, 7232–7241. [CrossRef]

115. Newton, A.C. Protein Kinase C: Structural and Spatial Regulation by Phosphorylation, Cofactors, and Macromolecular Interactions. *Chem. Rev.* **2001**, *101*, 2353–2364. [CrossRef]

116. Geribaldi-Doldán, N.; Gómez-Oliva, R.; Domínguez-García, S.; Nunez-Abades, P.; Castro, C. Protein Kinase C: Targets to Regenerate Brain Injuries? *Front. Cell Dev. Biol.* **2019**, *7*, 39. [CrossRef]

117. Marrocco, V.; Bogomolovas, J.; Ehler, E.; Dos Remedios, C.G.; Yu, J.; Gao, C.; Lange, S. PKC and PKN in Heart Disease. *J. Mol. Cell. Cardiol.* **2019**, *128*, 212–226. [CrossRef]

118. Newton, A.C. Protein Kinase C: Perfectly Balanced. *Crit. Rev. Biochem. Mol. Biol.* **2018**, *53*, 208–230. [CrossRef]

119. Lai, D.; Yu, S.; van Ofwegen, L.; Totzke, F.; Proksch, P.; Lin, W. 9,10-Secosteroids, Protein Kinase Inhibitors from the Chinese Gorgonian *Astrogorgia* sp. *Bioorg. Med. Chem.* **2011**, *19*, 6873–6880. [CrossRef]

120. Zhang, J.-R.; Li, P.-L.; Tang, X.-L.; Qi, X.; Li, G.-Q. Cytotoxic Tetraprenylated Alkaloids from the South China Sea Gorgonian *Euplexaura robusta*. *Chem. Biodivers.* **2012**, *9*, 2218–2224. [CrossRef]

121. Sorek, H.; Rudi, A.; Benayahu, Y.; Ben-Califa, N.; Neumann, D.; Kashman, Y. Nuttingins A-F and Malonganenones D-H, Tetraprenylated Alkaloids from the Tanzanian Gorgonian *Euplexaura nuttingi*. *J. Nat. Prod.* **2007**, *70*, 1104–1109. [CrossRef]

122. Jiang, W.; Wang, D.; Wilson, B.A.P.; Voeller, D.; Bokesch, H.R.; Smith, E.A.; Lipkowitz, S.; O'Keefe, B.R.; Gustafson, K.R. Sinularamides A-G, Terpenoid-Derived Spermidine and Spermine Conjugates with Casitas B-Lineage Lymphoma Proto-Oncogene B (Cbl-b) Inhibitory Activities from a *Sinularia* sp. Soft Coral. *J. Nat. Prod.* **2021**, *84*, 1831–1837. [CrossRef] [PubMed]

123. Coval, S.J.; Patton, R.W.; Petrin, J.M.; James, L.; Rothofsky, M.L.; Lin, S.L.; Patel, M.; Reed, J.K.; McPhail, A.T.; Bishop, W.R. A Cembranolide Diterpene Farnesyl Protein Transferase Inhibitor from the Marine Soft Coral *Lobophytum cristagalli*. *Bioorg. Med. Chem. Lett.* **1996**, *6*, 909–912. [CrossRef]

124. Whalen, K.E.; Lane, A.L.; Kubanek, J.; Hahn, M.E. Biochemical Warfare on the Reef: The Role of Glutathione Transferases in Consumer Tolerance of Dietary Prostaglandins. *PLoS ONE* **2010**, *5*, e8537. [CrossRef] [PubMed]

125. Liu, Y.-C.; Gu, H. Cbl and Cbl-b in T-Cell Regulation. *Trends Immunol.* **2002**, *23*, 140–143. [CrossRef] [PubMed]

126. Jafari, D.; Mousavi, M.J.; Keshavarz Shahbaz, S.; Jafarzadeh, L.; Tahmasebi, S.; Spoor, J.; Esmaeilzadeh, A. E3 Ubiquitin Ligase Casitas B Lineage Lymphoma-b and Its Potential Therapeutic Implications for Immunotherapy. *Clin. Exp. Immunol.* **2021**, *204*, 14–31. [CrossRef]

127. Paolino, M.; Choidas, A.; Wallner, S.; Pranjic, B.; Uribesalgo, I.; Loeser, S.; Jamieson, A.M.; Langdon, W.Y.; Ikeda, F.; Fededa, J.P.; et al. The E3 Ligase Cbl-b and TAM Receptors Regulate Cancer Metastasis via Natural Killer Cells. *Nature* **2014**, *507*, 508–512. [CrossRef]

128. Zhang, F.L.; Casey, P.J. Protein Prenylation: Molecular Mechanisms and Functional Consequences. *Annu. Rev. Biochem.* **1996**, *65*, 241–269. [CrossRef]

129. Lobell, R.B.; Omer, C.A.; Abrams, M.T.; Bhimnathwala, H.G.; Brucker, M.J.; Buser, C.A.; Davide, J.P.; de Solms, S.J.; Dinsmore, C.J.; Ellis-Hutchings, M.S.; et al. Evaluation of Farnesyl:Protein Transferase and Geranylgeranyl:Protein Transferase Inhibitor Combinations in Preclinical Models. *Cancer Res.* **2001**, *61*, 8758–8768.

130. Head, J.; Johnston, S.R. New Targets for Therapy in Breast Cancer: Farnesyltransferase Inhibitors. *Breast Cancer Res.* **2004**, *6*, 262. [CrossRef]

131. Hayes, J.D.; Flanagan, J.U.; Jowsey, I.R. Glutathione Transferases. *Annu. Rev. Pharmacol. Toxicol.* **2005**, *45*, 51–88. [CrossRef]

132. O'Brien, M.L.; Tew, K.D. Glutathione and Related Enzymes in Multidrug Resistance. *Eur. J. Cancer* **1996**, *32*, 967–978. [CrossRef]

133. Mahajan, S.; Atkins, W.M. The Chemistry and Biology of Inhibitors and Pro-Drugs Targeted to Glutathione S-Transferases. *Cell. Mol. Life Sci. CMLS* **2005**, *62*, 1221–1233. [CrossRef]

134. Seufferheld, M.J.; Kim, K.M.; Whitfield, J.; Valerio, A.; Caetano-Anollés, G. Evolution of Vacuolar Proton Pyrophosphatase Domains and Volutin Granules: Clues into the Early Evolutionary Origin of the Acidocalcisome. *Biol. Direct* **2011**, *6*, 50. [CrossRef]

135. Segami, S.; Asaoka, M.; Kinoshita, S.; Fukuda, M.; Nakanishi, Y.; Maeshima, M. Biochemical, Structural and Physiological Characteristics of Vacuolar H+-Pyrophosphatase. *Plant Cell Physiol.* **2018**, *59*, 1300–1308. [CrossRef]

136. Hirono, M.; Ojika, M.; Mimura, H.; Nakanishi, Y.; Maeshima, M. Acylspermidine Derivatives Isolated from a Soft Coral, *Sinularia* sp., Inhibit Plant Vacuolar H(+)-Pyrophosphatase. *J. Biochem.* **2003**, *133*, 811–816. [CrossRef]

137. Halling, P.; Fitzpatrick, P.F.; Raushel, F.M.; Rohwer, J.; Schnell, S.; Wittig, U.; Wohlgemuth, R.; Kettner, C. An Empirical Analysis of Enzyme Function Reporting for Experimental Reproducibility: Missing/Incomplete Information in Published Papers. *Biophys. Chem.* **2018**, *242*, 22–27. [CrossRef]

138. Copeland, R.A. *Evaluation of Enzyme Inhibitors in Drug Discovery: A Guide for Medicinal Chemists and Pharmacologists*, 2nd ed.; John Wiley & Sons: Hoboken, NJ, USA, 2013.

139. Copeland, R.A. *Enzymes, A Practical Introduction to Structure, Mechanism, and Data Analysis*, 2nd ed.; Wiley-VCH: New York, NY, USA, 2000; ISBN 0-471-22063-9.

140. Copeland, R.A. Evaluation of Enzyme Inhibitors in Drug Discovery: A Guide for Medicinal Chemists and Pharmacologists. *Methods Biochem. Anal.* **2005**, *46*, 1–265.

141. Lankatillake, C.; Luo, S.; Flavel, M.; Lenon, G.B.; Gill, H.; Huynh, T.; Dias, D.A. Screening Natural Product Extracts for Potential Enzyme Inhibitors: Protocols, and the Standardisation of the Usage of Blanks in α-Amylase, α-Glucosidase and Lipase Assays. *Plant Methods* **2021**, *17*, 3. [CrossRef]

142. Christopeit, T.; Øverbø, K.; Danielson, U.H.; Nilsen, I.W. Efficient Screening of Marine Extracts for Protease Inhibitors by Combining FRET Based Activity Assays and Surface Plasmon Resonance Spectroscopy Based Binding Assays. *Mar. Drugs* **2013**, *11*, 4279–4293. [CrossRef]

143. Hanada, K.; Tamai, M.; Yamagishi, M.; Ohmura, S.; Sawada, J.; Tanaka, I. Isolation and Characterization of E–64, a New Thiol Protease Inhibitor. *Agric. Biol. Chem.* **1978**, *42*, 523–528. [CrossRef]

144. Bennett, S.E.; Schimerlik, M.I.; Mosbaugh, D.W. Kinetics of the Uracil-DNA Glycosylase/Inhibitor Protein Association. Ung Interaction with Ugi, Nucleic Acids, and Uracil Compounds. *J. Biol. Chem.* **1993**, *268*, 26879–26885. [CrossRef] [PubMed]

145. Zhao, Y.; Jin, Y.; Wei, S.-S.; Lee, W.-H.; Zhang, Y. Purification and Characterization of an Irreversible Serine Protease Inhibitor from Skin Secretions of *Bufo andrewsi*. *Toxicon Off. J. Int. Soc. Toxinol.* **2005**, *46*, 635–640. [CrossRef] [PubMed]

146. Faller, B.; Bieth, J.G. Kinetics of the Interaction of Chymotrypsin with Eglin c. *Biochem. J.* **1991**, *280 (Pt 1)*, 27–32. [CrossRef]

147. Lineweaver, H.; Burk, D. The Determination of Enzyme Dissociation Constants. *ACS Publ.* **1934**, *56*, 658–666. [CrossRef]

148. Dixon, M. The Determination of Enzyme Inhibitor Constants. *Biochem. J.* **1953**, *55*, 170–171. [CrossRef]

149. Cortés, A.; Cascante, M.; Cárdenas, M.L.; Cornish-Bowden, A. Relationships between Inhibition Constants, Inhibitor Concentrations for 50% Inhibition and Types of Inhibition: New Ways of Analysing Data. *Biochem. J.* **2001**, *357*, 263–268. [CrossRef]

150. Morrison, J.F. Kinetics of the Reversible Inhibition of Enzyme-Catalysed Reactions by Tight-Binding Inhibitors. *Biochim. Biophys. Acta* **1969**, *185*, 269–286. [CrossRef]
151. Reytor Gonzalez, M.L.; Del Rivero Antigua, M.A. Reviewing the Experimental and Mathematical Factors Involved in Tight Binding Inhibitors Ki Values Determination: The Bi-Functional Protease Inhibitor SmCI as a Test Model. *Biochimie* **2021**, *181*, 86–95. [CrossRef]
152. Baell, J.B.; Holloway, G.A. New Substructure Filters for Removal of Pan Assay Interference Compounds (PAINS) from Screening Libraries and for Their Exclusion in Bioassays. *J. Med. Chem.* **2010**, *53*, 2719–2740. [CrossRef]
153. Baell, J.B.; Nissink, J.W.M. Seven Year Itch: Pan-Assay Interference Compounds (PAINS) in 2017—Utility and Limitations. *ACS Chem. Biol.* **2018**, *13*, 36–44. [CrossRef]
154. Baell, J.B. Feeling Nature's PAINS: Natural Products, Natural Product Drugs, and Pan Assay Interference Compounds (PAINS). *J. Nat. Prod.* **2016**, *79*, 616–628. [CrossRef]
155. Babaoglu, K.; Simeonov, A.; Irwin, J.J.; Nelson, M.E.; Feng, B.; Thomas, C.J.; Cancian, L.; Costi, M.P.; Maltby, D.A.; Jadhav, A.; et al. Comprehensive Mechanistic Analysis of Hits from High-Throughput and Docking Screens against Beta-Lactamase. *J. Med. Chem.* **2008**, *51*, 2502–2511. [CrossRef]
156. Jadhav, A.; Ferreira, R.S.; Klumpp, C.; Mott, B.T.; Austin, C.P.; Inglese, J.; Thomas, C.J.; Maloney, D.J.; Shoichet, B.K.; Simeonov, A. Quantitative Analyses of Aggregation, Autofluorescence, and Reactivity Artifacts in a Screen for Inhibitors of a Thiol Protease. *J. Med. Chem.* **2010**, *53*, 37–51. [CrossRef]
157. Aldrich, C.; Bertozzi, C.; Georg, G.I.; Kiessling, L.; Lindsley, C.; Liotta, D.; Merz, K.M.; Schepartz, A.; Wang, S. The Ecstasy and Agony of Assay Interference Compounds. *J. Chem. Inf. Model.* **2017**, *57*, 387–390. [CrossRef]
158. Feng, B.Y.; Simeonov, A.; Jadhav, A.; Babaoglu, K.; Inglese, J.; Shoichet, B.K.; Austin, C.P. A High-Throughput Screen for Aggregation-Based Inhibition in a Large Compound Library. *J. Med. Chem.* **2007**, *50*, 2385–2390. [CrossRef]
159. Coan, K.E.D.; Shoichet, B.K. Stoichiometry and Physical Chemistry of Promiscuous Aggregate-Based Inhibitors. *J. Am. Chem. Soc.* **2008**, *130*, 9606–9612. [CrossRef]

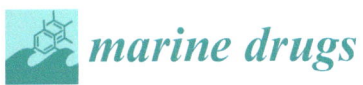

Article

Effect of Phlorotannins from Brown Algae *Costaria costata* on α-N-Acetylgalactosaminidase Produced by Duodenal Adenocarcinoma and Melanoma Cells

Irina Bakunina [1,*], Tatiana Imbs [1], Galina Likhatskaya [1], Valeria Grigorchuk [2], Anastasya Zueva [1], Olesya Malyarenko [1]and Svetlana Ermakova [1]

[1] G.B. Elyakov Pacific Institute of Bioorganic Chemistry, Far Eastern Branch, Russian Academy of Sciences, 159 Pr-t 100-let Vladivostoka Str., 690022 Vladivostok, Russia
[2] Federal Scientific Center of the East Asia Terrestrial Biodiversity, Far Eastern Branch, Russian Academy of Sciences, 159 Pr-t 100-let Vladivostoka Str., 690022 Vladivostok, Russia
* Correspondence: bakun@list.ru

Abstract: The inhibitor of human α-N-acetylgalactosaminidase (α-NaGalase) was isolated from a water–ethanol extract of the brown algae *Costaria costata*. Currently, tumor α-NaGalase is considered to be a therapeutic target in the treatment of cancer. According to NMR spectroscopy and mass spectrometric analysis, it is a high-molecular-weight fraction of phlorethols with a degree of polymerization (DP) equaling 11–23 phloroglucinols (CcPh). It was shown that CcPh is a direct inhibitor of α-NaGalases isolated from HuTu 80 and SK-MEL-28 cells (IC$_{50}$ 0.14 ± 0.008 and 0.12 ± 0.004 mg/mL, respectively) and reduces the activity of this enzyme in HuTu 80 and SK-MEL-28 cells up to 50% at concentrations of 15.2 ± 9.5 and 5.7 ± 1.6 μg/mL, respectively. Molecular docking of the putative DP-15 oligophlorethol (P15OPh) and heptaphlorethol (PHPh) with human α-NaGalase (PDB ID 4DO4) showed that this compound forms a complex and interacts directly with the Asp 156 and Asp 217 catalytic residues of the enzyme in question. Thus, brown algae phlorethol CcPh is an effective marine-based natural inhibitor of the α-NaGalase of cancer cells and, therefore, has high therapeutic potential.

Keywords: α-N-acetylgalactosaminidase; α-NaGalase; inhibitor; phlorotannins; brown algae; *Costaria costata*; carcinoma; melanoma; cancer cells

Citation: Bakunina, I.; Imbs, T.; Likhatskaya, G.; Grigorchuk, V.; Zueva, A.; Malyarenko, O.; Ermakova, S. Effect of Phlorotannins from Brown Algae *Costaria costata* on α-N-Acetylgalactosaminidase Produced by Duodenal Adenocarcinoma and Melanoma Cells. *Mar. Drugs* 2023, *21*, 33. https://doi.org/10.3390/md21010033

Academic Editors: Francesc Xavier Avilés and Isel Pascual

Received: 10 December 2022
Revised: 26 December 2022
Accepted: 27 December 2022
Published: 30 December 2022

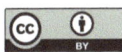

1. Introduction

α-N-Acetylgalactosaminidase (α-NaGalase) (EC 3.2.1.49) removes α-linked residues of N-acetylgalactosaminide from the non-reducing ends of various complex carbohydrates and glycoconjugates. Glycolipids, glycopeptides, and glycoproteins; blood group A erythrocyte antigens [1–3]; lipopolysaccharides of the cell walls; and capsules of bacteria [4–6] are physiological substrates for α-NaGalase. This enzyme is widespread in the organs and tissues of mammals, bacteria, and fungi.

Human α-NaGalase is a lysosomal enzyme encoded by the sole NAGA gene localized to chromosome 22q13→qter [7]. This enzyme's structure, mechanism of action, and role in the human body have been studied in detail [8,9]. According to the structural classification of carbohydrate-active enzymes (CAZy), this enzyme belongs to the 27 family of glycoside hydrolases (GH27) [10]. It is produced by all cancer cells and accumulates in the blood plasma of cancer patients [11]. This enzyme, which is released from cancer cells, is active at pH 6.0–6.8 and has endo-type activity, hydrolyzing the O-glycosidic linkage between α-N-acetylgalactosamine and serine or threonine in glycoproteins [12]. These properties of the enzyme prevent macrophage activation in cancer patients via the deglycosylation of the vitamin D$_3$-binding protein, which is the precursor of the macrophage-activating factor (GcMAF) [13,14]. The level of enzyme activity and number of its forms increase in blood serum, especially at the initial stage of the disease and the stage of metastasis [15]. A high level of the enzyme activity leads to immunosuppression in patients with advanced cancer [16]. Thus, α-NaGalase, as an immunosuppressive agent in cancer patients, is considered to be a potential therapeutic target in cancer treatment.

The activity of this aggressive enzyme can be suppressed in various ways. Knockdown of the NAGA gene with a transfection reagent in EPG85.257RDB cells leads to an increase in the rate of late apoptosis and to augmentative and regressive effects on cell death and migration [17]. A study of the effects of Naga-shRNA downregulation in the MCF-7 (human breast carcinoma) and A2780 (human ovarian carcinoma) cell lines showed significant inhibition of the migratory and invasive properties of cancer cell lines [18]. However, the epigenetic modification of the NAGA gene by DNA hypermethylation reduced the expression of α-NaGalase and increased chemoresistance to cisplatin in ovarian cancer [19]. Previously, we have shown that the treatment of DLD-1 adenocarcinoma cells with fucoidan from the brown alga *Fucus evanescens* reduces the production of this enzyme [20]. Some aaptamines and makaluvamines isolated from marine sponges showed no direct inhibitory effect on cancer-associated α-NaGalase; however, isoaaptamine, 9-demethylaaptamine, damirone B, and makaluvamine H reduced the expression of the enzyme in the human colorectal adenocarcinoma cell line DLD-1 at a concentration 5 μM [21].

The polyphenolic compounds of brown algae constitute a class of oligomeric and polymeric phlorotannins. They consist of phloroglucinol (1,3,5-trihydroxybenzene) as a basic unit linked in different ways. The increased interest in these compounds over the last few years has arisen due to their wide range of biological activities. A number of reviews have summarized the results of comprehensive studies of phlorotannins in relation to their biological significance, isolation, structural features, and action, for which the latter mainly comprises antioxidant, antitumor, antidiabetic, and anti-inflammatory activities [22–25]. An especially interesting finding was that eckol stimulated the innate and adaptive immune responses responsive to tumor surveillance in mice with a sarcoma activating the phagocytic system [26]. We previously showed that the impurity of phenols plays a key role in the antioxidant activity exhibited by fucoidan from the brown alga *F. evanescens* [27]. The polyphenolic impurities contained in fucoidan fractions of brown algae *F. evanescens* reduced the protection of sea urchin embryogenesis and caused the appearance of a large number of embryos with morphological abnormalities [28]. Previous studies have described the direct inhibitory effects of phlorotannins on hyaluronidase [29], lipoxygenase [30], the glycosidases of marine mollusks [31], amylase, lipase and trypsin [32], reverse transcriptase, protease [33], and the central nervous system-related enzymes acetyl- and butyryl-cholinesterases, monoaminoxidases, β-secretase, and tyrosinase [34].

This article aimed to study the effects of phlorotannins from the brown algae *C. costata* on α-NaGalase produced by duodenal adenocarcinoma HuTu 80 and melanoma SK-MEL-28 cell lines, namely, the suppression or increase in the activity of α-NaGalase in cancer cells, as well as the direct inhibition or activation of isolated enzymes.

2. Results

2.1. Biochemical and Catalytic Properties of α-NaGalases

Isolation and Purification of α-NaGalase from Cell Lysates

The protein fractions enriched with α-NaGalase activity were isolated from the cell lysates of duodenal adenocarcinoma HuTu 80 and melanoma SK-MEL-28 cell lines in accordance with procedures described previously [20,21]. The following study of the biochemical characteristics of α-NaGalase is necessary for the investigation of phlorotannins' effects on the enzyme's activity.

The effects of pH on the enzyme's activity are shown on Figure 1.

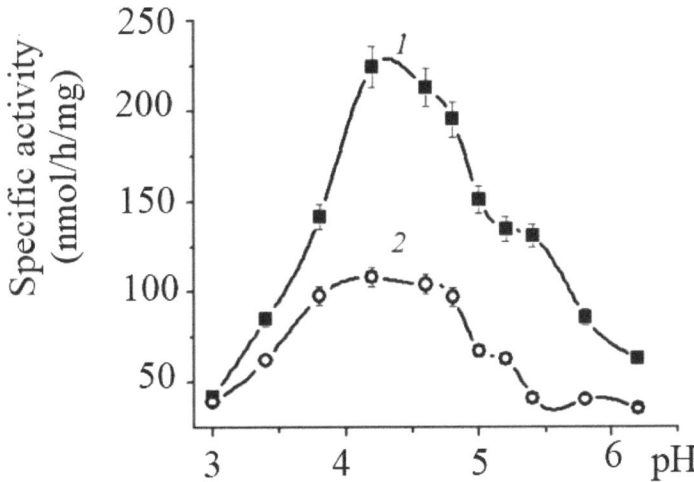

Figure 1. Effects of pH on the specific activity of α-NaGalases from HuTu 80 (1) and SK-MEL-28 (2) cell lines. Solution of 0.05 M sodium citrate buffer.

The enzymes of both cell lines exhibit maximum activity in the pH range from 4.0 to 5.5. The specific activity of HuTu 80 α-NaGalase exceeded the activity of the SK-MEL-28 enzyme by almost threefold.

To determine the Michaelis–Menten constant (K_m) and the maximum reaction rate (V_{max}) of the α-NaGalase of both cell lines, the concentration of the pNPNAGal substrate was varied from 0.07 to 9.0 mM in a solution of Na citrate with pH 4.5.

This experiment showed that the K_m values of the HuTu 80 and SK-MEL-28 enzymes differ slightly, but the V_{max} value of HuTu 80 α-NaGalase was almost three times higher than the V_{max} value of the SK-MEL-28 enzyme (Table 1). The high K_m values and low V_{max} values of the studied enzymes probably characterize their low affinity for the commercial chromogenic standard substrate.

Table 1. Catalytic parameters K_m and V_{max} of α-NaGalases [1] from HuTu 80 and SK-MEL-28 cell lines.

Cell Lines	K_m (mM)	V_{max} (nmol/h/mL)
HuTu 80	4.20 ± 0.14	411.2 ± 6.5
SK-MEL-28	6.90 ± 0.43	138.8 ± 4.8

[1] For p-NPNAGal as substrate in 0.05 M Na citrate buffer pH 4.5.

2.2. Phlorotannins of Brown Algae C. costata

2.2.1. Brown Alga Collection and Phlorotannins' Isolation

The fraction of phlorotannins (CcPh) was isolated from the water–ethanol extract of the brown algae *C. costata* using sequential liquid extraction with organic solvents and chromatography on silica gel, polychrome-1, and C-18 as described earlier with some modifications [35]. The CcPh fraction was characterized by nuclear magnetic resonance (NMR) spectroscopy and mass spectrometry, as described below.

2.2.2. Nuclear Magnetic Resonance Analysis

The ^{1}H NMR spectrum of the CcPh fraction showed a distribution of ^{1}H signals between 5.8 and 6.3 ppm, which is typical for polyphenols. Observations in experiments with HMBC (Figure 2, Table 2) confirmed the presence of phlorotannin structures.

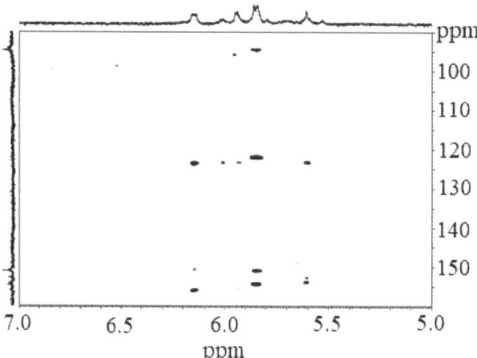

Figure 2. Fragmented HMBC spectrum of the CcPh fraction.

Table 2. HMBC * assignments of the CcPh fraction of *C. costata*.

Structure		^{13}C (δ in ppm)	^1H (δ in ppm)
Unsubstituted benzene carbons		94.3	5.86–5.83
		93.8	5.94; 5.61
		94.5	6.16
Diaryl–ether bond (ether linkage)		123.6	6.13–6.17
		123.5	5.93
		123.6	6.01
		123.5	5.59–5.62
		122.4	5.83–5.86
Benzene carbon bearing hydroxylated groups		156.0	6.13–6.17
		153.9	5.59–5.62
		152.9	5.59–5.62
		150.9	6.13–6.17
		151.1	5.83–5.86
		154.0	5.83–5.86
		154.6	5.83–5.86

* CcPh were dissolved in DMSO-d with tetramethylsilane as the internal standard.

The HMBC spectrum showed characteristic carbon atom resonances at 93.8–94.5 ppm corresponding to unsubstituted benzene carbons; signals in the range of 122.0 to 123.6 ppm corresponded to diaryl–ether bonds (phloroglucinol units connected by a simple ether); and signals between 150.9 and 156.0 ppm were characteristic of benzene carbon-bearing hydroxylated groups.

However, signals at 100–105 ppm and 142–148 ppm were not present. This fact indicates the absence of aryl–aryl carbon atoms, as well as the presence of additional OH functions other than 1,3,5-OH groups. Thus, fucolic type units and fugalol type units are absent in the studied sample. It can be concluded that this polymer belongs to the phlorethol class of the phlorotannins.

2.2.3. Mass Spectra Analysis

The molecular weight of the CcPh fraction was determined by ESI–MS. Negative ESI–MS measurements showed the mixture of pseudomolecule ions of CcPh at m/z 744 to m/z 1364 $[M − 2H]^{-2}$. The degree of phloroglucinol polymerization ranged from 12 to 22 phloroglucinol units in the CcPh fraction, with the most abundant phlorethols containing between 15 and 18 phloroglucinol units (m/z 930 to m/z 1116 $[M – 2H]^{-2}$) (Table 3, Figure 3)

Table 3. The data concerning elemental compositions, monoisotopic masses, and ions of the CcPh *.

Degree of Polymerization	$[M - 2H]^{-2}$		Signal Strength (%)	Elemental Composition	Monoisotopic Mass (Da)
	m/z Measured	*m/z* Calculated			
11	682.0898	682.0888	6	$C_{66}H_{46}O_{33}$	1366.1921
12	744.0940	744.0968	12	$C_{72}H_{50}O_{36}$	1490.2082
13	806.1019	806.1048	30	$C_{78}H_{54}O_{39}$	1614.2242
14	868.1105	868.1129	46	$C_{84}H_{58}O_{42}$	1738.2403
15	930.1183	930.1209	66	$C_{90}H_{62}O_{45}$	1862.2563
16	992.1262	992.1289	99	$C_{96}H_{66}O_{48}$	1986.2724
17	1054.1332	1054.1369	99	$C_{102}H_{70}O_{51}$	2110.2884
18	1116.1430	1116.1449	74	$C_{108}H_{74}O_{54}$	2234.3044
19	1178.1483	1178.1530	60	$C_{114}H_{78}O_{57}$	2358.3205
20	1240.1588	1240.1610	50	$C_{120}H_{82}O_{60}$	2482.3365
21	1302.1652	1302.1690	30	$C_{126}H_{86}O_{63}$	2606.3526
22	1364.1746	1364.1770	16	$C_{132}H_{90}O_{66}$	2730.3686
23	1426.1839	1426.1851	6	$C_{138}H_{94}O_{69}$	2854.3847

* ESI–MS spectra were detected in negative ion mode HRMS at each degree of polymerization (DP), representing the predominant charge state detected under the experimental conditions described. The strength of signals expressed as a percentage (%) of intensity (100% = 550).

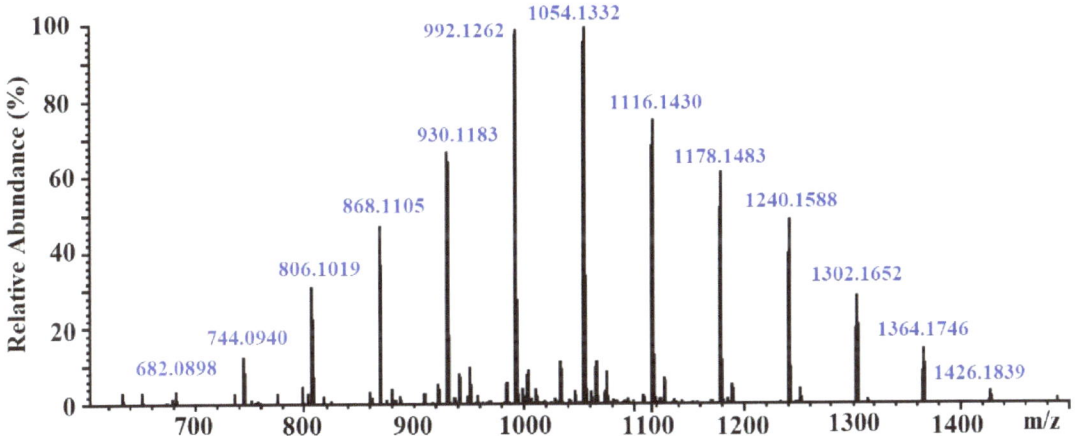

Figure 3. ESI–MS spectra, operating in negative mode (ES-), of phlorethols fraction CcPh from *Costaria costata*.

2.3. The Effect of the Phlorethol CcPh on α-NaGalases in Cancer Cells

2.3.1. Cytotoxic Effect of CcPh fraction on Human Duodenal Carcinoma HuTu 80 and Melanoma SK-MEL-28 Cells

For the first step, the effects of non-toxic CcPh concentrations on the viability of human HuTu 80 and SK-MEL-28 cells were tested by an MTS assay. It was shown that the concentrations of CcPh that caused a 50% reduction in cell viability (IC_{50}) were 92 ± 3 μg/mL and 102 ± 5 μg/mL for the HuTu 80 and SK-MEL-28 cells, respectively. Phlorethol CcPh was non-cytotoxic up to 40 μg/ml for both cell lines.

2.3.2. The Inhibitory Potency of the CcPh for α-NaGalases in Cancer Cells

Figure 4 shows the effect of the phlorethol CcPh on the production of the enzyme α-NaGalase by the HuTu 80 and SK-MEL-28 cancer cells.

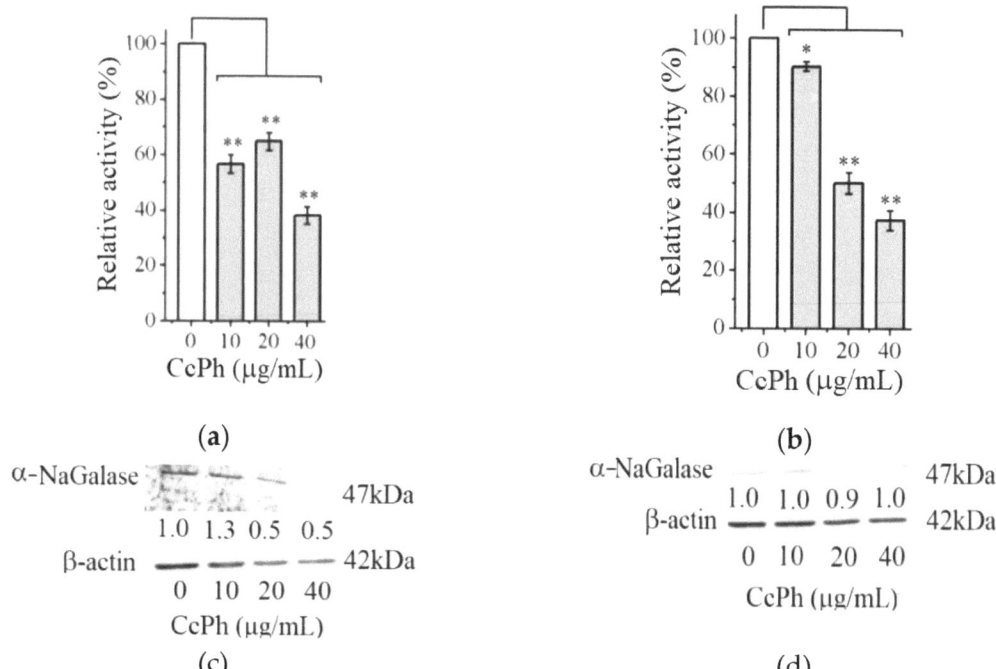

Figure 4. Relative activity of α-NaGalase of lysates after treatment of duodenal cancer cells HuTu 80 (**a**) and melanoma SK-MEL-28 (**b**) with 10, 20, and 40 μg/mL of the CcPh compared to the enzyme of untreated cells as positive control (0). Relative activity of α-NaGalase was defined as $A/A_0 \times 100$ (%), where A and A_0 are the specific activities of α-NaGalase of the samples and the control experiment (0), respectively. The results of the α-NaGalase protein expression assay conducted via Western blot analysis are as follows: α-NaGalase protein expression was significantly decreased by CcPh compared to controls for HuTu 80 (**c**) and SK-MEL-28 (**d**). Data are shown as means $\pm$ standard deviation (SD) of values from three independent experiments. Student's *t*-test was used to evaluate the data with the following significance levels: * $p < 0.05$ and ** $p < 0.01$. Corresponding signal intensities were determined in a densitometrical manner and normalized to total protein (β-actin) in each lane and are given below for each data point.

As can be seen from Figure 4, the activity of the α-NaGalases in the lysates of the treated cancer cells of both cancer lines decreases with an increase in the CcPh concentration up to 40 μg/mL (Figure 4a,b). The CcPh fraction reduces α-NaGalase activity by 50% in the HuTu 80 and SK-MEL-28 cells at concentrations (IC_{50}) of 15.2 ± 9.5 and 5.7 ± 1.6 μg/mL, respectively. However, it should be noted that this compound is an inhibitor of enzyme biosynthesis only in the HuTu 80 cancer cells (Figure 4c) and not in the SK-MEL-28 cancer cells (Figure 4d). According to the results of the Western blotting analysis, the level of α-NaGalase protein after the dose-dependent treatment with CcPh decreased in the HuTu 80 cells (Figure 4c) but did not change in the SK-MEL-28 cells (Figure 4d).

2.4. The Phlorethol CcPh as Direct Inhibitors of α-NaGalases

The potency of CcPh as a direct inhibitor was studied by a standard end-point assay. Figure 5 shows the dose–response curves regarding the inhibition of HuTu 80 α-NaGalase (1) and SK-MEL-28 α-NaGalase (2) by CcPh at final concentrations from 0 to 1.67 mg/mL. The IC_{50} values evaluated from the coefficients of the sigmoid curves with nonlinear regressions were 0.14 ± 0.008 and 0.12 ± 0.004 mg/mL.

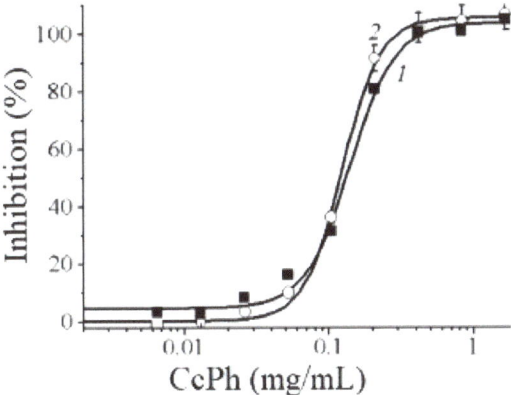

Figure 5. Dose–response curves of HuTu 80- (1) and SK-MEL-28-related (2) α-NaGalases inhibition after preincubation with CcPh for 30 min, followed by addition of substrate and 4 h incubation with enzyme and substrate. Inhibition (%) are plotted against concentration of CcPh on a logarithmic scale.

To determine the reversibility of the action of CcPh action towards the α-NaGalase activity, we carried out the dialysis of the inactivated enzymes. The activity of the enzymes did not recover after dialysis against the buffer solution for 60 h, but the enzyme in the absence of the inhibitor retained 100% activity during this dialysis process. However, the time-dependence of the IC_{50} values was not observed after the preincubation of CcPh with these enzymes for 5, 20, 60, and 120 min (data not shown). Thus, it was shown that CcPh is a fast-binding, irreversible inhibitor of α-NaGalase.

2.5. Theoretical Models of Human α-NaGalase Complexes with Oligophlorethols

2.5.1. Theoretical Models of Putative Heptaphlorethol

The putative structure of the linear oligomer, termed heptaphlorethol (PHPh), which consists of seven monomeric units (phloroglucinol) linked by aryl–ether bonds, was generated using the Molecule Build module of the MOE 2020.09 program. The 2D-structure of PHPh and its optimized 3D-structure are shown on Figure 6.

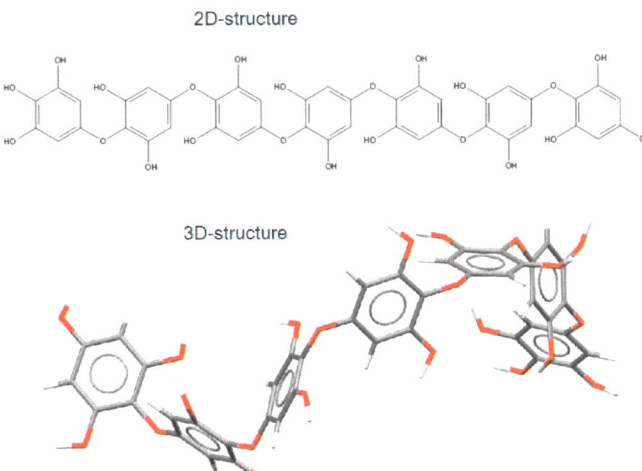

Figure 6. The 2D- and 3D-structures of PHPh (top and bottom picture, respectively) of putative linear oligomer consisting of seven monomeric units (phloroglucinol) linked by aryl–ether bonds.

2.5.2. Theoretical Model of the Putative Oligophlorethol Complexes with Human α-NaGalase

To support the active-site-directed nature of α-NaGalase inactivation and assess the possible binding sites for oligophlorethols, molecular docking was performed on α-NaGalase's active center. The active center of the α-NaGalase is located in the central $(\beta/\alpha)_8$ domain, in which Asp 156 and Asp217 are the catalytic nucleophile and acid/base residues, respectively. The molecular docking of the putative PHPh with α-NaGalase showed that the compound formed a complex with the active site of the enzyme. The key interactions of this inhibitor with the active site of the α-NaGalase are shown in Figures 7 and 8. The molecular docking of PHPh with α-NaGalase showed that the compound forms a complex with the active site of the enzyme. The flexible PHPh molecule fills the pit around the active site's pocket by forcefully adhering to the surface of the protein.

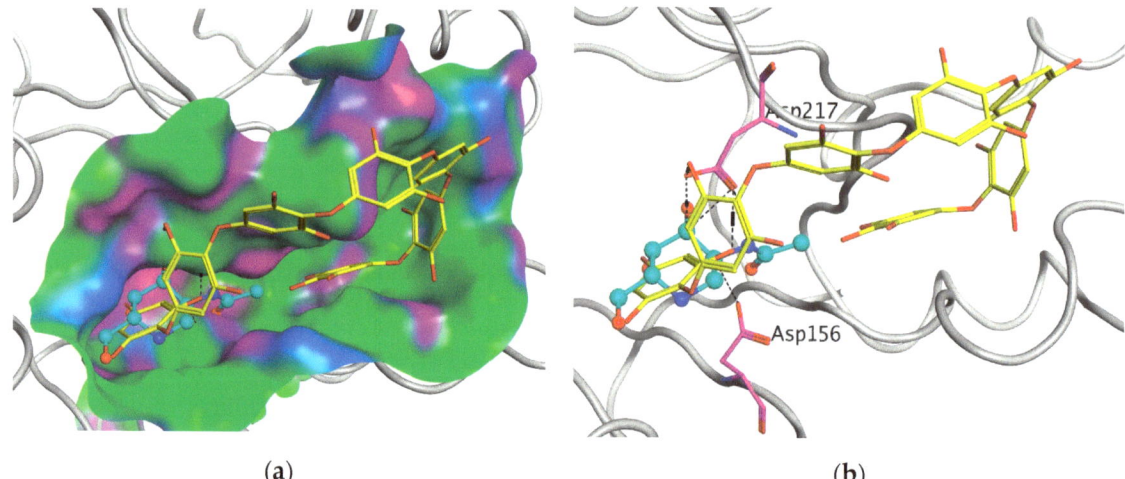

(a)   (b)

Figure 7. Molecular docking of human lysosomal α-NaGalase (PDB ID 4DO4) with PHPh. (**a**) Molecular surface of α-NaGalase binding site is shown in green (hydrophobic), pink (H-Bonding), and blue (mildly Polar). PHPh is shown as sticks (yellow) and iminosugar 2-acetamido-1,2-dideoxy-D-galactonojirimycin (DGNJAc) is shown as a ball-and-stick diagram (turquoise). Oxygen atoms are shown in red. (**b**) Localization of the inhibitor DGNJAc and heptaphlorethol in the active site of the human lysosomal α-NaGalase. Catalytic residues Asp 156 and 217 are shown in pink. The structure of α-NaGalase is shown as a backbond in gray.

The terminal phloroglucinol residue enters the active site and occupies the catalytic site between Asp 156 and Asp 217. This can be seen from the superposition of α-NaGalase complexes with PHPh and the potent inhibitor of the enzyme 2-acetamido-1,2-dideoxy-D-galactonojirimycin (DGJNAc) (Figure 7a,b). The complex of the PHPh with α-NaGalase's active center is stabilized by hydrogen bonds of hydroxyl groups with polar, acidic sidechains and basic backbones (Figure 8a). As can be seen from the superposition of the structures of the complexes PHPh and DGNJAc with the active center of the enzyme (Figure 7), the binding sites of the PHPh and DGNJAc overlap. This indicates the active-site-directed nature of the α-NaGalase's inactivation by the compound. Furthermore, PHPh directly interacts with catalytic residue Asp 217, and its terminal phloroglucinol residue locat-ed deep in the active center blocks the substrate's entrance into the pocket of the active center towards the catalytic residues Asp 156 and Asp 217 (Figure 7a,b).

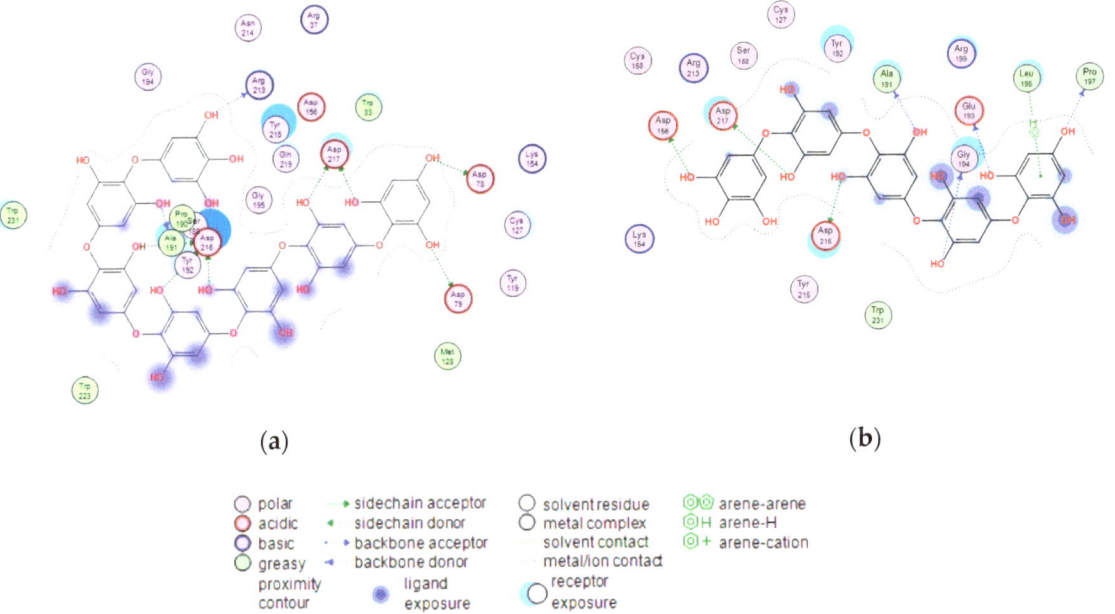

(**a**)   (**b**)

○ polar	◆ sidechain acceptor	○ solvent residue
○ acidic	◆ sidechain donor	○ metal complex
○ basic	·▸ backbone acceptor	solvent contact
○ greasy	◂ backbone donor	metal/ion contact
proximity	ligand	receptor
contour	exposure	exposure

arene-arene
arene-H
arene-cation

Figure 8. 2D-diagram of contacts of the complexes of human lysosomal α-NaGalase (PDB ID 4DO4) with PHPh (**a**), and fragment of P15OPh (**b**).

The molecular docking of the P15OPh with α-NaGalase showed that only five monomer units of the compound form complexes with the active site of the enzyme. The remaining section of the molecule is located on the surface of the protein globule outside the active center. The model of the 3D structure of the complex of this compound with α-NaGalase is not shown. However, a 2D-diagram of the key interactions of the fragment consisting of five monomer units with the active site of α-NaGalase is shown in Figure 8b. The fragment did not present better interaction than DGNJAc, but it is also located in the active site of the enzyme and forms hydrogen bonds with catalytic residues (Table 4).

Table 4. Binding energy and hydrogen bonds of P15OPh fragment and DGJNAc with α-NaGalase.

P15OPh fragment								
	Ligand			Receptor		Interaction	Distance	E (kcal/mol)
O	1	O	Pro	197	(A)	H-donor	2.66	−1.1
O	6	O	Glu	193	(A)	H-donor	2.63	−2.3
O	19	O	Gly	194	(A)	H-donor	2.65	−2.8
O	32	O	Ala	191	(A)	H-donor	2.79	−2.8
O	40	OD1	Asp	216	(A)	H-donor	2.54	−1.0
O	45	OD1	Asp	217	(A)	H-donor	2.57	−5.5
O	59	OD2	Asp	156	(A)	H-donor	2.52	−3.0
6-ring		CB	Leu	196	(A)	pi-H	4.31	−0.6

Table 4. *Cont.*

				DGJNAc				
	Ligand			Receptor		Interaction	Distance	E (kcal/mol)
N2	7	OD1	Asp	217	(A)	H-donor	2.81	−6.4
O4	17	OD1	Asp	78	(A)	H-donor	2.62	−3.4
O6	24	OD2	Asp	797	(A)	H-donor	2.73	−2.8
N5	26	OD2	Asp	156	(A)	H-donor	2.74	−17.3
C1	29	OD2	Asp	217	(A)	H-donor	3.55	−0.8
O7	1	OG	Ser	188	(A)	H-acceptor	2.63	−2.6
O3	13	NZ	Lys	154	(A)	H-acceptor	2.75	−7.0
O3	13	NH1	Arg	213	(A)	H-acceptor	3.07	−1.3
N5	26	OD2	Asp	156	(A)	ionic	2.74	-6.4

3. Discussion

Elevated levels of the α-NaGalase enzyme are a well-known feature of cancer cells; moreover, the ability to metastasize, disrupt programmed cell death, and exhibit drug resistance are the most obvious features of cancer cells. Currently, data on the correlation of the activity or expression of α-NaGalase genes responsible for carcinogenesis are beginning to appear in the literature. A study of the effects of Naga-shRNA suppression on the human breast carcinoma cell line MCF-7 and the human ovarian carcinoma cell line A2780 showed significant inhibition of the migratory and invasive properties of cancer cells [18]. Jafari et al. also found that after silencing α-NaGalase in the cells of human gastric adenocarcinoma, α-NaGalase downregulation had augmentative and regressive effects on cell death and migration, but no significant difference in daunorubicin resistance was observed [17]. In this paper, we studied the effects of brown algae-isolated high-molecular-weight phlorethols CcPh on the regulation of cancer-associated α-NaGalase activity.

It is known that brown algae synthesize several classes of phlorotannins, which differ with respect to the types of linkages between their phloroglucinol units. Fucols and phlorethols only consist of aryl–aryl or aryl–ether bonds, respectively, whereas fucophlorethols contain both types of linkages. Fuhalols are composed of ether-linked phloroglucinol units, with some of them containing additional hydroxyl groups other than the 1,3,5 OH functions originally present on the phloroglucinol moiety. Eckols are characterized by the presence of dibenzodioxin elements with structures of the benzofuran type in some cases [36]. It should be noted that phlorotannins have a large mass range, namely, from 126 Da to >100 kDa [36]. The molecular weight of the CcPh was determined by ESI–MS in the negative ion mode and consisted of a mixture of pseudomolecule ions at m/z 744 to m/z 1364 $[M - 2H]^{-2}$. The most abundant phlorethols contained between 15 and 18 phloroglucinol units (m/z 930 to m/z 1116 $[M - 2H]^{-2}$) (Table 3). Doubly charged masses are the main components in this spectrum. According to Melanson et al., with an increasing phlorotannin size, there is a greater probability of the appearance of multiple charge sites. Larger phlorotannins can be detected, as they appear as multiply charged ions under electrospray ionization conditions, gaining one negative charge for every ionized hydroxyl group (loss of H) [37]. Our mass-spectrometric analysis shows that the CcPh fraction is represented by phlorethols from 11 to 23 degrees of the polymerization of phloroglucinol, differing by one monomeric unit (Figure 3, Table 3). At present, the separation of long, condensed phlorotannins is a difficult task and is complicated by an increase in the number of isomers with an increasing polymer length.

Previously, it was shown that phlorethols CcPh (Mw_m = 2520 Da) isolated from brown algae C. costata at non-toxic concentrations inhibited the human colorectal cells HCT-116 and HT-29's colony formation ability in vitro and significantly enhanced their sensitivity to low, non-toxic X-ray irradiation [38]. The same fraction of CcPh irreversibly inactivated the recombinant enzyme endo-α-1,4-L-fucanase (EC 3.2.1.212) from the marine bacterium *Formosa alga* KMM 3553^T (IC_{50} = 39 µg/mL) [35]. Another fraction of phlorotannins from the brown algae *F. evanescens* inhibited recombinant endo-α-1,4-L-fucanase (IC_{50} = 22 µg/mL) [35] and α-L-fucosidase (IC_{50} = 29 µg/mL) from the marine bacterium *Formosa alga* KMM 3553^T, as well as a native endo-fucanase (in which the interval of inhibiting concentrations was 30–80 µg/mL) from the marine mollusk *Patinopecten yessoensis* and β-glucosidase (IC_{50} = 100 µg/mL) from the marine mollusk *Littorina sitkata* [39].

To study the effect of CcPh on the activity of α-NaGalase, we chose the human duodenal adenocarcinoma HuTu 80 and melanoma SK-MEL-28 cell lines and used two assays: the first was the treatment of cells with the CcPh fraction (in vitro), while the second was the direct treatment of α-NaGalase isolated from cell lysates with the CcPh fraction. Consequently, we observed a decrease in the α-NaGalase activity of the HuTu 80 and SK-MEL-28 cell lines after the treatment of the cells with CcPh. A similar effect was detected after the action of the brown algae fucoidan towards DLD-1 colorectal adenocarcinoma cells [20]. The marine sponge metabolites isoaaptamine, 9-demethylaaptamine, damiron B, and macaluvamine H also reduced the enzyme activity in the DLD-1 cell line from 100% to 64, 57, 52, and 50%, respectively, at a concentration of 5 µM [21]. However, neither fucoidan nor the marine sponge metabolites (the aaptamine and macaluvamine classes of alkaloids) directly inhibited α-NaGalase. Notably, the marine sponge-derived highly anti-cancer-active polybrominated diphenyl ethers [40,41] had no direct inhibitory effects on the cancer cell-associated α-NaGalase of the lines RPMI-7951 (ATCC #no. HTB-66^{TM}), MDA-MB-231 (ATCC #no.HTB-26^{TM}), DLD-1 (ATCC #no.CCL-221), HT-29 (ATCC #no.HTB-38^{TM}), HCT-116 (ATCC #no.CCL-247), and SK-MEL-28 (ATCC #no. HTB-72^{TM}), as well as the murine healthy epidermal cell line JB6 Cl 41 (ATCC #no. CRL-2010^{TM}) [42]. At present, there is very little information concerning the inhibitors of GH27 family α-N-acetylgalactosaminidase. Clark et al. [43] showed that the iminosugar 2-acetamido-1,2-dideoxy-D-galactonojirimycin (DGJNAc) can inhibit, stabilize, and chaperone human α-NaGalase both in vitro and in vivo. Ayers et al [44] showed that galacto-iteamine, an unnatural analog of the alkaloid iteamine (o-aminobenzyl α-D-glucopyranoside) isolated from the sole plant *Itea virginica* L. inflorescence, was a weak direct inhibitor of α-NaGalase in chicken liver.

4. Materials and Methods

4.1. Materials and Reagents

Human duodenal carcinoma HuTu 80 (ATCC #no.HTB-40^{TM}) and melanoma SK-MEL-28 (ATCC #no. HTB-72^{TM}) cancer cells were obtained from the American Type Culture Collection (Manassas, VA, USA). Minimum Essential Medium (MEM) and Dulbecco's Modified Eagle's Medium (DMEM), phosphate-buffered saline (PBS), L-glutamine, penicillin–streptomycin solution, and trypsine were purchased from Sigma-Aldrich (St. Louis, MO, USA), while fetal bovine serum (FBS) was purchased from Biowest (Ranch, FL, USA), agar was purchased from Becton (Le Point-de-Claix, France), sodium hydrocarbonate (NaHCO$_3$) was purchased from BioloT (St. Petersburg, Russia), p-nitrophenyl-N-acetyl-α-D-galactosaminide (p-NPNAGal) and Bradford reagent were purchased from Sigma-Aldrich (St. Louis, MO, USA), and recombinant protein markers for SDS-PAGE-electrophoresis were purchased from BioRad (1000 Alfred Nobel Drive, Hercules, CA, USA). The 3-(4,5-Dimethylthiazol-2-yl)-5-(3-carboxymethoxyphenyl)-2-(4-sulfophenyl)-2H-tetrazolium (MTS) samples were purchased from Promega (Fitchburg, WI, USA). Blotting Grade Bloker Non-Fat Dry Milk was purchased from BioRad (Hercules, CA, USA), primary NAGA Rabbit polyclonal antibody (PA5-97299) was purchased from Invitrogen (Rockford, IL, USA), Goat Anti-mouse IgG HRP-linked antibody was purchased from Sigma-Aldrich (St. Louis, MO, USA), and Anti-rabbit IgG and HRP-linked antibodies were purchased from Cell Signaling Technologies (Danvers, MA, USA). Polychrome-1 was purchased from Reakhim (Moscow, Russia), Sephadex^{TM} LH-20 was purchased from GE Healthcare (Bio-Sciences, Uppsala, Sweden), C-18 silica gel column was purchased from Sigma-Aldrich (St. Louis, MO, USA), and Sorbfil plates for TLC were purchased from ZAO Sorbopolimer (Krasnodar, Russia).

4.2. Experimental Equipment

Microplate spectrophotometer (BioTek Instruments, Highland Park, Winooski, VT, USA) was used for measuring optical density at 400 nm (D400). Ultrasonic homogenizer Bandelin Sonopuls (Bandelin electronic GmbH & Co., Berlin, Germany) was used for homogenization of cells' biomass. GenBAflex-tubes 6–8 kDa (Scienova GmbH, Wildenbruchstabe, Jena, Germany) were used for dialysis. ^{1}H NMR and ^{13}C NMR spectra were recorded on a Bruker AVANCE DRX-500 NMR spectrometer at 500 and 125 MHz, respectively. Mini-PROTEAN Tetra Handcast Systems (Bio-Rad, Hercules, CA, USA) were used for SDS-PAG electrophoresis. GS-800 Calibrated Densitometr (Bio-Rad, Hercules, CA, USA) was used for gel visualization. Semi-dry transblot instrument from Bio-Rad (Hercules, CA, USA) and polyvinylidene difluoride membranes (PVDF) from Millipore (Billerica, MA, USA) were used for Western blot analysis. ChemiDoc M.D. Universal Hood III Gel Documentation System (Bio-Rad, Hercules, CA, USA) was used to visualize blots.

4.3. Brown Alga Phlorotannin Inverstigation

4.3.1. Brown Alga Collection and Phlorotannins' Isolation

The brown alga *C. costata* (Turn.) Saund (order Laminariales) was collected in Peter the Great Bay, Sea of Japan, in July 2020.

Phlorotannins were isolated from brown algae as described previously [35]. The fraction CcPh was characterized by nuclear magnetic resonance (NMR) spectroscopy and mass spectrometry as described below. Freshly collected brown alga *C. costata* (7000 g) was rinsed with fresh water, cleaned to remove epiphytes, dried with filter paper, crushed, and extracted with EtOH (96%, 10 L) for 30 days at room temperature. The extract was filtered, and an aliquot of 4.5 L was concentrated in vacuum to 1.3 L. The concentrate was extracted sequentially with hexane (3 × 1000 mL), CHCl$_3$ (3 × 1000 mL), and EtOAc (3 × 1000 mL). The EtOAc extract was evaporated until reaching dryness. The obtained residue (1000 mg) was separated by chromatography using a column of silica gel (1500 × 150 mm) into 10 fractions (1–10) that were eluted sequentially by C$_6$H$_6$ (fraction 1) and C$_6$H$_6$–EtOAc (stepwise gradient, 10:1–1:1 (fractions 2–5), EtOAc (fraction 6) (409 mg), CHCl$_3$ (fraction 7), CHCl$_3$–EtOH 1:1 (fractions 8), and EtOH (fraction 9). Fraction 6 was separated over Polychrome-1 using H$_2$O–EtOH (stepwise gradient) into five fractions (6.1–6.5). Fraction 6.3, eluted by H$_2$O–EtOH (2.5:1, 133 mg), was separated over a column of silica gel 100C-18 using H$_2$O–EtOH (stepwise gradient 0–96 in 5% steps) to fraction 6.3.20 (24.6 mg), which was eluted by EtOH (20%). Fraction 6.3.20 was separated over a column of sephadex LH-20 using 50% aqueous acetone into 4 fractions. Fraction 6.3.20.4 (10 mg), named CcPh, was used in the experiment.

Column fractions were analyzed by TLC on Sorbfil plates that were sprayed with FeCl$_3$ solution (50%), followed by heating to 70 °C. R$_f$ values were determined using Me$_2$CO:C$_6$H$_6$:H$_2$O:HCO$_2$H (90:30:8:5 drops).

4.3.2. Nuclear Magnetic Resonance Analysis

The NMR spectra of the CcPh fractions dissolved in DMSO-d were obtained on a Bruker Avance-III 500 HD spectrometer (Bruker, Karlsruhe, Germany) at an operating frequency of 500 MHz and at 35 °C with tetramethylsilane used as an internal standard.

4.3.3. Mass Spectra Analysis

The high-resolution mass spectrometry (HRMS) data were collected using a hybrid ion trap–time-of-flight mass-spectrometer (LCMS-IT-TOF, Shimadzu, Japan). The mass spectra were recorded, applying negative ion electrospray ionization (ESI) mode with a resolution of 12,000. The following operating settings were used: the range of *m/z* detection was 300–2500, the drying gas (N$_2$) pressure was 150 kPa, the nebulizer gas flow rate was 1.5 L/min, the ion source potential was 4.5 kV, the detector voltage was 1.65 kV, and the n temperatures for curved desolvation line (CDL) and heat block were 200 °C. The mass accuracy was below 4 ppm. Data were acquired and processed using the Shimadzu

LCMS Solution software (v.3.60.361). Masses of phlorethols were calculated using the respective chemical formula of a typical phlorethol, $C_{6n}H_{4n+2}O_{3n}$, where n is the number of phloroglucinol units.

4.4. Cell Culturing

Human duodenal carcinoma HuTu 80 and melanoma SK-MEL-28 cancer cells were grown in monolayer in Minimum Essential Medium (MEM) and Dulbecco's Modified Eagle's Medium (DMEM), respectively, with addition of 10% FBS and 1% penicillin-streptomycin solution. The cell cultures were maintained at 37 °C in humidified atmosphere containing 5% CO_2

4.4.1. Cytotoxic Activity Assays

Cancer cells (8×10^3/200 μL) were seeded in 96-well plates for 24 h at 37 °C in a 5% CO_2 incubator. The cells were treated with phlorethol CcPh at concentrations ranging from 0 to 200 μg for an additional 24 h. Subsequently, cells were incubated with 15 μL of MTS reagent for 3 h, and the absorbance in each well was measured at 490/630 nm using a microplate reader. All the experiments were repeated three times, and the mean absorbance values were calculated.

4.4.2. Preparation of Cell Lysate

Every 3–4 days, HuTu 80 and SK-MEL-28 cells were rinsed in phosphate-buffered saline (PBS), detached from the tissue culture flask by 1X trypsin/EDTA solution, harvested with appropriate medium, and centrifuged at 500 rpm for 3 min. The culture media were discarded, and cell pellets were resuspended in 0.02% EDTA/15 mM Tris (pH 7.0) solution and frozen at -80 °C.

4.4.3. Treatment of Cells by Phlorethol CcPh

HuTu 80 and SK-MEL-28 cells (5×10^5 cells/dish) were seeded in 60 mm dishes. After 24 h, the cells were treated with a medium containing different concentrations of phlorethol CcPh (0, 10, 20, and 40 μg/mL). After 24 h, the cells were harvested, as described in Section 4.4.2., "Preparation of cells lysate". After each treatment of the cells with phlorethol CcPh, cell lysates were prepared, the target enzyme was extracted, and its specific activity was determined, as described below in the Section 4.5.2.

4.5. Biochemical and Catalytic Properties of α-NaGalases

4.5.1. Isolation and Purification of α-NaGalase from Cell Lysates

The frozen lysates of the cancer cells in the 15 mM Tris buffer, which were maintained at pH 7.0 and kept in 0.02% EDTA, were defrosted and sonicated 10 times at 20 s intervals with a break of 1 min in ice bath. To remove the cellular detritus, the cell homogenate was centrifuged at 4 °C and 10,000 rpm for 30 min. The supernatant proteins were precipitated with 70% ammonium sulfate and kept overnight at 4 °C to form a pellet. The protein pellet was collected by centrifugation (at 4 °C and 10,000 rev/min for 30 min) and dissolved in 0.05 M sodium citrate buffer at pH 5.0. The extract was dialyzed against the same buffer and centrifuged to separate the insoluble precipitate. The supernatant was used in further work as partly purified enzyme in the enzyme's activity essays. The purification quality was controlled by 12% Laemmli-SDS-PAGE [45].

4.5.2. Enzyme Assay

The activity α-NaGalase was determined by increasing the amount of p-nitrophenol (pNP). To assay the α-NaGalase activity, 10 μL of cell extract and 90 μL of substrate pNPNA-Gal (8.8 mM) in 0.05 M sodium citrate buffer, at pH 4.5, were placed in cells of 96-well plates and incubated at 37 °C for 5 h. The reactions were stopped by the addition of 200 μL of 1 M Na_2CO_3 solution. Absorbance of pNP was measured at 400 nm. Results were read with a computer program, Gen5, and processed with Excel software. The unit of standard activity

(U) was defined as the amount of the enzyme catalyzing the formation of 1 nmol of pNP (ε_{400} = 18,300 M^{-1} cm^{-1}) per 1 h under the conditions indicated by Formula (1):

$$U = \frac{\Delta D \times V \times 1000}{18.3 \times v \times \tau},\tag{1}$$

where ΔD = (D_{400} of the enzymatic reaction – D_{400} of the blank), V is the total volume of the reaction mixture (300 μL), v is the volume of the enzyme solution aliquot (10 μL), τ is the reaction time (h), and 1000 is the conversion factor in nmol.

Specific activity (A) was calculated as the standard enzyme activity per 1 mg of protein. All calculations were based on reactions with consumption of 10% of the chromogenic substrate. The protein concentrations were estimated by the Bradford method with BSA as a standard [46].

4.5.3. pH Optimum of α-NaGalases Action

To determine the pH optimum of the enzyme, the mixture contained 10 μL of the enzyme solution (after the last stage of purification) and 90 μL of the substrate in a solution of 0.05 M Na–citrate buffer at pH 3.0–6.2 (initial concentration 3 mg/mL). Enzyme activity was determined after 5 h incubation at 37 °C, as described above.

4.5.4. Catalytic Properties of α-NaGalases

To determine the K_m and V_{max} values of α-NaGgalase, a substrate solution of various concentrations was added to 10 μL of the enzyme solution (stock solution of protein was 1.2 and 0.8 mg/mL for HuTu 80 and SK-MEL-28 α-NaGalase, respectively) and incubated at 37 °C for 5 h. The final substrate concentrations in the incubation mixture were 0.07, 0.14, 0.28, 0.56, 1.13, 2.25, 4.50, and 9.0 mM. Reactions were stopped by adding 200 μL of Na$_2$CO$_3$. Activity was determined as described above. The Michaelis–Menten constants, K_m and V_{max}, were determined from the non-linear regression coefficients using the Michaelis–Menten equation (Origin 8.1 software).

4.6. The Inhibitory Potency of the Phlorethol CcPh

For this experiment, 8 μL of enzyme (349 and 60 U/mL for HuTu 80 and SK-MEL-28 α-NaGalase, respectively) in 0.05 M sodium citrate buffer solution (pH 4.5) was preincubated for 30 min at 20 °C with 2 μL of water-soluble test compound at various concentrations (from 0 to 1.67 mg/mL in a probe) to facilitate enzyme and inhibitor's interaction. The enzyme reaction was initiated by adding 90 μL of the substrate pNPNAGal (8.8 and 14 mM for HuTu 80 and SK-MEL-28 α-NaGalase, respectively) in the appropriate buffer solution. After 5 h, the reaction was stopped by adding 200 μL of 1 M Na$_2$CO$_3$. The amount of pNP was quantified by spectrophotometric detection at 400 nm. A mixture containing phlorethol CcPh at the appropriate concentration was used to compensate for the absorption at 400 nm by these compounds. Inhibition I (%), was calculated as follows (2):

$$I = \frac{Ao - Ai}{Ao} \times 100\tag{2}$$

where Ao is a specific activity of the enzyme in the absence of an inhibitor, calculated as described above. Ai is the specific activity of the enzyme in presence of an inhibitor, calculated as follows (3):

$$Ai = \frac{(D400\ reaction - D400\ blank - D400\ CcPh) \times V \times 1000}{18.3 \times v \times \tau \times mg\ of\ protein},\tag{3}$$

where $D_{400\ CcPh}$ is the absorbance of CcPh at the appropriate concentration.

The IC_{50} values were determined from the non-linear regression coefficients of the Hill's equation using OriginLab software (version 8.1).

The Irreversibility of α-NaGalase Inhibition by Phlorethol CcPh

To determine the reversibility of the α-NaGalase inhibition by CcPh, 10 μL (10 mg/mL) of aqueous solution of phlorethol CcPh was added to 40 μL of the enzyme in 0.05 M sodium citrate buffer solution (pH 4.5). The remaining reaction mixture was dialyzed against 1 L of the 0.05 M sodium citrate buffer solution for 60 h at 4 °C. The buffer was changed 3 times during the dialysis. The enzymatic activity was determined as described above. A sample of α-NaGalase treated with H_2O in the absence of the inhibitor was dialyzed and used as a control for determination of the initial activity. The experiment was carried out in two replicates. The degree of inhibition was calculated as above.

4.7. Relative Protein α-NaGalase Quantification in Lysates and Extracts of Cancer Cells by Western Blot Analysis

After HuTu 80 and SK-MEL-28 cells (6×10^5) were cultured in a 7 cm dish overnight, they were treated with 10, 20, or 40 μg/mL of phlorethol CcPh for an additional 24 h. After treatment, the cells were harvested by 1X trypsin/EDTA solution and lysed with lysis buffer containing 0.88% NaCl, 50 mM Tris-HCl (pH 7.6), 1% NP-40, 0.25% $NaClO_2$, 1 mM PMSF, and 1 mM Na_3VO_4, and then disrupted with sonication at 10 kHz 3 times for 10 s on ice. The suspension was centrifuged for 15 min at 13000 g and 4 °C. The resulting supernatant was used for Western blot analysis. Protein content was determined by Lowry assay [47]. Lysates were loaded onto 12% SDS-PAG and electrophoresed at a constant potential (100 V, 60 mA) in the discontinuous buffer system according to Laemmli-SDS-PAGE protocol. Separated proteins were electrophoretically transferred to polyvinylidene difluoride membranes (PVDF). The membranes were blocked with 5% non-fat milk for 1 h and then incubated with the respective specific primary antibody (β-actin and α-NaGalase at 1:1000 dilution) at 4 °C overnight. Protein bands were visualized using an enhanced chemiluminescence reagent (ECL Plus, GE Healthcare, Marlborough, MA, USA) after hybridization with Goat Anti-mouse IgG HRP-linked antibody (for b-actin) and Anti-rabbit IgG HRP-linked antibody (for α-NaGalase) (1:10,000 diluted). Band density was quantified via Quantity One 4.6 software (BioRad, Hercules, CA, USA).

4.8. Data Analysis

All figures shown in this study are representative of at least three independent experiments with similar results. Statistical differences were evaluated using the Student's *t*-test and considered significant at * $p < 0.05$ and ** $p < 0.01$.

4.9. Molecular Docking of Phlorethol CcPh with Human α-NaGalase

The 3D-structures of the putative linear oligomers consisting of fifteen (P15OPh) or seven (PHPh) monomeric units (phloroglucinol) linked by aryl-ether bonds were built using the Molecule Build module of the Molecular Operating Environment package version 2020.09 (MOE, 2020.09; Chemical Computing Group ULC, Montreal, QC, Canada). The structures of P15OPh and PHPh were optimized using the Amber10:EHT forcefield. The crystal structure of human α-NaGalase (PDB ID 4DO4) [43] protonated at pH 5.0 was used for molecular docking via Docking module of the MOE 2020.09. Contact analysis of P15OPh was performed for a fragment smaller than 100 atoms (pentaphlorethol), since the Ligand Interaction module of the MOE program has a limitation for a ligand size of less than 100 atoms. The structures of 30 complexes were calculated with the London dG score, and the 5 most energetically advantageous complexes were optimized with the GBVI/WSA dG score. Contact analysis was carried out using the Ligand Interaction module of the MOE program.

5. Conclusions

The present study demonstrates the procedure for the purification of phlorotannin from the brown algae *C. costata* and its structural characterization by NMR spectroscopy and high-resolution mass spectrometry analysis. The phlorotannin profile contains several linear, inseparable compounds with many isomer forms and degrees of polymerization, from 11 to 23 phloroglucinol units, which bind with aryl–ether bonds, thereby revealing typical characteristics of phlorethols. The CcPh fraction decreased the activity of α-NaGalase in the HuTu 80 duodenal adenocarcinoma and SK-MEL-28 melanoma cell lines, and irreversibly inactivated the isolated enzymes. It was shown in silico that the oligophlorethols bind tightly to the active site of human lysosomal α-NaGalase. The terminal residues of oligophlorethols enter the active site and occupy the catalytic center between Asp 156 and Asp 217. This indicates that the inactivation of α-NaGalase by the CcPh inhibitor is directed to the active site. Thus, it can be concluded that the CcPh phlorethol fraction isolated from the brown algae *C. costata* is an effective marine-based natural inhibitor of cancer cell-associated, immunosuppressive α-NaGalase, which has immunomodulatory properties. This work constitutes an important contribution to understanding one of the aspects of the anticancer activity of this group of marine compounds. Based on these results, we suggest that phlorethol CcPh has high pharmaceutical and therapeutic potential.

Author Contributions: Conceptualization, I.B. and S.E.; methodology, I.B., O.M. and S.E.; validation, S.E., T.I. and I.B.; investigation: isolation of enzymes, kinetic experiments—I.B., cell cultivation and treatment of cells—S.E. and O.M., isolation and purification of phlorethol CcPh—T.I., spectral analyses—V.G., PAGE and Western blotting analyses A.Z.; bioinformatics analysis and computer modeling of protein-inhibitor complex structures: G.L.; data curation, S.E. and I.B.; writing—original draft preparation, I.B., T.I., A.Z. and G.L. writing—review and editing, I.B., S.E. and T.I.; supervision, S.E.; project administration, I.B.; funding acquisition, I.B. All authors have read and agreed to the published version of the manuscript.

Funding: This research was funded by RFBR (Russian Foundation for Basic Research), grant number 20-04-00591.

Institutional Review Board Statement: Not applicable.

Informed Consent Statement: Not applicable.

Data Availability Statement: Not applicable.

Conflicts of Interest: The authors declare no conflict of interest.

References

1. Clausen, H.; Hakomori, S.-I. ABH and related histo-blood group antigens; immunochemical differences in carrier isotypes and their distribution. *Vox Sang.* **1989**, *56*, 1–20. [CrossRef]
2. Wu, A.M.; Wu, J.H.; Chen, Y.Y.; Tsai, M.S.; Herp, A. Forssman pentasaccharide and polyvalent Galβ1→4GlcNAc as major ligands with affinity for Caragana arborescens agglutinin. *FEBS Lett.* **1999**, *463*, 223–230. [CrossRef]
3. Nakajima, H.; Kurosaka, A.; Fujisawa, A.; Kawasaki, T.; Matsuyana, M.; Nagayo, T.; Yamashina, I. Isolation and characterization of a glycoprotein from a human rectal adenocarcinoma. *J. Biochem.* **1983**, *93*, 651–659. [CrossRef]
4. Wu, A.M. Carbohydrate structural units in glycosphingolipids as receptors for Gal and GalNAc reactive lectins. *Neurochem. Res.* **2002**, *27*, 593–600. [CrossRef] [PubMed]
5. Kenne, L.; Lindberg, B. Bacterial Polysaccharides. In *The Polysaccharides*; Aspinoll, G.O., Ed.; Academic Press: New York, NY, USA, 1983; Volume 2, pp. 287–363.
6. Tomshich, S.V.; Isakov, V.V.; Komandrova, N.A.; Shevchenko, L.S. Structure of the O-specific polysaccharide of the marine bacterium *Arenibacter palladensis* KMM 3961$^\text{T}$ containing 2-acetamido-2-deoxy-L-galacturonic acid. *Biochemistry* **2012**, *77*, 87–91. [CrossRef]
7. Wang, A.M.; Desnick, R.J. Structural organization and complete sequence of the human α-N-acetylgalactosaminidase gene: Homology with the α-galactosidase A gene provides evidence for evolution from a common ancestral gene. *Genomics* **1991**, *10*, 133–142. [CrossRef] [PubMed]
8. Garman, S.C.; Hannick, L.; Zhu, A.; Garboczi, D.N. The 1.9 A° Structure of α-N-Acetylgalactosaminidase: Molecular Basis of Glycosidase Deficiency Diseases. *Structure* **2002**, *10*, 425–434. [CrossRef] [PubMed]
9. Clark, N.E.; Garman, S.C. The 1.9 Å structure of human α-N-acetylgalactosaminidase: The molecular basis of Schindler and Kanzaki diseases. *J. Mol. Biol.* **2009**, *393*, 435–447. [CrossRef]
10. Lombard, V.; Ramulu, H.G.; Drula, E.; Coutinho, P.M.; Henrissat, B. The carbohydrate-active enzymes database (CAZy) in 2013. *Nucleic Acids Res.* **2014**, *42*, D490–D495. [CrossRef] [PubMed]
11. Albracht, S.P.J. Immunotherapy with GcMAF revisited-A critical overview of the research of Nobuto Yamamoto. *Cancer Treat. Res. Commun.* **2022**, *31*, 100537. [CrossRef]

12. Mohamad, S.B.; Nagasawa, H.; Uto, Y.; Hori, H. Tumor cell alpha-N-acetylgalactosaminidase activity and its involvement in GcMAF-related macrophage activation. *Comp. Biochem. Physiol. A Mol. Integr. Physiol.* **2002**, *132*, 1–8. [CrossRef] [PubMed]

13. Yamamoto, N.; Naraparaju, V.R.; Asbell, S.O. Deglycosylation of serum vitamin D_3-binding protein leads to immunosuppression in cancer patients. *Cancer Res.* **1996**, *56*, 2827–2831. [PubMed]

14. Greco, M.; De Mitri, M.; Chiriacò, F.; Leo, G.; Brienza, E.; Maffia, M. Serum proteomic profile of cutaneous malignant melanoma and relation to cancer progression: Association to tumor derived alpha-N-acetylgalactosaminidase activity. *Cancer Lett.* **2009**, *283*, 222–229. [CrossRef] [PubMed]

15. Albracht, S.P.J.; van Pelt, J. Multiple exo-glycosidases in human serum as detected with the substrate DNP-α-GalNAc. II. Three α-N-acetylgalactosaminidase-like activities in the pH 5 to 8 region. *BBA Clin.* **2017**, *8*, 90–96. [CrossRef]

16. Saburi, E.; Tavakol-Afshari, J.; Biglari, S.; Mortazavi, Y. Is α-N-acetylgalactosaminidase the key to curing cancer? A mini-review and hypothesis. *JBUON* **2017**, *22*, 1372–1377.

17. Jafari, M.; Rahimi, N.; Jami, M.-S.; Chaleshtori, M.H.; Elahian, F.; Mirzaei, S.A. Silencing of α-N-acetylgalactosaminidase in the gastric cancer cells amplified cell death and attenuated migration, while the multidrug resistance remained unchanged. *Cell Biol. Int.* **2022**, *46*, 255–264. [CrossRef] [PubMed]

18. Saburi, E.; Tavakolafshari, J.; Mortazavi, Y.; Biglari, A.; Mirzaei, S.A.; Nadri, S. shRNA-mediated downregulation of α-N-Acetylgalactosaminidase inhibits migration and invasion of cancer cell lines. *Iran J. Basic. Med. Sci.* **2017**, *20*, 1021–1028.

19. Ha, Y.-N.; Sung, H.Y.; Yang, S.-D.; Chae, Y.J.; Ju, W.; Ahn, J.-H. Epigenetic modification of α-N-acetylgalactosaminidase enhances cisplatin resistance in ovarian cancer. *Korean J. Physiol. Pharmacol.* **2018**, *22*, 43–51. [CrossRef]

20. Bakunina, I.Y.; Chadova, O.A.; Malyarenko, O.S.; Ermakova, S.P. The Effect of fucoidan from the brown alga *Fucus evanescence* on the activity of α-N-acetylgalactosaminidase of human colon carcinoma cells. *Mar. Drugs* **2018**, *16*, 155. [CrossRef]

21. Utkina, N.K.; Likhatskaya, G.N.; Malyarenko, O.S.; Ermakova, S.P.; Balabanova, L.A.; Slepchenko, L.M.; Bakunina, I.Y. Effects of sponge-derived alkaloids on activities of the bacterial α-D-galactosidase and human cancer cell α-N-Acetylgalactosaminidase. *Biomedicines* **2021**, *9*, 510. [CrossRef]

22. Erpela, F.; Mateosb, R.; Pérez-Jiménezb, J.; Pérez-Correaa, J.R. Phlorotannins: From isolation and structural characterization, to the evaluation of their antidiabetic and anticancer potential. *Food Res. Int.* **2020**, *137*, 109589. [CrossRef] [PubMed]

23. Mekini, I.G.; Skroza, D.; Šimat, V.; Hamed, I.; Cagalj, M.; Perkovi, Z.P. Phenolic Content of Brown Algae (Pheophyceae) Species: Extraction, Identification, and Quantification. *Biomolecules* **2019**, *9*, 244.

24. Khan, F.; Jeong, G.-J.; Sajjad, M.; Khan, A.; Tabassum, N.; Kim, Y.-M. Seaweed-derived phlorotannins: A review of multiple biological roles and action mechanisms. *Mar. Drugs* **2022**, *20*, 384. [CrossRef] [PubMed]

25. Shrestha, S.; Zhang, W.; Smid, S.D. Phlorotannins: A review on biosynthesis, chemistry and bioactivity. *Food Biosci.* **2021**, *39*, 100832. [CrossRef]

26. Zhang, M.Y.; Guo, J.; Hu, X.M.; Zhao, S.Q.; Li, S.L.; Wang, J. An in vivo antitumor effect of eckol from marine brown algae by improving the immune response. *Food Funct.* **2019**, *10*, 4361–4371. [CrossRef]

27. Imbs, T.I.; Skriptsova, A.V.; Zvyagintseva, T.N. Antioxidant activity of fucose-containing sulfated polysaccharides obtained from *Fucus evanescens* by different extraction methods. *J. Appl. Phycol.* **2015**, *27*, 545–553. [CrossRef]

28. Kiseleva, M.I.; Imbs, T.I.; Avilov, S.A.; Bakunina, I.Y. The effects of polyphenolic impurities in fucoidan samples from the brown alga *Fucus distichus* subsp. *evanescens* (C. Agardh) H.T. Powell, 1957 on the embryogenesis in the sea urchin *Strongylocentrotus intermedius* (A. Agassiz, 1864) and on the embryotoxic action of cucumarioside. *Rus. J. Mar. Biol.* **2021**, *47*, 290–299.

29. Shibata, T.; Fujimoto, K.; Nagayama, K.; Yamaguchi, K.; Nakamura, T. Inhibitory activity of brown algal phlorotannins against hyaluronidase. *Int. J. Food Sci. Technol.* **2002**, *37*, 703–709. [CrossRef]

30. Shibata, T.; Nagayama, K.; Tanaka, R.; Yamaguchi, K.; Nakamura, T. Inhibitory effects of brown algal phlorotannins on secretory phospholipase A2s, lipoxygenases and cyclooxygenases. *J. Appl. Phycol.* **2003**, *15*, 61–66. [CrossRef]

31. Shibata, T.; Yamaguchi, K.; Nagayama, K.; Kawaguchi, S.; Nakamura, T. Inhibitory activity of brown algal phlorotannins against glycosidases from the viscera of the turban shell *Turbo cornutus*. *Eur. J. Phycol.* **2002**, *37*, 493–500. [CrossRef]

32. Lee, S.-H.; Li, Y.; Karadeniz, F.; Kim, M.-M.; Kim, S.-K. α-Glucosidase and α-amylase inhibitory activities of phloroglucinal derivatives from edible marine brown alga, *Ecklonia cava*. *J. Sci. Food Agric.* **2009**, *89*, 1552–1558. [CrossRef]

33. Ahn, M.-J.; Yoon, K.-D.; Min, S.-Y.; Lee, J.S.; Kim, J.H.; Kim, T.G.; Kim, S.H.; Kim, N.-G.; Huh, H.; Kim, J. Inhibition of HIV-1 reverse transcriptase and protease by phlorotannins from the brown alga *Ecklonia cava*. *Biol. Pharm. Bull.* **2004**, *27*, 544–547. [CrossRef]

34. Barbosa, M.; Valentão, P.; Andrade, P.B. Polyphenols from brown seaweeds (Ochrophyta, Phaeophyceae): Phlorotannins in the pursuit of natural alternatives to tackle neurodegeneration. *Mar. Drugs* **2020**, *18*, 654. [CrossRef] [PubMed]

35. Imbs, T.I.; Silchenko, A.S.; Fedoreev, S.A.; Isakov, V.V.; Ermakova, S.P.; Zvyagintseva, T.N. Fucoidanase inhibitory activity of phlorotannins from brown algae. *Algal Res.* **2018**, *32*, 54–59. [CrossRef]

36. Martinez, J.H.I.; Castaneda, H.G.T. Preparation and chromatographic analysis of plorotannins. *J. Chrom. Sci.* **2013**, *51*, 825–838. [CrossRef] [PubMed]

37. Melanson, J.E.; MacKinnon, S.L. Characterization of phlorotannins from brown algae by LC-HRMS. In *Natural Products from Marine Algae: Methods and Protocol, Methods in Molecular Biology*; Stengel, D.B., Connan, S., Eds.; Springer Science + Business Media: New York, NY, USA, 2015; Volume 1308, pp. 253–267.

38. Malyarenko, O.S.; Imbs, T.I.; Ermakova, S.P. In vitro anticancer and radiosensitizing activities of phlorethols from the brown alga *Costaria costata*. *Molecules* **2020**, *25*, 3208. [CrossRef] [PubMed]
39. Silchenko, A.S.; Imbs, T.I.; Zvyagintseva, T.N.; Fedoreev, S.A.; Ermakova, S.P. Brown alga metabolites–inhibitors of marine organism fucoidan hydrolases. *Chem. Nat. Compd.* **2017**, *53*, 345–350. [CrossRef]
40. Utkina, N.K.; Likhatskaya, G.N.; Balabanova, L.A.; Bakunina, I.Y. Sponge-derived polybrominated diphenyl ethers and dibenzo-*p*-dioxins, irreversible inhibitors of the bacterial α-D-galactosidase. *Environ. Sci. Process. Impacts* **2019**, *21*, 1754–1763. [CrossRef]
41. Utkina, N.K.; Denisenko, V.A. New polybrominated diphenyl ether from the marine sponge *Dysidea herbacea*. *Chem. Nat. Compd.* **2006**, *42*, 606–607. [CrossRef]
42. Utkina, N.K.; Ermakova, S.P.; Bakunina, I.Y. Effects of sponge-derived polybrominated diphenyl ethers on human cancer cell α-N-acetylgalactosaminidase and bacterial α-D-galactosidase and their antioxidant activity. *Environ. Sci. Adv.* 2022; *in press*. [CrossRef]
43. Clark, N.E.; Metcalf, M.C.; Best, D.; Fleet, G.W.J.; Garman, S.C. Pharmacological chaperones for human α-N-acetylgalactosaminidase. *Proc. Natl. Acad. Sci. USA* **2012**, *109*, 17400–17405. [CrossRef]
44. Ayers, B.J.; Hollinshead, J.; Saville, A.W.; Nakagawa, S.; Adachi, I.; Kato, A.; Izumori, K.; Bartholomew, B.; Fleet, G.W.J.; Nash, R.; et al. The first alkaloid isolated from *Itea virginica* L. inflorescence. *Phytochemistry* **2014**, *100*, 126–131. [CrossRef] [PubMed]
45. Laemmli, V.K. Cleavage of structural proteins during of the head of bacteriophage T4. *Nature* **1970**, *227*, 680–685. [CrossRef]
46. Bradford, M.M. A rapid and sensitive method for the quantitation of microgram quantities of protein utilizing the principle of protein-dye binding. *Anal. Biochem.* **1976**, *72*, 248–254. [CrossRef] [PubMed]
47. Lowry, O.H.; Rosebrough, N.J.; Farr, A.L.; Randall, R.J. Protein measurement with the Folin phenol reagent. *J. Biol. Chem.* **1951**, *193*, 265–275. [CrossRef] [PubMed]

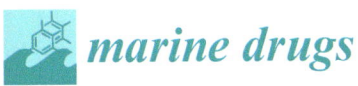

Review

β-Lactams from the Ocean

Jed F. Fisher and Shahriar Mobashery

Department of Chemistry & Biochemistry, 354 McCourtney Hall, University of Note Dame, Notre Dame, IN 46656–5670, USA; jfisher1@nd.edu (J.F.F.); mobashery@nd.edu (S.M.)

Abstract: The title of this essay is as much a question as it is a statement. The discovery of the β-lactam antibiotics—including penicillins, cephalosporins, and carbapenems—as largely (if not exclusively) secondary metabolites of terrestrial fungi and bacteria, transformed modern medicine. The antibiotic β-lactams inactivate essential enzymes of bacterial cell-wall biosynthesis. Moreover, the ability of the β-lactams to function as enzyme inhibitors is of such great medical value, that inhibitors of the enzymes which degrade hydrolytically the β-lactams, the β-lactamases, have equal value. Given this privileged status for the β-lactam ring, it is therefore a disappointment that the exemplification of this ring in marine secondary metabolites is sparse. It may be that biologically active marine β-lactams are there, and simply have yet to be encountered. In this report, we posit a second explanation: that the value of the β-lactam to secure an ecological advantage in the marine environment might be compromised by its close structural similarity to the β-lactones of quorum sensing. The steric and reactivity similarities between the β-lactams and the β-lactones represent an outside-of-the-box opportunity for correlating new structures and new enzyme targets for the discovery of compelling biological activities.

Keywords: enzyme inhibitors; PBP, penicillin-binding protein; β-lactonase; salinosporamide; AHL; *N*-acylhomoserine lactone; quorum quenching

Citation: Fisher, J.F.; Mobashery, S. β-Lactams from the Ocean. *Mar. Drugs* **2023**, *21*, 86. https://doi.org/10.3390/md21020086

Received: 21 December 2022
Revised: 21 January 2023
Accepted: 24 January 2023
Published: 25 January 2023

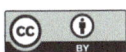

1. Introduction

The discovery of antibacterial antibiotics revolutionized the practice of medicine [1,2]. Among the seminal structures isolated during the golden age of antibacterial discovery—the two decades following the realization in 1943 of the clinical efficacy of the penicillins—were bacitracin, polymyxins, vancomycin, and cephalosporins. These structures (including the penicillins) share three attributes: they are still used in modern medicine, their mechanism is the inhibition of the proper assembly of the bacterial cell envelope [3,4], and they originate as secondary metabolites of terrestrial organisms. This latter attribute has engendered (on multiple occasions) the question: might marine organisms also offer unique and transformative antibacterial structures? The potential value of marine organisms as a source of compelling, biologically active structures is no longer a premise, but a fact. Indeed, the impressive list of antitumor-antibiotic structures isolated from marine sources (didemnin, gephromycin, gliotoxin, grincamycin, ilimaquinone, lamellarin, largazole, lurbinectedin, meridianin, peloruside, phorbazole, plinabulin, staurosporine, trodusquemine, withanolide . . .) exemplifies both unique chemical structure and exceptional biological activity [5–7]. While the experience with another marine antitumor antibiotic (bryostatin) has underscored the extraordinary difficulty of translating exceptional in vitro activity to clinical relevance [8–10], it has also proven that marine-derived structures are "privileged" in that their structural diversification can uncover new clinical utilities [11,12]. Given that the future for antibacterial discovery is structured to counter infections caused by multi-drug-resistant bacteria, chemical entities that have privilege are prized. Recognition that the biosynthetic source of these marine structures is in many cases marine bacteria is complemented by a growing understanding of what bacteria to culture and how to genetically manipulate the bacteria. These questions regarding marine bacteria, as in the case of marine *Streptomyces* [13–16], may address the difficulty of understanding the ecological role of "antibiotic" secondary metabolites [17,18], so as to enable activation of their biosynthetic gene clusters. Practical solutions to this challenge were discussed recently with reference to lasonolide A, another as yet promising marine antitumor antibiotic [19,20].

The structural focus is the β-lactam ring—the four-membered cyclic amide substructure—of penicillin (Figure 1). The β-lactam ring confers the antibacterial biological activity, not just to the penicillins but to the other clinically important structural sub-classes which together comprise the diverse β-lactam antibiotic family. These sub-classes include cephalosporins, cephamycins, clavulanic acid, nocardicins, monobactams, and carbapenems [21]. All of these β-lactams are enzyme inhibitors. Most pathogenic bacteria contain a cell wall that is made biosynthetically from glycan strands, which have peptide stems on their alternate saccharides [22]. In the final stage of cell-wall biosynthesis, these stems are cross-linked so as to conjoin adjacent glycan strands. Cross-linking is the result of acyl transfer from one stem to the nucleophilic serine of the transpeptidase enzyme catalyst, followed by the transfer of the acyl moiety to an amine functional group of the adjacent glycan strand. Linkage of adjacent glycan strands across the surface of the bacterium creates an encasing cell-wall polymer, called the peptidoglycan. β-Lactams inactivate the transpeptidase enzymes of peptidoglycan biosynthesis [23]. Their β-lactam ring is recognized as structural mimetics of the endogenous stem peptide and acylates the active-site serine with the concomitant opening of the β-lactam ring. As the resulting acyl-enzyme is sterically incompetent for acyl-transfer [24], the catalytic activity of these transpeptidase enzymes—termed historically as "penicillin-binding proteins" (PBPs)—is lost. This loss of activity is bactericidal when bacteria are growing actively.

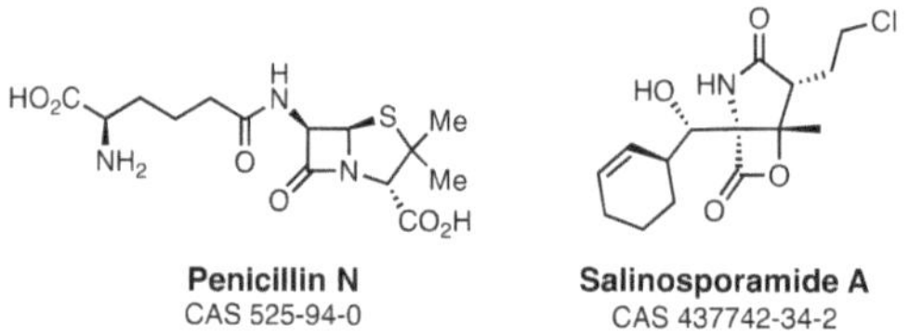

Penicillin N
CAS 525-94-0

Salinosporamide A
CAS 437742-34-2

Figure 1. Structures of the terrestrial-derived β-lactam antibacterial antibiotic penicillin N and the marine-derived β-lactone antitumor antibiotic salinosporamide A.

The marine antitumor antibiotic salinosporamide A (Figure 1) offers a structural counterpoint to the β-lactam sub-structure. Salinosporamide A (Marizomib®) is currently in late-stage clinical evaluation for brain cancer [25,26]. Its structural core is a β-lactone ring. In a mechanism similar to the β-lactams, its β-lactone is opened by the active-site threonine of the human 20S proteasome to give an acyl-enzyme species [27,28]. An ensuing second intramolecular ring-closing reaction displaces the chlorine as a chloride-leaving group and renders the acylation irreversible [29]. The biosynthetic complexity of the penicillins and the salinosporamides is comparable. Given that marine organisms biosynthesize the latter, do they also synthesize the former?

In this essay, we address the following questions. Do marine organisms biosynthesize notable inhibitors of bacterial cell-wall biosynthesis? Do marine organisms biosynthesize classical antibacterial β-lactams? Do marine organisms biosynthesize (other) β-lactams? Is there a relationship between the β-lactam functional group and the β-lactone functional group, and the observation from the marine environment that marine bacteria have numerous β-lactam-hydrolyzing enzymes?

2. Do Marine Organisms Biosynthesize Exceptional Inhibitors of Bacterial Cell-Wall Biosynthesis?

At present, no marine structure having both the efficacy and safety to justify its clinical use has been identified. None of the structures shown in Figures 2 and 3 meet this standard. All of the exploratory antibacterial antibiotics in current clinical trials have terrestrial origin [30–32]. However, the distinction between the marine and terrestrial origins of natural products must be done cautiously. While there are numerous examples of structurally and biologically unprecedented marine secondary metabolites (for example, the list of marine-derived antitumor antibiotics presented above), the two realms have substantial structural overlap [33]. Moreover, as is seen with respect to the antimicrobial evaluation of terrestrial secondary metabolites, the antimicrobial evaluation of marine secondary metabolites likewise identifies innumerable structures possessing modest to good antibacterial activity [34]. Inventories of these structures are published regularly [15,35–48]. Within these inventories are found structures that are truly distinctive, often in the multiple aspects of their biosynthesis, ring construction, and biological activity.

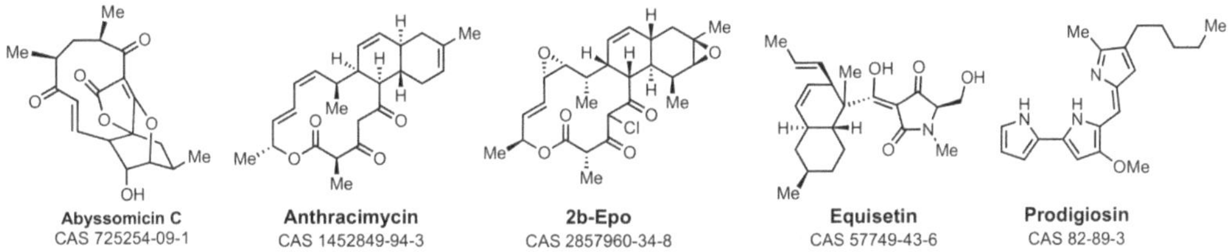

Figure 2. Distinctive marine-derived antibiotic structures with mechanisms other than interference with the enzymes of bacterial cell-wall biosynthesis.

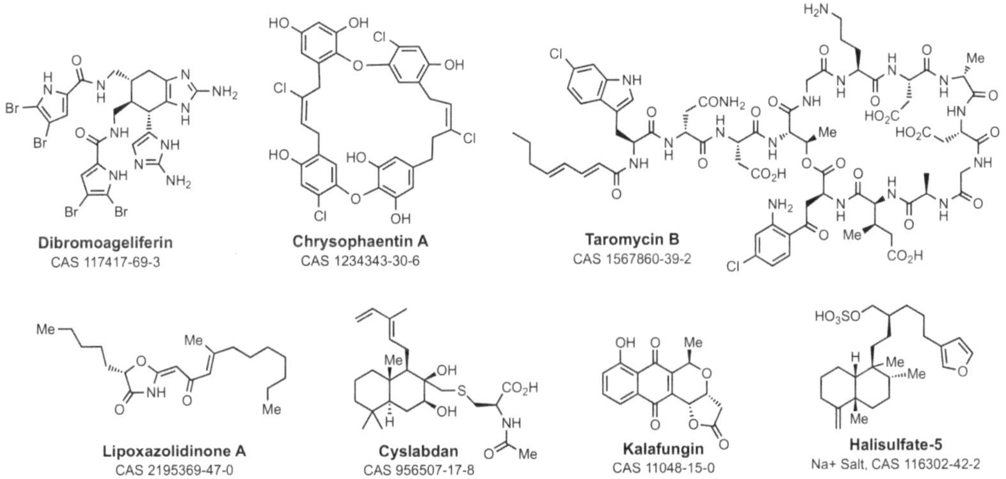

Figure 3. Distinctive marine-derived antibiotic structures with mechanisms involving inhibition of bacterial proteins. Dibromoageliferin, chrysophaentin A, taromycin B, lipoxazolidinone A, and cyslabdan inhibit key proteins involved in the synthesis of the bacterial cell envelope. Kalafungin and halisulfate-5 are inhibitors of the β-lactam antibiotic-resistance enzymes of bacteria, the β-lactamases.

The structures in Figure 2 exemplify distinctive marine-derived antibacterials. The abyssomicin family of macrolactones (more than thirty spirotetronate structures, exemplified here by abyssomicin C) is encountered as secondary metabolites of marine *Streptomyces* [49–54]. The abyssomicins have attracted extensive synthetic (notably, evaluation of the property of many members of this family, including abyssomicin C, to show room-temperature atropisomers) and biosynthetic studies. Abyssomicin C has potent Gram-positive (*Staphylococcus aureus*) antibacterial and antimycobacterial (*Mycobacterium tuberculosis*) activities (both, MIC 5 mg·L^{-1}). In addition, the abyssomicins show human cell-line cytotoxicity. The enzyme target of the abyssomicins is 4-amino-4-deoxychorismate synthase (PabB), the enzyme catalyst for the synthesis of 4-aminobenzoic acid from chorismite [55]. Loss of PabB activity blocks folate coenzyme biosynthesis [50,53]. PabB inactivation by abyssomicin is initiated by the conjugate addition of the thiol of its catalytic cysteine to the enone of abyssomycin to give the enolate [55]. Intramolecular trapping of this enolate by the butenolide sub-structure of abyssomycin gives the stable, final covalent structure of inactivated PabB [56]. This mechanistic sequence is conceptually similar to the salinosporamides against their different enzyme target.

Anthracimycin is a macrolide isolated from marine *Streptomyces* (but now also a terrestrial secondary metabolite) [57,58]. Anthracimycin also has engendered chemical interest. Its biosynthesis (and that of a cognate secondary metabolite, chlorotonil) is visualized as involving a spontaneous (while during PKS assembly) intramolecular [4 + 2] cycloaddition [59–62]. Anthracimycin shows in vitro MIC values of ≤ 0.25 mg·L^{-1} against all strains of *S. aureus* [63]. Notwithstanding a fundamental difference with respect to stereochemistry (Figure 3, compare the ring stereochemistry of anthramycin to that 2b-Epo), comparable antibacterial as well as antimalarial activities are found for chlorotonil derivatives. Culture of the chlorotonil-producing myxobacterium *Sorangium cellulosum* on a >150 L scale secured multi-gram quantities of chlorotonil. Its chemical stabilization (by reductive mono-dechlorination) followed by bis-epoxidation (to improve the water solubility to 16 μM) gave structure 2b-Epo, retaining essentially the full breadth of biological activities [64]. Structure 2b-Epo has in vitro MIC values of <0.05 mg·L^{-1} against several Gram-positive bacteria (including an MIC$_{90}$ of 0.1 mg·L^{-1} against methicillin-resistant *S. aureus*), oral safety in mice at 50 mg·kg^{-1} attaining serum concentrations above the MIC for the activity for 24 h, and efficacy in the *S. aureus* mouse neutropenic thigh infection assay at i.v. 2×5 mg·kg^{-1} dosing [64]. Its mechanism is not yet known. Equisetin exemplifies a structure with a breadth of biological activities, among which is the inhibition of bacterial acetyl-CoA carboxylase resulting in failed fatty acid biosynthesis [65]. Its own biosynthesis involves an enzyme-catalyzed ring-forming Diels–Alder cycloaddition [66,67]. Equisitin has potent Gram-positive antibacterial activity [68,69] and shows pronounced synergy with polymyxins against pathogenic Gram-negative bacteria [68,70]. Marine bacteria have significant potential as producing organisms of the tripyrrole prodiginines [71]. The prodiginines (represented by prodigiosin) demonstrate a breadth of biological activities, also including pronounced synergy with polymyxins against pathogenic Gram-negative bacteria [72–75].

The structures in Figure 3 exemplify a second set of distinctive marine-sponge-derived antibiotics. This figure shows structures that act to inhibit different targets within bacterial cell-wall biosynthesis. Dibromoageliferin represents one structure within the large and diverse class of bromopyrrole-imidazolamine structures (including also the sceptrins, the oroidins, and the nagelamides) [34]. As a class, these structures show potent Gram-positive and Gram-negative antibacterial activity [76–78]. They interfere with multiple stages of cell-envelope biosynthesis, including membrane integrity, assembly of the cytoskeleton, and peptidoglycan integrity [79,80]. The alga-derived chrysophaetins target the FtsZ protein of the Gram-positive cytoskeleton [81–83]. Taromycin A is recognized immediately as a marine-derived cognate structure of the Gram-positive antibiotic, daptomycin [84,85]. Daptomycin interferes with bacterial peptidoglycan biosynthesis by complexation with its biosynthetic intermediates [86,87]. Daptomycin is used increasingly in the clinic against serious Gram-positive bacterial infections. The marine origin of dibromoageliferin, chrysophaetin A, and taromycin A is attested to by their halo substituents.

Labdanes are secondary metabolites of both terrestrial and marine *Streptomyces* [88–90]. Although weakly antibacterial against methicillin-resistant *S. aureus* (MRSA, MIC 32–64 mg·L^{-1}), as an inhibitor of the FEM enzymes unique to *S. aureus* [91], cyslabdan synergy reduces the in vitro MIC of carbapenems against MRSA by up to 1,000-fold (in the presence of 10 mg·L^{-1} cyslabdan, the MIC of imipenem is reduced from 16 mg·L^{-1} to 0.015 mg·L^{-1}). The potentiation of the MICs of β-lactams was much less (32-fold for penicillins, 4–32-fold for cephalosporins) [92], implicating a high correlation between the specific PBP inactivated by the β-lactam and synergistic inhibition of the FEM enzymes by cyslabdan. β-Lactam synergy was observed with a marine-derived cyslabdan (isolated from a different marine *Streptomyces*) across a panel of Gram-positive and Gram-negative bacteria. The basis for the synergy was attributed (in part) to the inhibition of the β-lactam-hydrolyzing (β-lactamase) activity of the panel [93]. Remarkably, this interpretation has not received subsequent verification, possibly as a result of the separation between laboratories having access to the marine-derived structure, and laboratories with the ability to carry out a rigorous mechanistic study using enzymes from notable bacterial pathogens. Synthetic access to cyslabdan structures is, however, established [94]. Lipoxazolidinones are a class of marine-derived Gram-positive antibiotics [95,96]. They have several outstanding attributes: potent Gram-positive antibacterial activity (MRSA strains, MIC ≤ 2 mg·L^{-1}), dual mechanisms of action (inhibition of both peptidoglycan and protein biosynthesis) with low frequency of resistance mutation, and accessibility to synthetic modification, with the possibility of expansion of their antibacterial activity to Gram-negative bacteria [97]. The relationship between their structure to their molecular mechanism is not known. Their oxazolidinone ring suggests the possibility of target acylation, as seen for the β-lactams and the salinosporamides (but not a mechanistic aspect of the better-known oxazolidinone Gram-positive antibiotics, exemplified by linezolid).

The two final structures in Figure 3 are marine-derived inhibitors of β-lactam antibiotic resistance enzymes of bacteria, the β-lactamases. Kalafungin (isolated from marine *Streptomyces*) is a weak (IC$_{50}$ = 225 μM) inhibitor of Gram-positive β-lactamases [98]. Halisulfate-5 is a more potent inhibitor (K_i = 6 μM) of the clinically much more relevant AmpC β-lactamases of Gram-negative bacteria [99]. The crystal structure of the halisulfate-5·AmpC complex opens the opportunity for structure-based design. Recognition that marine sources produce inhibitors of these β-lactamases (as assessed in an in vitro assay) suggests two conclusions: that marine organisms might biosynthesize β-lactams, and that these β-lactamases are present as a resistance mechanism to these β-lactams. As we discuss, neither conclusion has decisive experimental support.

3. Do Marine Organisms Biosynthesize The Classical Antibacterial β-Lactams?

It is uncertain whether marine organisms biosynthesize classic β-lactam antibiotics. A momentous event in the history of the β-lactams was the isolation by Brotzu in 1945—from the Mediterranean Sea, near a sewage outfall located at Cagliari, Sardinia—of the *Cephalosporium acremonium* fungus, which biosynthesizes cephalosporin C. Notwithstanding the singular importance of his discovery, no antibacterial β-lactam has been isolated since from a marine source. The subsequent β-lactam sub-families—nocardicins, clavulanic acid, monobactams, and carbapenems—discovered over the course of ensuing decades are secondary metabolites of terrestrial bacteria. While numerous biologically active secondary metabolites are isolated from marine *Penicillium* fungi, none is a β-lactam [45,100]. A 2003 analysis of the genomic DNA of the marine fungus *Kallichroma tethys* identified two genes (*pcbAB* and *pcbC*) encoding proteins homologous to the penicillin biosynthetic enzymes of *Acremonium chrysogenum* [101]. While circumstantial evidence suggested that these genes were regulated and expressed, no antibiotic was identified in its culture. This observation has not been pursued. This absence of interest may reflect the remarkable accomplishment of the industrial-scale production of penicillins and cephalosporins from the antecedents of their original producing fungi. It would appear that there is no commercial need for a marine-derived producing organism of these antibiotics. If this explanation is correct, the result is unfortunate. Contrary to the surmise that the β-lactam represents a challenging functional group for biosynthesis, the biosynthetic pathways leading to the individual β-lactam sub-families are astonishingly diverse [102–104]. Nature has devised multiple pathways for the biosynthesis of β-lactam. Moreover, with the exception of nocardicins, each β-lactam sub-family has achieved a dramatic impact in the chemotherapy of bacterial infections. If a marine producer of a new sub-family of the antibiotic β-lactams is discovered, this discovery could be equally transformative.

4. Do Marine Organisms Biosynthesize β-lactams?

Marine organisms biosynthesize other β-lactams. However, the structural exemplification is sparse (Figure 4). Antibiotic X372A was isolated in 1975 from a marine *Streptomyces* bacterium [105]. Its Gram-positive and Gram-negative antibacterial activity is the result of an ATP-dependent inhibition of glutamine synthetase, and not from inhibition of bacterial cell-wall synthesis. The mechanism of this inhibition, as studied with the related β-lactam structure tabtoxinine-β-lactam ("tobacco wildfire toxin") biosynthesized by terrestrial *Pseudomonas* bacteria [106,107], does not involve the opening of its β-lactam ring [108,109]. Chartelline B was isolated in 1987 (as one of several related structures) from the marine bryozoan *Chartella papyracea*. It is not described as yet as having a biological activity [110]. Monamphilectine A was isolated (as one of several related structures) in 2010 from a Caribbean *Hymeniacidon* sp. sponge [111]. The isocyanide-containing monamphilectines have potent in vitro activity against the malaria-causing *Plasmodium falciparum* parasite [112]. The molecular target is not known.

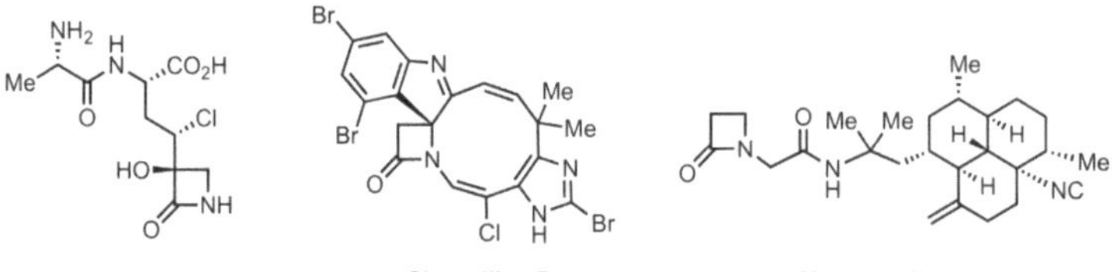

Antibiotic X372A
CAS 54922-56-4

Chartelline B
CAS 110271-21-1

Monamphilectine A
CAS 1256166-32-1

Figure 4. Structures of the marine-derived β-lactams.

5. Does the Marine Environment Contain β-lactam-degrading Enzymes?

A prominent role for marine-biosynthesized, β-lactam-containing enzyme inhibitors is not yet supported. To this date, three β-lactam-containing natural products are identified as biosynthesized by marine organisms. None is an inhibitor of bacterial cell-wall biosynthesis. To date, marine organisms biosynthesize several compounds that are adjuvants of the antibiotic activity of the terrestrial β-lactams (and possibly, other antibiotics), and several structures that inhibit in vitro the resistance enzymes, which hydrolytically degrade terrestrial-derived β-lactam antibiotics. These few examples could be interpreted to signify that the β-lactam functional group lacks significance within marine biology. Such an interpretation might follow the expectation that within the marine environment, the enzyme catalysts capable of the hydrolytic degradation of the terrestrial β-lactam antibiotics are not necessary and thus are uncommon. The evidence that this conclusion is incorrect is overwhelming. The oceans teem with such enzymes.

Two reasons support the prevalence of β-lactam-degrading enzymes in marine environments. The first reason is the copious and undisciplined use of antibiotics in human and animal medicine. The result is a profound "anthropogenic pollution" of the marine environment [113]. Antibiotic-resistance genes in the marine environment are now pervasive [114–119]. While the enzymes of antibiotic resistance—both terrestrial and marine [120,121]—are ancient, anthropogenic pollution has catalyzed their distribution. In anthropogenic-polluted marine environments, antibiotic-resistance enzymes are necessary for the survival of indigenous bacteria.

The basis for a second reason begins with the reminder that a principal basis for the resistance of bacteria to β-lactam antibiotics is the production of hydrolytic enzymes. These enzymes divide between those using an active-site serine nucleophile (Class A, C, and D) and those using zinc-ion catalysis (Class B, the metallo-β-lactamases). The serine β-lactamases are related evolutionarily to the penicillin-binding proteins of cell-wall biosynthesis, again with an ancient evolutionary separation of the β-lactamases from the penicillin-binding proteins [122,123]. The penicillin-binding protein motif is found additionally in esterase enzymes [124,125] and in biosynthetic transpeptidases [126,127].

Moreover, some of these esterases hydrolyze β-lactam antibiotics [128,129]. This mechanistic promiscuity underscores a fundamental difficulty in using in vitro enzymatic activity as a basis for enzyme nomenclature or presupposing a catalytic purpose for the enzyme. The magnitude of this difficulty is further emphasized by yet another aspect of bacterial ecology, that of quorum sensing [130]. Indeed, the recognition of quorum sensing as a phenomenon was made first with respect to the initiation of bioluminescence by marine *Vibrio* bacteria [131,132]. Quorum sensing offers a possible second reason for the extensive presence of β-lactam-hydrolyzing enzymes in the marine environment.

The context to understand this possible relationship begins with the chemical structures of the two ring systems introduced already: the β-lactams and the β-lactones. These rings have commonalities beyond ring size. β-Lactone structures are successful affinity probes of the penicillin-binding proteins (PBPs) [133–135]. The product of Class D β-lactamase hydrolysis of carbapenems is a β-lactone [136,137]. To these two rings may be added the isoxazolidin-3-one ring. This ring is encountered in lactivicin, which is also an inhibitor of the penicillin-binding proteins and the serine β-lactamases [138,139]. Each of these three rings (Panel A in Figure 5) is imbued with particular reactivity for the acylation of a nucleophile [139–142], and this reactivity is used to inhibit an array of enzymes [143]. The fourth ring of Panel A in Figure 5—dihydrofuran-2(3*H*)-one—while having lower intrinsic reactivity due to the absence of ring strain—is the ring system of the *N*-acylhomoserine lactone (AHL) class of quorum-sensing elicitors [130–132,144]. AHL quorum sensing does not use enzyme acylation. As quorum sensing correlates frequently with virulence, the identification of inhibitors of quorum sensing is an important objective [145,146]. While the favored *N*-acyl moiety is bacterial species-dependent (the AHL depicted in Panel B in Figure 5 is the AHL used to initiate marine *Vibrio* bioluminescence), the homoserine lactone ring is common to the AHL class of structures. One common transformation to abolish AHL signaling (a process termed quorum quenching) is the hydrolysis of the AHL amide with the release of the fatty acid. A second common transformation to achieve quorum quenching is hydrolytic ring-opening of the lactone. This reaction is catalyzed by the AHL lactonases (as further shown in Panel B in Figure 5). AHL lactonases are ubiquitous in marine bacteria [147]. The similarity between the hydrolytic reaction catalyzed by the AHL lactonases, and the hydrolytic reaction catalyzed by the β-lactamases, is evident (Panel B in Figure 5). This similarity challenges the classification of the serine-dependent enzymes and the metal-dependent enzymes found in marine bacteria. When such enzymes are purified and annotated as β-lactamases (and often as having an ancient heritage) [148–152], is the basis for their heritage that of β-lactam resistance or that of quorum quenching [153]? Selleck et al. suggest credibly that lactonase/lactamase promiscuity may offer an evolutionary advantage [153].

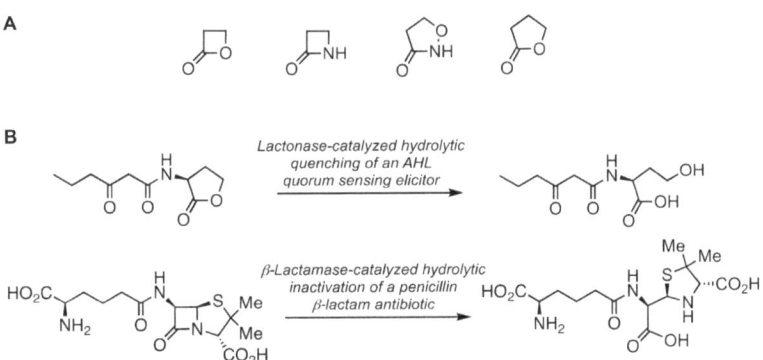

Figure 5. Panel (**A**), small rings activated for acyl-transfer. Panel (**B**), a comparison of the hydrolytic reactions catalyzed by the AHL quorum-quenching β-lactonases (upper reaction) and the β-lactamases (lower reaction).

One example merits further comment. A class A β-lactamase produced by a bacterium at 1050 m below the surface of the Pacific Ocean turns over penicillins at or near the diffusion limit. This level of catalytic competence cannot be adventitious, implying a directed evolution for the purpose [149]. In light of the fact that the gene sequence for this enzyme shares the same GC content as the other genes within the genome of this bacterium, the anthropogenic origin in this case was ruled out. This enzyme was argued as the first bona fide β-lactam-resistance enzyme from a marine source. The antibiotic-resistance enzyme could be perceived as a countermeasure against organisms that produce β-lactam antibiotics within the niche in the depths of the ocean.

The intrinsic reactivity of β-lactones has been exploited to identify other antibacterial enzyme targets [141,154]. Several synthetic β-lactones were examined for their quorum-sensing activity. One β-lactone cognate structure (Figure 6, 1421598-00-6) lacked activity as an autoinducer of *Pseudomonas aeruginosa* quorum sensing [155]. A second β-lactone (Figure 6, 2021255-49-0) inhibits *Vibrio* quorum sensing, but also as a result of enzyme inactivation within the fatty-acid biosynthetic pathway and not within quorum pathways [156]. Antibacterial β-lactones act by inactivation of the ClpP protease of Gram-positive bacteria [157–159], and have been used to interrogate the biological mechanism of AHL-structure type eukaryotic human immune modulation [155,160,161]. Lastly, sub-structure searching of the AHL β-lactone structure returns as close structures salinosporamide (Figure 1) and obafluorin (Figure 6, a secondary metabolite of *Pseudomonas fluorescens*) [162]. The Gram-positive and Gram-negative antibacterial activity of obafluorin was identified recently as the result of the inhibition of bacterial threonyl-tRNA synthetase [163,164]. The structural similarity among obafluorin, salinosporamide, the AHL autoinducers, and obafluorin was noted previously [165]. To our knowledge, neither salinosporamide nor obafluorin has been examined for enzyme inhibition within the quorum or cell-wall biosynthesizing pathways.

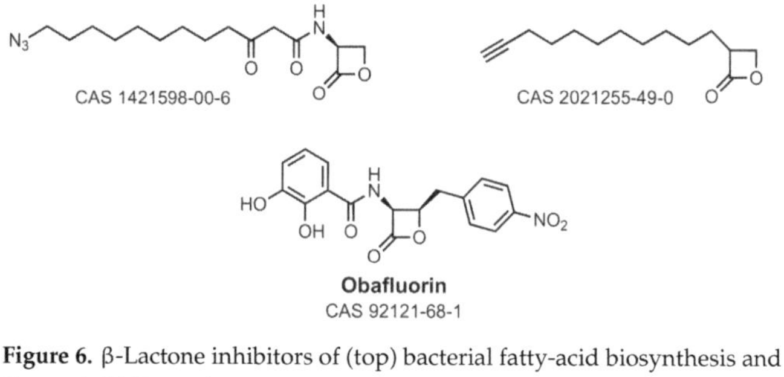

CAS 1421598-00-6

CAS 2021255-49-0

Obafluorin
CAS 92121-68-1

Figure 6. β-Lactone inhibitors of (top) bacterial fatty-acid biosynthesis and bottom (obafluorin) of threonyl-tRNA synthetase.

In this essay, we discuss evidence to support the possibility that promiscuity with respect to the substrate—β-lactone or β-lactam—for marine β-lactonases/β-lactamases may explain (in part) a diminished advantage for a marine fungus or bacterium to produce a β-lactam antibiotic. A similarity in the chemical reactivity of the β-lactone and β-lactam may suggest value to examining marine β-lactones as new inhibitors of cell-wall biosynthesis. Both suggestions fit within "outside-the-box" approaches [166] to ensure a future for antibacterial discovery [167]. Further evidence is needed to support this possibility. Such support could inaugurate a new research field in the area of marine antimicrobial drugs.

Author Contributions: J.F.F. and S.M.: writing. All authors have read and agreed to the published version of the manuscript.

Funding: Financial support of the authors is provided by the National Institutes of Health grants GM131685, AI148217, and AI104987.

Data Availability Statement: Not applicable.

Conflicts of Interest: The authors declare no conflict of interest.

References

1. Kardos, N.; Demain, A.L. Penicillin: The medicine with the greatest impact on therapeutic outcomes. *Appl. Microbiol. Biotechnol.* **2011**, *92*, 677–687. [CrossRef]
2. Ramírez-Rendon, D.; Passari, A.K.; Ruiz-Villafán, B.; Rodríguez-Sanoja, R.; Sánchez, S.; Demain, A.L. Impact of novel microbial secondary metabolites on the pharma industry. *Appl. Microbiol. Biotechnol.* **2022**, *106*, 1855–1878. [CrossRef]
3. Walsh, C.T.; Wencewicz, T.A. Prospects for new antibiotics: A molecule-centered perspective. *J. Antibiot.* **2014**, *67*, 7–22. [CrossRef]
4. Page, J.E.; Walker, S. Natural products that target the cell envelope. *Curr. Opin. Microbiol.* **2021**, *61*, 16–24. [CrossRef]
5. Gerwick, W.H.; Moore, B.S. Lessons from the past and charting the future of marine natural products drug discovery and chemical biology. *Chem. Biol.* **2012**, *19*, 85–98. [CrossRef] [PubMed]
6. Jiménez, C. Marine natural products in medicinal chemistry. *ACS Med. Chem. Lett.* **2018**, *9*, 959–961. [CrossRef] [PubMed]
7. Ren, X.; Xie, X.; Chen, B.; Liu, L.; Jiang, C.; Qian, Q. Marine natural products: A potential source of anti-hepatocellular carcinoma drugs. *J. Med. Chem.* **2021**, *64*, 7879–7899. [CrossRef]
8. Wender, P.A.; Quiroz, R.V.; Stevens, M.C. Function through synthesis-informed design. *Acc. Chem. Res.* **2015**, *48*, 752–760. [CrossRef] [PubMed]
9. Figuerola, B.; Avila, C. The phylum *Bryozoa* as a promising source of anticancer drugs. *Mar. Drugs* **2019**, *17*, 477. [CrossRef] [PubMed]
10. Wu, R.; Chen, H.; Chang, N.; Xu, Y.; Jiao, J.; Zhang, H. Unlocking the drug potential of the bryostatin family: Recent advances in product synthesis and biomedical applications. *Chem. Eur. J.* **2020**, *26*, 1166–1195. [CrossRef]
11. Wender, P.A.; Sloane, J.L.; Luu-Nguyen, Q.H.; Ogawa, Y.; Shimizu, A.J.; Ryckbosch, S.M.; Tyler, J.H.; Hardman, C. Function-oriented synthesis: Design, synthesis, and evaluation of highly simplified bryostatin analogues. *J. Org. Chem.* **2020**, *85*, 15116–15128. [CrossRef]
12. Abramson, E.; Hardman, C.; Shimizu, A.J.; Hwang, S.; Hester, L.D.; Snyder, S.H.; Wender, P.A.; Kim, P.M.; Kornberg, M.D. Designed PKC-targeting bryostatin analogs modulate innate immunity and neuroinflammation. *Cell Chem. Biol.* **2021**, *28*, 537–545. [CrossRef]
13. Jackson, S.A.; Crossman, L.; Almeida, E.L.; Margassery, L.M.; Kennedy, J.; Dobson, A.D.W. Diverse and abundant secondary metabolism biosynthetic gene clusters in the genomes of marine sponge derived *Streptomyces* spp. isolates. *Mar. Drugs* **2018**, *16*, 67. [CrossRef] [PubMed]
14. Tischler, D. A perspective on enzyme inhibitors from marine organisms. *Mar. Drugs* **2020**, *18*, 431. [CrossRef] [PubMed]
15. Duan, Z.; Liao, L.; Chen, B. Complete genome analysis reveals secondary metabolite biosynthetic capabilities of *Streptomyces* sp. R527F isolated from the Arctic Ocean. *Mar. Genomics* **2022**, *63*, 100949. [CrossRef]
16. Shi, S.; Cui, L.; Zhang, K.; Zeng, Q.; Li, Q.; Ma, L.; Long, L.; Tian, X. *Streptomyces marincola* sp. nov., a novel marine actinomycete, and its biosynthetic potential of bioactive natural products. *Front. Microbiol.* **2022**, *13*, 860308. [CrossRef] [PubMed]
17. Mlot, C. Microbiology. Antibiotics in nature: Beyond biological warfare. *Science* **2009**, *324*, 1637–1639. [CrossRef]
18. Davies, J.; Davies, D. Origins and evolution of antibiotic resistance. *Microbiol. Mol. Biol. Rev.* **2010**, *74*, 417–433. [CrossRef]
19. Uppal, S.; Metz, J.L.; Xavier, R.K.M.; Nepal, K.K.; Xu, D.; Wang, G.; Kwan, J.C. Uncovering lasonolide A biosynthesis using genome-resolved metagenomics. *mBio* **2022**, *13*, e0152422. [CrossRef]
20. Schmidt, E.W.; Lin, Z. Translating marine symbioses toward drug development. *mBio* **2022**, *13*, e0249922. [CrossRef]
21. Testero, S.A.; Llarrull, L.; Fisher, J.F.; Mobashery, S. β-Lactam antibiotics. *Burg. Med. Chem. Drug Discov. Dev.* **2021**, *7*, 1–188. [CrossRef]
22. De Benedetti, S.; Fisher, J.F.; Mobashery, S. Bacterial cell wall: Morphology and biochemistry: Chapter 18. In *Practical Handbook of Microbiology*, 4th ed.; Taylor and Francis: New York, NY, USA, 2021; pp. 167–204. [CrossRef]
23. Sauvage, E.; Kerff, F.; Terrak, M.; Ayala, J.A.; Charlier, P. The penicillin-binding proteins: Structure and role in peptidoglycan biosynthesis. *FEMS Microbiol. Rev.* **2008**, *32*, 234–258. [CrossRef]
24. Pratt, R.F. β-Lactamases: Why and how. *J. Med. Chem.* **2016**, *59*, 8207–8220. [CrossRef]
25. McCauley, E.P.; Piña, I.C.; Thompson, A.D.; Bashir, K.; Weinberg, M.; Kurz, S.L.; Crews, P. Highlights of marine natural products having parallel scaffolds found from marine-derived bacteria, sponges, and tunicates. *J. Antibiot.* **2020**, *73*, 504–525. [CrossRef]
26. Bauman, K.D.; Shende, V.V.; Chen, P.Y.; Trivella, D.B.B.; Gulder, T.A.M.; Vellalath, S.; Romo, D.; Moore, B.S. Enzymatic assembly of the salinosporamide γ-lactam-β-lactone anticancer warhead. *Nat Chem. Biol.* **2022**, *18*, 538–546. [CrossRef]
27. Gulder, T.A.; Moore, B.S. Salinosporamide natural products: Potent 20S proteasome inhibitors as promising cancer chemothera-peutics. *Angew. Chem. Int. Ed.* **2010**, *49*, 9346–9367. [CrossRef] [PubMed]
28. Della Sala, G.; Agriesti, F.; Mazzoccoli, C.; Tataranni, T.; Costantino, V.; Piccoli, C. Clogging the ubiquitin-proteasome machinery with marine natural products: Last decade update. *Mar. Drugs* **2018**, *16*, 467. [CrossRef] [PubMed]
29. Serrano-Aparicio, N.; Moliner, V.; Świderek, K. On the origin of the different reversible characters of salinosporamide A and homosalinosporamide A in the covalent inhibition of the human 20S proteasome. *ACS Catal.* **2021**, *11*, 11806–11819. [CrossRef]
30. Theuretzbacher, U.; Gottwalt, S.; Beyer, P.; Butler, M.; Czaplewski, L.; Lienhardt, C.; Moja, L.; Paul, M.; Paulin, S.; Rex, J.H.; et al. Analysis of the clinical antibacterial and antituberculosis pipeline. *Lancet Infect. Dis.* **2019**, *19*, e40–e50. [CrossRef] [PubMed]
31. Chahine, E.B.; Dougherty, J.A.; Thornby, K.A.; Guirguis, E.H. Antibiotic approvals in the last decade: Are we keeping up with resistance? *Ann. Pharmacother.* **2022**, *56*, 441–462. [CrossRef]

32. Prasad, N.K.; Seiple, I.B.; Cirz, R.T.; Rosenberg, O.S. Leaks in the pipeline: A failure analysis of Gram-negative antibiotic development from 2010 to 2020. *Antimicrob. Agents Chemother.* **2022**, *66*, e0005422. [CrossRef]
33. Voser, T.M.; Campbell, M.D.; Carroll, A.R. How different are marine microbial natural products compared to their terrestrial counterparts? *Nat. Prod. Rep.* **2022**, *39*, 7–19. [CrossRef]
34. Melander, R.J.; Basak, A.K.; Melander, C. Natural products as inspiration for the development of bacterial antibiofilm agents. *Nat. Prod. Rep.* **2020**, *37*, 1454–1477. [CrossRef] [PubMed]
35. Tortorella, E.; Tedesco, P.; Palma Esposito, F.; January, G.G.; Fani, R.; Jaspars, M.; de Pascale, D. Antibiotics from deep-sea microorganisms: Current discoveries and perspectives. *Mar. Drugs* **2018**, *16*, 355. [CrossRef] [PubMed]
36. Liu, M.; El-Hossary, E.M.; Oelschlaeger, T.A.; Donia, M.S.; Quinn, R.J.; Abdelmohsen, U.R. Potential of marine natural products against drug-resistant bacterial infections. *Lancet Infect. Dis.* **2019**, *19*, e237–e245. [CrossRef]
37. Wiese, J.; Imhoff, J.F. Marine bacteria and fungi as promising source for new antibiotics. *Drug Dev. Res.* **2019**, *80*, 24–27. [CrossRef]
38. Avila, C.; Angulo-Preckler, C. Bioactive compounds from marine heterobranchs. *Mar. Drugs* **2020**, *18*, 657. [CrossRef]
39. Barbosa, F.; Pinto, E.; Kijjoa, A.; Pinto, M.; Sousa, E. Targeting antimicrobial drug resistance with marine natural products. *Int. J. Antimicrob. Agents* **2020**, *56*, 106005. [CrossRef]
40. Bech, P.K.; Lysdal, K.L.; Gram, L.; Bentzon-Tilia, M.; Strube, M.L. Marine sediments hold an untapped potential for novel taxonomic and bioactive bacterial diversity. *mSystems* **2020**, *5*, e00782-20. [CrossRef] [PubMed]
41. Durães, F.; Szemerédi, N.; Kumla, D.; Pinto, M.; Kijjoa, A.; Spengler, G.; Sousa, E. Metabolites from marine-derived fungi as potential antimicrobial adjuvants. *Mar. Drugs* **2021**, *19*, 475. [CrossRef]
42. Nweze, J.A.; Mbaoji, F.N.; Huang, G.; Li, Y.; Yang, L.; Zhang, Y.; Huang, S.; Pan, L.; Yang, D. Antibiotics development and the potentials of marine-derived compounds to stem the tide of multidrug-resistant pathogenic bacteria, fungi, and protozoa. *Mar. Drugs* **2020**, *18*, 145. [CrossRef]
43. Willems, T.; De Mol, M.L.; De Bruycker, A.; De Maeseneire, S.L.; Soetaert, W.K. Alkaloids from marine fungi: Promising antimicrobials. *Antibiotics* **2020**, *9*, 340. [CrossRef]
44. Stincone, P.; Brandelli, A. Marine bacteria as source of antimicrobial compounds. *Crit. Rev. Biotechnol.* **2020**, *40*, 306–319. [CrossRef] [PubMed]
45. Gomes, N.G.M.; Madureira-Carvalho, Á.; Dias-da-Silva, D.; Valentão, P.; Andrade, P.B. Biosynthetic versatility of marine-derived fungi on the delivery of novel antibacterial agents against priority pathogens. *Biomed. Pharmacother.* **2021**, *140*, 111756. [CrossRef]
46. Srinivasan, R.; Kannappan, A.; Shi, C.; Lin, X. Marine bacterial secondary metabolites: A treasure house for structurally unique and effective antimicrobial compounds. *Mar. Drugs* **2021**, *19*, 530. [CrossRef] [PubMed]
47. Li, H.; Maimaitiming, M.; Zhou, Y.; Li, H.; Wang, P.; Liu, Y.; Schäberle, T.F.; Liu, Z.; Wang, C.Y. Discovery of marine natural products as promising antibiotics against *Pseudomonas aeruginosa*. *Mar. Drugs* **2022**, *20*, 192. [CrossRef]
48. Krishna MS, A.; Mohan, S.; Ashitha, K.T.; Chandramouli, M.; Kumaran, A.; Ningaiah, S.; Babu, K.S.; Somappa, S.B. Marine based natural products: Exploring the recent developments in the identification of antimicrobial agents. *Chem. Biodivers.* **2022**, *19*, e202200513. [CrossRef]
49. Huang, H.; Song, Y.; Li, X.; Wang, X.; Ling, C.; Qin, X.; Zhou, Z.; Li, Q.; Wei, X.; Ju, J. Abyssomicin monomers and dimers from the marine-derived *Streptomyces koyangensis* SCSIO 5802. *J. Nat. Prod.* **2018**, *81*, 1892–1898. [CrossRef] [PubMed]
50. Sadaka, C.; Ellsworth, E.; Hansen, P.R.; Ewin, R.; Damborg, P.; Watts, J.L. Review on abyssomicins: Inhibitors of the chorismate pathway and folate biosynthesis. *Molecules* **2018**, *23*, 1371. [CrossRef]
51. Braddock, A.A.; Theodorakis, E.A. Marine spirotetronates: Biosynthetic edifices that inspire drug discovery. *Mar. Drugs* **2019**, *17*, 232. [CrossRef]
52. Monjas, L.; Fodran, P.; Kollback, J.; Cassani, C.; Olsson, T.; Genheden, M.; Larsson, D.G.J.; Wallentin, C.J. Synthesis and biological evaluation of truncated derivatives of abyssomicin C as antibacterial agents. *Beilstein J. Org. Chem.* **2019**, *15*, 1468–1474. [CrossRef]
53. Fiedler, H.P. Abyssomicins—A 20-year retrospective view. *Mar. Drugs* **2021**, *19*, 299. [CrossRef] [PubMed]
54. Devine, A.J.; Parnell, A.E.; Back, C.R.; Lees, N.R.; Johns, S.T.; Zulkepli, A.Z.; Barringer, R.; Zorn, K.; Stach, J.E.M.; Crump, M.P.; et al. The role of cytochrome P450 AbyV in the final stages of abyssomicin C biosynthesis. *Angew. Chem. Int. Ed.* **2023**, *62*, e202213053. [CrossRef] [PubMed]
55. Keller, S.; Schadt, H.S.; Ortel, I.; Süssmuth, R.D. Action of atrop-abyssomicin C as an inhibitor of 4-amino-4-deoxychorismate synthase PabB. *Angew. Chem. Int. Ed.* **2007**, *46*, 8284–8286. [CrossRef]
56. Bihelovic, F.; Karadzic, I.; Matovic, R.; Saicic, R.N. Total synthesis and biological evaluation of (−)-*atrop*-abyssomicin C. *Org. Biomol. Chem.* **2013**, *11*, 5413–5424. [CrossRef] [PubMed]
57. Jang, K.H.; Nam, S.J.; Locke, J.B.; Kauffman, C.A.; Beatty, D.S.; Paul, L.A.; Fenical, W. Anthracimycin, a potent anthrax antibiotic from a marine-derived actinomycete. *Angew. Chem. Int. Ed.* **2013**, *52*, 7822–7824. [CrossRef]
58. Rodríguez, V.; Martín, J.; Sarmiento-Vizcaíno, A.; de la Cruz, M.; García, L.A.; Blanco, G.; Reyes, F. Anthracimycin B, a potent antibiotic against Gram-positive bacteria isolated from cultures of the deep-sea actinomycete *Streptomyces cyaneofuscatus* M-169. *Mar. Drugs* **2018**, *16*, 406. [CrossRef]
59. Alt, S.; Wilkinson, B. Biosynthesis of the novel macrolide antibiotic anthracimycin. *ACS Chem. Biol.* **2015**, *10*, 2468–2479. [CrossRef]
60. Jungmann, K.; Jansen, R.; Gerth, K.; Huch, V.; Krug, D.; Fenical, W.; Müller, R. Two of a kind–the biosynthetic pathways of chlorotonil and anthracimycin. *ACS Chem. Biol.* **2015**, *10*, 2480–2490. [CrossRef]

61. Harunari, E.; Komaki, H.; Igarashi, Y. Biosynthetic origin of anthracimycin: A tricyclic macrolide from *Streptomyces* sp. *J. Antibiot.* **2016**, *69*, 403–405. [CrossRef] [PubMed]
62. Liu, T.; Ren, Z.; Chunyu, W.X.; Li, G.D.; Chen, X.; Zhang, Z.T.; Sun, H.B.; Wang, M.; Xie, T.P.; Wang, M. Exploration of diverse secondary metabolites from *Streptomyces* sp. YINM00001, using genome mining and one strain many compounds approach. *Front. Microbiol.* **2022**, *13*, 831174. [CrossRef]
63. Hensler, M.E.; Jang, K.H.; Thienphrapa, W.; Vuong, L.; Tran, D.N.; Soubih, E.; Lin, L.; Haste, N.M.; Cunningham, M.L.; Kwan, B.P.; et al. Anthracimycin activity against contemporary methicillin-resistant *Staphylococcus aureus*. *J. Antibiot.* **2014**, *67*, 549–553. [CrossRef]
64. Hofer, W.; Oueis, E.; Fayad, A.A.; Deschner, F.; Andreas, A.; de Carvalho, L.P.; Hüttel, S.; Bernecker, S.; Pätzold, L.; Morgenstern, B.; et al. Regio- and stereoselective epoxidation and acidic epoxide opening of antibacterial and antiplasmodial chlorotonils yield highly potent derivatives. *Angew. Chem. Int. Ed.* **2022**, *61*, e202202816. [CrossRef] [PubMed]
65. Larson, E.C.; Lim, A.L.; Pond, C.D.; Craft, M.; Čavužić, M.; Waldrop, G.L.; Schmidt, E.W.; Barrows, L.R. Pyrrolocin C and equisetin inhibit bacterial acetyl-CoA carboxylase. *PLoS ONE* **2020**, *15*, e0233485. [CrossRef]
66. Fujiyama, K.; Kato, N.; Re, S.; Kinugasa, K.; Watanabe, K.; Takita, R.; Nogawa, T.; Hino, T.; Osada, H.; Sugita, Y.; et al. Molecular basis for two stereoselective Diels-Alderases that produce decalin skeletons. *Angew. Chem. Int Ed.* **2021**, *60*, 22401–22410. [CrossRef]
67. Chi, C.; Wang, Z.; Liu, T.; Zhang, Z.; Zhou, H.; Li, A.; Jin, H.; Jia, H.; Yin, F.; Yang, D. Crystal structures of Fsa2 and Phm7 catalyzing [4 + 2] cycloaddition reactions with reverse stereoselectivities in equisetin and phomasetin biosynthesis. *ACS Omega* **2021**, *6*, 12913–12922. [CrossRef] [PubMed]
68. Chen, S.; Liu, D.; Zhang, Q.; Guo, P.; Ding, S.; Shen, J.; Zhu, K.; Lin, W. A marine antibiotic kills multidrug-resistant bacteria without detectable high-level resistance. *ACS Infect. Dis.* **2021**, *7*, 884–893. [CrossRef]
69. Tian, J.; Chen, S.; Liu, F.; Zhu, Q.; Shen, J.; Lin, W.; Zhu, K. Equisetin targets intracellular *Staphylococcus aureus* through a host acting strategy. *Mar. Drugs* **2022**, *20*, 656. [CrossRef] [PubMed]
70. Zhang, Q.; Chen, S.; Liu, X.; Lin, W.; Zhu, K. Equisetin restores colistin sensitivity against multi-drug resistant Gram-negative bacteria. *Antibiotics* **2021**, *10*, 1263. [CrossRef] [PubMed]
71. Jeong, Y.; Kim, H.J.; Kim, S.; Park, S.Y.; Kim, H.; Jeong, S.; Lee, S.J.; Lee, M.S. Enhanced large-scale production of *Hahella chejuensis*-derived prodigiosin and evaluation of Its bioactivity. *J. Microbiol. Biotechnol.* **2021**, *31*, 1624–1631. [CrossRef]
72. Sakai-Kawada, F.E.; Ip, C.G.; Hagiwara, K.A.; Awaya, J.D. Biosynthesis and bioactivity of prodiginine analogs in marine bacteria, *Pseudoalteromonas*: A mini review. *Front. Microbiol.* **2019**, *10*, 1715. [CrossRef] [PubMed]
73. Mattingly, A.E.; Cox, K.E.; Smith, R.; Melander, R.J.; Ernst, R.K.; Melander, C. Screening an established natural product library identifies secondary metabolites that potentiate conventional antibiotics. *ACS Infect. Dis.* **2020**, *6*, 2629–2640. [CrossRef]
74. He, S.; Li, P.; Wang, J.; Zhang, Y.; Lu, H.; Shi, L.; Huang, T.; Zhang, W.; Ding, L.; He, S. Discovery of new secondary metabolites from marine bacteria *Hahella* based on an omics strategy. *Mar. Drugs* **2022**, *20*, 269. [CrossRef] [PubMed]
75. Siwawannapong, K.; Nemeth, A.M.; Melander, R.J.; Rong, J.; Davis, J.R.; Taniguchi, M.; Carpenter, M.E.; Lindsey, J.S.; Melander, C. Simple dipyrrin analogues of prodigiosin for use as colistin adjuvants. *ChemMedChem* **2022**, *17*, e202200286. [CrossRef] [PubMed]
76. Wang, B.; Waters, A.L.; Sims, J.W.; Fullmer, A.; Ellison, S.; Hamann, M.T. Complex marine natural products as potential epigenetic and production regulators of antibiotics from a marine *Pseudomonas aeruginosa*. *Microb. Ecol.* **2013**, *65*, 1068–1075. [CrossRef]
77. Pech-Puch, D.; Pérez-Povedano, M.; Martinez-Guitian, M.; Lasarte-Monterrubio, C.; Vázquez-Ucha, J.C.; Bou, G.; Rodríguez, J.; Beceiro, A.; Jimenez, C. In vitro and in vivo assessment of the efficacy of bromoageliferin, an alkaloid isolated from the sponge *Agelas dilatata*, against *Pseudomonas aeruginosa*. *Mar. Drugs* **2020**, *18*, 326. [CrossRef]
78. Freire, V.F.; Gubiani, J.R.; Spencer, T.M.; Hajdu, E.; Ferreira, A.G.; Ferreira, D.A.S.; de Castro Levatti, E.V.; Burdette, J.E.; Camargo, C.H.; Tempone, A.G.; et al. Feature-based molecular networking discovery of bromopyrrole alkaloids from the marine sponge *Agelas dispar*. *J. Nat. Prod.* **2022**, *85*, 1340–1350. [CrossRef]
79. Bernan, V.S.; Roll, D.M.; Ireland, C.M.; Greenstein, M.; Maiese, W.M.; Steinberg, D.A. A study on the mechanism of action of sceptrin, an antimicrobial agent isolated from the South Pacific sponge *Agelas mauritiana*. *J. Antimicrob. Chemother.* **1993**, *32*, 539–550. [CrossRef] [PubMed]
80. Rodriguez, A.D.; Lear, M.J.; La Clair, J.J. Identification of the binding of sceptrin to MreB via a bidirectional affinity protocol. *J. Am. Chem. Soc.* **2008**, *130*, 7256–7258. [CrossRef]
81. Keffer, J.L.; Huecas, S.; Hammill, J.T.; Wipf, P.; Andreu, J.M.; Bewley, C.A. Chrysophaentins are competitive inhibitors of FtsZ and inhibit Z-ring formation in live bacteria. *Bioorg. Med. Chem.* **2013**, *21*, 5673–5678. [CrossRef] [PubMed]
82. Davison, E.K.; Bewley, C.A. Antimicrobial chrysophaentin analogs identified from laboratory cultures of the marine microalga *Chrysophaeum taylorii*. *J. Nat. Prod.* **2019**, *82*, 148–153. [CrossRef]
83. Fullenkamp, C.R.; Hsu, Y.P.; Quardokus, E.M.; Zhao, G.; Bewley, C.A.; VanNieuwenhze, M.; Sulikowski, G.A. Synthesis of 9-dechlorochrysophaentin A enables studies revealing bacterial cell wall biosynthesis inhibition phenotype in *B. subtilis*. *J. Am. Chem. Soc.* **2020**, *142*, 16161–16166. [CrossRef]
84. Yamanaka, K.; Reynolds, K.A.; Kersten, R.D.; Ryan, K.S.; Gonzalez, D.J.; Nizet, V.; Dorrestein, P.C.; Moore, B.S. Direct cloning and refactoring of a silent lipopeptide biosynthetic gene cluster yields the antibiotic taromycin A. *Proc. Natl. Acad. Sci. USA* **2014**, *111*, 1957–1962. [CrossRef] [PubMed]

85. Baltz, R.H. Genome mining for drug discovery: Cyclic lipopeptides related to daptomycin. *J. Ind. Microbiol. Biotechnol.* **2021**, *48*, kuab020. [CrossRef]

86. Wood, T.M.; Zeronian, M.R.; Buijs, N.; Bertheussen, K.; Abedian, H.K.; Johnson, A.V.; Pearce, N.M.; Lutz, M.; Kemmink, J.; Seirsma, T.; et al. Mechanistic insights into the C55-P targeting lipopeptide antibiotics revealed by structure-activity studies and high-resolution crystal structures. *Chem. Sci.* **2022**, *13*, 2985–2991. [CrossRef]

87. Taylor, S.D. A decade of research on daptomycin. *Synlett* **2022**, *33*, 1695–1706. [CrossRef]

88. Tomoda, H. New approaches to drug discovery for combating MRSA. *Chem. Pharm. Bull.* **2016**, *64*, 104–111. [CrossRef]

89. Ikeda, H.; Shin-Ya, K.; Nagamitsu, T.; Tomoda, H. Biosynthesis of mercapturic acid derivative of the labdane-type diterpene, cyslabdan that potentiates imipenem activity against methicillin-resistant *Staphylococcus aureus*: Cyslabdan is generated by mycothiol-mediated xenobiotic detoxification. *J. Ind. Microbiol. Biotechnol.* **2016**, *43*, 325–342. [CrossRef] [PubMed]

90. Guzmán-Trampe, S.M.; Ikeda, H.; Vinuesa, P.; Macías-Rubalcava, M.L.; Esquivel, B.; Centeno-Leija, S.; Tapia-Cabrera, S.M.; Mora-Herrera, S.I.; Ruiz-Villafán, B.; Rodríguez-Sanoja, R. Production of distinct labdane-type diterpenoids using a novel cryptic labdane-like cluster from *Streptomyces thermocarboxydus* K155. *Appl. Microbiol. Biotechnol.* **2020**, *104*, 741–750. [CrossRef] [PubMed]

91. Koyama, N.; Tokura, Y.; Münch, D.; Sahl, H.G.; Schneider, T.; Shibagaki, Y.; Ikeda, H.; Tomoda, H. The nonantibiotic small molecule cyslabdan enhances the potency of β-lactams against MRSA by inhibiting pentaglycine interpeptide bridge synthesis. *PLoS ONE* **2012**, *7*, e48981. [CrossRef]

92. Fukumoto, A.; Kim, Y.P.; Hanaki, H.; Shiomi, K.; Tomoda, H.; Omura, S. Cyslabdan, a new potentiator of imipenem activity against methicillin-resistant *Staphylococcus aureus*, produced by *Streptomyces* sp. K04-0144. II. Biological activities. *J. Antibiot.* **2008**, *61*, 7–10. [CrossRef]

93. Shanthi, J.; Senthil, A.; Gopikrishnan, V.; Balagurunathan, R. Characterization of a potential β-lactamase inhibitory metabolite from a marine Streptomyces sp. PM49 active against multidrug-resistant pathogens. *Appl. Biochem. Biotechnol.* **2015**, *175*, 3696–3708. [CrossRef] [PubMed]

94. Ohtawa, M.; Hishinuma, Y.; Takagi, E.; Yamada, T.; Ito, F.; Arima, S.; Uchida, R.; Kim, Y.P.; Ōmura, S.; Tomoda, H.; et al. Synthesis and structural revision of cyslabdan. *Chem. Pharm. Bull.* **2016**, *64*, 1370–1377. [CrossRef]

95. Mills, J.J.; Robinson, K.R.; Zehnder, T.E.; Pierce, J.G. Synthesis and biological evaluation of the antimicrobial natural product lipoxazolidinone A. *Angew. Chem. Int. Ed.* **2018**, *57*, 8682–8686. [CrossRef] [PubMed]

96. Valdes-Pena, M.A.; Massaro, N.P.; Lin, Y.C.; Pierce, J.G. Leveraging marine natural products as a platform to tackle bacterial resistance and persistence. *Acc. Chem. Res.* **2021**, *54*, 1866–1877. [CrossRef] [PubMed]

97. Robinson, K.R.; Mills, J.J.; Pierce, J.G. Expanded structure-activity studies of lipoxazolidinone antibiotics. *ACS Med. Chem. Lett.* **2019**, *10*, 374–377. [CrossRef] [PubMed]

98. Mary, T.R.J.; Kannan, R.R.; Iniyan, A.M.; Ranjith, W.A.C.; Nandhagopal, S.; Vishwakarma, V.; Vincent, S.G.P. β-Lactamase inhibitory potential of kalafungin from marine *Streptomyces* in *Staphylococcus aureus* infected zebrafish. *Microbiol. Res.* **2021**, *244*, 126666. [CrossRef]

99. Jeong, B.G.; Na, J.H.; Bae, D.W.; Park, S.B.; Lee, H.S.; Cha, S.S. Crystal structure of AmpC BER and molecular docking lead to the discovery of broad inhibition activities of halisulfates against β-lactamases. *Comput. Struct. Biotechnol. J.* **2021**, *19*, 145–152. [CrossRef]

100. Liu, S.; Su, M.; Song, S.J.; Jung, J.H. Marine-derived *Penicillium* species as producers of cytotoxic metabolites. *Mar. Drugs* **2017**, *15*, 329. [CrossRef]

101. Kim, C.F.; Lee, S.K.; Price, J.; Jack, R.W.; Turner, G.; Kong, R.Y. Cloning and expression analysis of the *pcbAB-pcbC* β-lactam genes in the marine fungus *Kallichroma tethys*. *Appl. Environ. Microbiol.* **2003**, *69*, 1308–1314. [CrossRef]

102. Hamed, R.B.; Gomez-Castellanos, J.R.; Henry, L.; Ducho, C.; McDonough, M.A.; Schofield, C.J. The enzymes of β-lactam biosynthesis. *Nat. Prod. Rep.* **2013**, *30*, 21–107. [CrossRef]

103. Townsend, C.A. Convergent biosynthetic pathways to β-lactam antibiotics. *Curr. Opin. Chem. Biol.* **2016**, *35*, 97–108. [CrossRef] [PubMed]

104. Rabe, P.; Kamps, J.J.A.G.; Schofield, C.J.; Lohans, C.T. Roles of 2-oxoglutarate oxygenases and isopenicillin N synthase in β-lactam biosynthesis. *Nat. Prod. Rep.* **2018**, *35*, 735–756. [CrossRef] [PubMed]

105. Scannell, J.P.; Pruess, D.L.; Blount, J.F.; Ax, H.A.; Kellett, M.; Weiss, F.; Demny, T.C.; Williams, T.H.; Stempel, A. Antimetabolites produced by microorganisms. XII. (*S*)-Alanyl-3-[α(*S*)-chloro-3-(*S*)-hydroxy-2-oxo-3-azetidinylmethyl]-(*S*)-alanine, a new β-lactam containing natural product. *J. Antibiot.* **1975**, *28*, 1–6. [CrossRef]

106. Manning, M.E.; Danson, E.J.; Calderone, C.T. Functional chararacterization of the enzymes TabB and TabD involved in tabtoxin biosynthesis by *Pseudomonas syringae*. *Biochem. Biophys. Res. Commun.* **2018**, *496*, 212–217. [CrossRef]

107. Lyu, J.; Ushimaru, R.; Abe, I. Characterization of enzymes catalyzing the initial steps of the β-lactam tabtoxin biosynthesis. *Org. Lett.* **2022**, *24*, 3337–3341. [CrossRef] [PubMed]

108. Hart, K.M.; Reck, M.; Bowman, G.R.; Wencewicz, T.A. Tabtoxinine-β-lactam is a "stealth" β-lactam antibiotic that evades β-lactamase-mediated antibiotic resistance. *Med. Chem. Commun.* **2016**, *7*, 118–127. [CrossRef]

109. Patrick, G.J.; Fang, L.; Schaefer, J.; Singh, S.; Bowman, G.R.; Wencewicz, T.A. Mechanistic basis for ATP-dependent inhibition of glutamine synthetase by tabtoxinine-β-lactam. *Biochemistry* **2018**, *57*, 117–135. [CrossRef]

110. Anthoni, U.; Bock, K.; Chevolot, L.; Larsen, C.; Nielsen, P.H.; Christophersen, C. Marine alkaloids. 13. Chartellamide A and B, halogenated β-lactam indole-imidazole alkaloids from the marine bryozoan Chartella papyracea. *J. Org. Chem.* **1987**, *52*, 5638–5639. [CrossRef]

111. Avilés, E.; Rodríguez, A.D. Monamphilectine A, a potent antimalarial β-lactam from marine sponge *Hymeniacidon* sp: Isolation, structure, semisynthesis, and bioactivity. *Org. Lett.* **2010**, *12*, 5290–5293. [CrossRef]

112. Avilés, E.; Prudhomme, J.; Le Roch, K.G.; Rodríguez, A.D. Structures, semisyntheses, and absolute configurations of the antiplasmodial α-substituted β-lactam monamphilectines B and C from the sponge *Svenzea flava. Tetrahedron* **2015**, *71*, 487–494. [CrossRef] [PubMed]

113. Duff, J.P.; AbuOun, M.; Bexton, S.; Rogers, J.; Turton, J.; Woodford, N.; Irvine, R.; Anjum, M.; Teale, C. Resistance to carbapenems and other antibiotics in *Klebsiella pneumoniae* found in seals indicates anthropogenic pollution. *Vet. Rec.* **2020**, *187*, 154. [CrossRef] [PubMed]

114. Hatosy, S.M.; Martiny, A.C. The ocean as a global reservoir of antibiotic resistance genes. *Appl. Environ. Microbiol.* **2015**, *81*, 7593–7599. [CrossRef]

115. Elbehery, A.H.; Leak, D.J.; Siam, R. Novel thermostable antibiotic resistance enzymes from the Atlantis II Deep Red Sea brine pool. *Microb. Biotechnol.* **2017**, *10*, 189–202. [CrossRef]

116. Tan, L.; Li, L.; Ashbolt, N.; Wang, X.; Cui, Y.; Zhu, X.; Xu, Y.; Yang, Y.; Mao, D.; Luo, Y. Arctic antibiotic resistance gene contamination, a result of anthropogenic activities and natural origin. *Sci. Total Environ.* **2018**, *621*, 1176–1184. [CrossRef]

117. Blanco-Picazo, P.; Roscales, G.; Toribio-Avedillo, D.; Gómez-Gómez, C.; Avila, C.; Ballesté, E.; Muniesa, M.; Rodríguez-Rubio, L. Antibiotic resistance genes in phage particles from antarctic and mediterranean seawater ecosystems. *Microorganisms* **2020**, *8*, 1293. [CrossRef]

118. Cuadrat, R.R.C.; Sorokina, M.; Andrade, B.G.; Goris, T.; Dávila, A.M.R. Global ocean resistome revealed: Exploring antibiotic resistance gene abundance and distribution in TARA Oceans samples. *Gigascience* **2020**, *9*, giaa046. [CrossRef] [PubMed]

119. He, L.; Huang, X.; Zhang, G.; Yuan, L.; Shen, E.; Zhang, L.; Zhang, X.H.; Zhang, T.; Tao, L.; Ju, F. Distinctive signatures of pathogenic and antibiotic resistant potentials in the hadal microbiome. *Environ. Microbiome* **2022**, *17*, 19. [CrossRef]

120. Perry, J.; Waglechner, N.; Wright, G. The prehistory of antibiotic resistance. *Cold Spring Harb. Perspect. Med.* **2016**, *6*, a025197. [CrossRef]

121. Wright, G.D. Environmental and clinical antibiotic resistomes, same only different. *Curr. Opin. Microbiol.* **2019**, *51*, 57–63. [CrossRef]

122. Massova, I.; Mobashery, S. Kinship and diversification of bacterial penicillin-binding proteins and β-lactamases. *Antimicrob. Agents Chemother.* **1998**, *42*, 1–17. [CrossRef]

123. Modi, T.; Risso, V.A.; Martinez-Rodriguez, S.; Gavira, J.A.; Mebrat, M.D.; Van Horn, W.D.; Sanchez-Ruiz, J.M.; Ozkan, S.B. Hinge-shift mechanism as a protein design principle for the evolution of β-lactamases from substrate promiscuity to specificity. *Nat. Commun.* **2021**, *12*, 1852. [CrossRef] [PubMed]

124. Kwon, S.; Yoo, W.; Kim, Y.O.; Kim, K.K.; Kim, T.D. Molecular characterization of a novel family VIII esterase with β-lactamase activity (PsEstA) from *Paenibacillus* sp. *Biomolecules* **2019**, *9*, 786. [CrossRef]

125. Ryu, B.H.; Ngo, T.D.; Yoo, W.; Lee, S.; Kim, B.Y.; Lee, E.; Kim, K.K.; Kim, T.D. Biochemical and structural analysis of a novel esterase from *Caulobacter crescentus* related to penicillin-rinding protein (PBP). *Sci. Rep.* **2016**, *6*, 37978. [CrossRef] [PubMed]

126. Zhou, Y.; Lin, X.; Xu, C.; Shen, Y.; Wang, S.-P.; Liao, H.; Li, L.; Deng, H.; Lin, H.-W. Investigation of penicillin binding protein (PBP)-like peptide cyclase and hydrolase in surugamide non-ribosomal peptide biosynthesis. *Cell Chem. Biol.* **2019**, *26*, 737–744. [CrossRef] [PubMed]

127. Matsuda, K.; Kobayashi, M.; Kuranaga, T.; Takada, K.; Ikeda, H.; Matsunaga, S.; Wakimoto, T. SurE is a trans-acting thioesterase cyclizing two distinct non-ribosomal peptides. *Org. Biomol. Chem.* **2019**, *17*, 1058–1061. [CrossRef]

128. Cea-Rama, I.; Coscolín, C.; Gonzalez-Alfonso, J.L.; Raj, J.; Vasiljević, M.; Plou, F.J.; Ferrer, M.; Sanz-Aparicio, J. Crystal structure of a family VIII β-lactamase fold hydrolase reveals the molecular mechanism for its broad substrate scope. *FEBS J.* **2022**, *289*, 6714–6730. [CrossRef]

129. Jeon, J.H.; Lee, H.S.; Lee, J.H.; Koo, B.S.; Lee, C.M.; Lee, S.H.; Kang, S.G.; Lee, J.H. A novel family VIII carboxylesterase hydrolysing third- and fourth-generation cephalosporins. *Springerplus* **2016**, *5*, 525. [CrossRef]

130. Schuster, M.; Sexton, D.J.; Diggle, S.P.; Greenberg, E.P. Acyl-homoserine lactone quorum sensing: From evolution to application. *Annu. Rev. Microbiol.* **2013**, *67*, 43–63. [CrossRef]

131. Xavier, K.B.; Bassler, B.L. LuxS quorum sensing: More than just a numbers game. *Curr. Opin. Microbiol.* **2003**, *6*, 191–197. [CrossRef]

132. Ng, W.L.; Bassler, B.L. Bacterial quorum-sensing network architectures. *Annu. Rev. Genet.* **2009**, *43*, 197–222. [CrossRef]

133. Sharifzadeh, S.; Brown, N.W.; Shirley, J.D.; Bruce, K.E.; Winkler, M.E.; Carlson, E.E. Chemical tools for selective activity profiling of bacterial penicillin-binding proteins. *Methods Enzymol.* **2020**, *638*, 27–55. [CrossRef]

134. Brown, N.W.; Shirley, J.; Marshall, A.; Carlson, E. Comparison of bioorthogonal β-lactone activity-based probes for selective labeling of penicillin-binding proteins. *ChemBioChem* **2021**, *22*, 193–202. [CrossRef] [PubMed]

135. Flanders, P.L.; Contreras-Martel, C.; Brown, N.W.; Shirley, J.D.; Martins, A.; Nauta, K.N.; Dessen, A.; Carlson, E.E.; Ambrose, E.A. Combined structural analysis and molecular dynamics reveal penicillin-binding protein inhibition mode with β-lactones. *ACS Chem. Biol.* **2022**, *17*, 3110–3120. [CrossRef] [PubMed]

136. Aertker, K.M.J.; Chan, H.T.H.; Lohans, C.T.; Schofield, C.J. Analysis of β-lactone formation by clinically observed carbapenemases informs on a novel antibiotic resistance mechanism. *J. Biol. Chem.* **2020**, *295*, 16604–16613. [CrossRef] [PubMed]
137. Lohans, C.T.; van Groesen, E.; Kumar, K.; Tooke, C.L.; Spencer, J.; Paton, R.S.; Brem, J.; Schofield, C. A new mechanism for β-lactamases: Class D enzymes degrade 1β-methyl carbapenems via lactone formation. *Angew. Chem. Int. Ed.* **2018**, *57*, 1282–1285. [CrossRef]
138. Macheboeuf, P.; Fischer, D.S.; Brown Jr., T.; Zervosen, A.; Luxen, A.; Joris, B.; Dessen, A.; Schofield, C.J. Structural and mechanistic basis of penicillin-binding protein inhibition by lactivicins. *Nat. Chem. Biol.* **2007**, *3*, 565–569. [CrossRef]
139. Brown Jr., T.; Charlier, P.; Herman, R.; Schofield, C.J.; Sauvage, E. Structural basis for the interaction of lactivicins with serine β-lactamases. *J. Med. Chem.* **2010**, *53*, 5890–5894. [CrossRef] [PubMed]
140. Kluge, A.F.; Petter, R.C. Acylating drugs: Redesigning natural covalent inhibitors. *Curr. Opin. Chem. Biol.* **2010**, *14*, 421–427. [CrossRef]
141. Böttcher, T.; Sieber, S.A. β-Lactams and β-lactones as activity-based probes in chemical biology. *Med. Chem. Commun.* **2012**, *3*, 408–417. [CrossRef]
142. Wiedemann, E.N.; Mandl, F.A.; Blank, I.D.; Ochsenfeld, C.; Ofial, A.R.; Sieber, S.A. Kinetic and theoretical studies of β-lactone reactivity—A quantitative scale for biological application. *ChemPlusChem* **2015**, *80*, 1673–1679. [CrossRef] [PubMed]
143. Mazur, M.; Maslowiec, D. Antimicrobial activity of lactones. *Antibiotics* **2022**, *11*, 1327. [CrossRef]
144. Liu, J.; Fu, K.; Wu, C.; Qin, K.; Li, F.; Zhou, L. "In-Group" communication in marine *Vibrio*: A review of *N*-acyl homoserine lactones-driven quorum sensing. *Front. Cell. Infect. Microbiol.* **2018**, *8*, 139. [CrossRef]
145. Majik, M.S.; Gawas, U.B.; Mandrekar, V.K. Next generation quorum sensing inhibitors: Accounts on structure activity relationship studies and biological activities. *Bioorg. Med. Chem.* **2020**, *28*, 115728. [CrossRef]
146. Polaske, T.J.; Gahan, C.G.; Nyffeler, K.E.; Lynn, D.M.; Blackwell, H.E. Identification of small molecules that strongly inhibit bacterial quorum sensing using a high-throughput lipid vesicle lysis assay. *Cell Chem. Biol.* **2022**, *29*, 605–614. [CrossRef] [PubMed]
147. Borges, A.; Simões, M. Quorum sensing inhibition by marine bacteria. *Mar. Drugs* **2019**, *17*, 427. [CrossRef] [PubMed]
148. Weng, S.-F.; Chao, Y.-F.; Lin, J.-W. Identification and characteristic analysis of the *ampC* gene encoding β-lactamase from *Vibrio fischeri*. *Biochem. Biophys. Res. Commun.* **2004**, *314*, 838–843. [CrossRef] [PubMed]
149. Toth, M.; Smith, C.; Frase, H.; Mobashery, S.; Vakulenko, S. An antibiotic-resistance enzyme from a deep-sea bacterium. *J. Am. Chem. Soc.* **2010**, *132*, 816–823. [CrossRef]
150. Pietra, F. On 3LEZ, a deep-sea halophilic protein with in vitro class-A β-lactamase activity: Molecular-dynamics, docking, and reactivity simulations. *Chem. Biodivers.* **2012**, *9*, 2659–2684. [CrossRef] [PubMed]
151. Jiang, X.W.; Cheng, H.; Huo, Y.Y.; Xu, L.; Wu, Y.H.; Liu, W.H.; Tao, F.F.; Cui, X.J.; Zheng, B.W. Biochemical and genetic characterization of a novel metallo-β-lactamase from marine bacterium *Erythrobacter litoralis* HTCC 2594. *Sci. Rep.* **2018**, *8*, 803. [CrossRef]
152. Kieffer, N.; Guzmán-Puche, J.; Poirel, L.; Kang, H.J.; Jeon, C.O.; Nordmann, P. ZHO-1, an intrinsic MBL from the environmental Gram-negative species *Zhongshania aliphaticivorans*. *J. Antimicrob. Chemother.* **2019**, *74*, 1568–1571. [CrossRef] [PubMed]
153. Selleck, C.; Pedroso, M.M.; Wilson, L.; Krco, S.; Knaven, E.G.; Miraula, M.; Mitić, N.; Larrabee, J.A.; Brück, T.; Clark, A. Structure and mechanism of potent bifunctional β-lactam- and homoserine lactone-degrading enzymes from marine microorganisms. *Sci. Rep.* **2020**, *10*, 12882. [CrossRef]
154. Gersch, M.; Kreuzer, J.; Sieber, S.A. Electrophilic natural products and their biological targets. *Nat. Prod. Rep.* **2012**, *29*, 659–682. [CrossRef] [PubMed]
155. Garner, A.L.; Yu, J.; Struss, A.K.; Kaufmann, G.F.; Kravchenko, V.V.; Janda, K.D. Immunomodulation and the quorum sensing molecule 3-oxo-C12-homoserine lactone: The importance of chemical scaffolding for probe development. *Chem. Commun.* **2013**, *49*, 1515–1517. [CrossRef]
156. Zhao, W.; Lorenz, N.; Jung, K.; Sieber, S.A. Mechanistic analysis of aliphatic β-lactones in *Vibrio harveyi* reveals a quorum sensing independent mode of action. *Chem. Commun.* **2016**, *52*, 11971–11974. [CrossRef] [PubMed]
157. Bottcher, T.; Sieber, S.A. β-Lactones as specific inhibitors of ClpP attenuate the production of extracellular virulence factors of *Staphylococcus aureus*. *J. Am. Chem. Soc.* **2008**, *130*, 14400–14401. [CrossRef]
158. Gersch, M.; Gut, F.; Korotkov, V.S.; Lehmann, J.; Bottcher, T.; Rusch, M.; Hedberg, C.; Waldmann, H.; Klebe, G.; Sieber, S.A. The mechanism of caseinolytic protease (ClpP) inhibition. *Angew. Chem. Int. Ed.* **2013**, *52*, 3009–3014. [CrossRef]
159. Krysiak, J.; Stahl, M.; Vomacka, J.; Fetzer, C.; Lakemeyer, M.; Fux, A.; Sieber, S.A. Quantitative map of β-lactone-induced virulence regulation. *J. Proteome Res.* **2017**, *16*, 1180–1192. [CrossRef]
160. Delago, A.; Gregor, R.; Dubinsky, L.; Dandela, R.; Hendler, A.; Krief, P.; Rayo, J.; Aharoni, A.; Meijler, M.M. A bacterial quorum sensing molecule elicits a general stress response in *Saccharomyces cerevisiae*. *Front. Microbiol.* **2021**, *12*, 632658. [CrossRef]
161. Rayo, J.; Gregor, R.; Jacob, N.T.; Dandela, R.; Dubinsky, L.; Yashkin, A.; Aranovich, A.; Thangaraj, M.; Ernst, O.; Barash, E.; et al. Immunoediting role for major vault protein in apoptotic signaling induced by bacterial *N*-acyl homoserine lactones. *Proc. Natl. Acad. Sci. USA* **2021**, *118*, e2012529118. [CrossRef]
162. Kreitler, D.F.; Gemmell, E.M.; Schaffer, J.E.; Wencewicz, T.A.; Gulick, A.M. The structural basis of N-acyl-α-amino-β-lactone formation catalyzed by a nonribosomal peptide synthetase. *Nat. Commun.* **2019**, *10*, 3432. [CrossRef] [PubMed]

163. Scott, T.A.; Batey, S.F.D.; Wiencek, P.; Chandra, G.; Alt, S.; Francklyn, C.S.; Wilkinson, B. Immunity-guided identification of threonyl-tRNA synthetase as the molecular target of obafluorin, a β-lactone antibiotic. *ACS Chem. Biol.* **2019**, *14*, 2663–2671. [CrossRef] [PubMed]

164. Travin, D.Y.; Severinov, K.; Dubiley, S. Natural Trojan horse inhibitors of aminoacyl-tRNA synthetases. *RSC Chem. Biol.* **2021**, *2*, 468–485. [CrossRef]

165. Schaffer, J.E.; Reck, M.R.; Prasad, N.K.; Wencewicz, T.A. β-Lactone formation during product release from a nonribosomal peptide synthetase. *Nat. Chem. Biol.* **2017**, *13*, 737–744. [CrossRef] [PubMed]

166. Lakemeyer, M.; Zhao, W.; Mandl, F.A.; Hammann, P.; Sieber, S.A. Thinking outside the box–novel antibacterials to tackle the resistance crisis. *Angew. Chem. Int. Ed.* **2018**, *57*, 14440–14475. [CrossRef]

167. Cook, M.A.; Wright, G.D. The past, present, and future of antibiotics. *Sci. Transl. Med.* **2022**, *14*, eabo7793. [CrossRef]

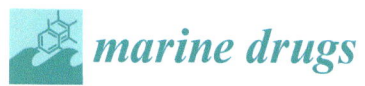

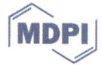

Article

Optimized Degradation and Inhibition of α-glucosidase Activity by *Gracilaria lemaneiformis* Polysaccharide and Its Production In Vitro

Xiaoshan Long [1,2,3], Xiao Hu [1,2,*], Shaobo Zhou [4], Huan Xiang [1,5], Shengjun Chen [1,5], Laihao Li [1,5], Shucheng Liu [3] and Xianqing Yang [1,2,*]

[1] Key Laboratory of Aquatic Product Processing, Ministry of Agriculture and Rural, South China Sea Fisheries Research Institute, Chinese Academy of Fishery Sciences, Guangzhou 510300, China; longxiaoshan1992@163.com (X.L.); xianghuan@scsfri.ac.cn (H.X.); chenshengjun@scsfri.ac.cn (S.C.); lilaihao@scsfri.ac.cn (L.L.)

[2] Co-Innovation Center of Jiangsu Marine Bio-Industry Technology, Jiangsu Ocean University, Lianyungang 222005, China

[3] College of Food Science and Technology, Guangdong Ocean University, Guangdong Provincial Key Laboratory of Aquatic Products Processing and Safety, Guangdong Provincial Engineering Technology Research Center of Marine Food, Guangdong Province Engineering Laboratory for Marine Biological Products, Zhanjiang 524088, China; Lsc771017@163.com

[4] School of Life Sciences, Institute of Biomedical and Environmental Science and Technology, University of Bedfordshire, Luton LU1 3JU, UK; shaobo.zhou@beds.ac.uk

[5] Collaborative Innovation Center of Provincial and Ministerial Co-construction for Marine Food Deep Processing, Dalian 116034, China

* Correspondence: huxiao@scsfri.ac.cn (X.H.); yangxq@scsfri.ac.cn (X.Y.)

Citation: Long, X.; Hu, X.; Zhou, S.; Xiang, H.; Chen, S.; Li, L.; Liu, S.; Yang, X. Optimized Degradation and Inhibition of α-glucosidase Activity by *Gracilaria lemaneiformis* Polysaccharide and Its Production In Vitro. *Mar. Drugs* **2022**, *20*, 13. https://doi.org/10.3390/md20010013

Academic Editor: Hitoshi Sashiwa

Received: 30 November 2021
Accepted: 20 December 2021
Published: 22 December 2021

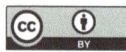
Abstract: *Gracilaria lemaneiformis* polysaccharide (GLP) exhibits good physiological activities, and it is more beneficial as it is degraded. After its degradation by hydrogen peroxide combined with vitamin C (H_2O_2-Vc) and optimized by Box–Behnken Design (BBD), a new product of GLP-HV will be generated. While using GLP as control, two products of GLP-H (H_2O_2-treated) and GLP-V (Vc-treated) were also produced. These products chemical characteristics (total sugar content, molecular weight, monosaccharide composition, UV spectrum, morphological structure, and hypolipidemic activity in vitro) were assessed. The results showed that the optimal conditions for H_2O_2-Vc degradation were as follows: H_2O_2-Vc concentration was 18.7 mM, reaction time was 0.5 h, and reaction temperature was 56 °C. The total sugar content of GLP and its degradation products (GLP-HV, GLP-H and GLP-V) were more than 97%, and their monosaccharides are mainly glucose and galactose. The SEM analysis demonstrated that H_2O_2-Vc made the structure loose and broken. Moreover, GLP, GLP-HV, GLP-H, and GLP-V had significantly inhibition effect on α-glucosidase, and their IC_{50} value were 3.957, 0.265, 1.651, and 1.923 mg/mL, respectively. GLP-HV had the best inhibition effect on α-glucosidase in a dose-dependent manner, which was the mixed type of competitive and non-competitive. It had a certain quenching effect on fluorescence of α-glucosidase, which may be dynamic quenching.

Keywords: *Gracilaria lemaneiformis*; polysaccharide; degradation optimization; chemical characteristics; hypolipidemic activity; α-glucosidase

1. Introduction

Gracilaria lemaneiformis belongs to *Rhodophyta* Phylum, *Gigartinales* Order, *Gracilariaceae* Family, and *Gracilaria* Genus, which is a kind of economic red algae, used as agar, feed, food, and drug resources [1,2]. The mariculture yield of *gracilaria* accounts for 10% of the algae production, second only to kelp. The main producing areas of *Gracilaria lemaneiformis* are the province of Fujian (75.5%), Guangdong (12.3%), and Shandong (12.3%) in China, and it is a traditional seaweed used both as medicine and food [3]. Polysaccharide is the main component of *Gracilaria lemaneiformis*, which has the physiological activities of hypoglycemic, hypolipidemic, hypotensive, anti-obesity, and antineoplastic effects [4–9]. However, the molecule and viscosity of *Gracilaria lemaneiformis* polysaccharide (GLP) are large, and the structure is complex, which is not conducive to the digestion and absorption in human body, and limits the application of polysaccharide. It has been said that polysaccharide with lower molecular weight presented better physiological effects after degradation [10–12]. Xu et al. [13] gained the degradation products of GLP with better tyrosinase inhibition and antioxidant abilities. Jin et al. [14] proved that oligosaccharides from *Gracilaria lemaneiformis* exhibited the protective effect on alcohol-induced hepatotoxicity.

It has been reported that degradation methods include physical [15–17] (ultrasonic, microwave, high temperature, high pressure, radiation), biological [12,18] (fermentation and enzyme), and chemical [11] (acid hydrolysis, reductant-oxidant) methods. The principle of physical degradation is to break the glyosidic bonds of polysaccharide by mechanical means, which has the advantages of being environmentally friendly, simple operation, controllable conditions, and low energy consumption. However, the degradation degree and the efficiency are low. It is usually used in combination with chemical methods [16]. Enzymes can selectively cut the specific glyosidic bond, which has the advantages of high efficiency and maintaining the structure of polysaccharide [19]. However, it has the disadvantages of specificity and high cost, which is unsuitable for a large number of degradations of polysaccharide [13]. Chemical degradation of polysaccharide mainly uses the chemical reagents to destroy glyosidic bonds to achieve the purpose of degradation, which is more rapid and low-cost [17]. In the acid degradation method, some inorganic acids, such as phosphoric acid and hydrochloric acid, are adopted to cause the glyosidic bond breakage, which degrade the polysaccharide into low molecular substances, and cause environmental pollution, resulting in by-products and low purity of degradation products [13]. Oxidants (such as H_2O_2) use free radicals to attack glyosidic bonds of polysaccharide to degrade, with non-toxic, convenient, inexpensive and without by-products, which is suitable to apply in the industry. Nevertheless, the sensitivity of glyosidic bonds at various positions of polysaccharide to H_2O_2 is different, therefore it is necessary to explore the conditions of H_2O_2 degradation, including H_2O_2 concentration, reaction time, temperature, etc., [20]. Alone, H_2O_2 treatment has a low oxidative degradation efficiency, while H_2O_2 can produce higher hydroxyl radicals with the assistance of other reagents (Vc, Cu^{2+} and Fe^{2+}) or means (ultrasound, microwave, radiation) [17]. Vc, Cu^{2+} and Fe^{2+} have strong reducibility that can react with H_2O_2 to produce HO^{2-} and OH^-. These free radicals degrade polysaccharide by attacking glyosidic bonds [16,21]. Chen et al. [10] adopted H_2O_2-Vc to degrade *Grateloupia livida* polysaccharide, and found that H_2O_2-Vc degradation is fast, effective, and beneficial to enhance the antioxidant activity of polysaccharide. It also has been found that the degradation of GLP treated by radiation-H_2O_2 promoted the better activity [11]. Compared with other methods, the effect of free radicals on the glyosidic bond is stronger, the degree of degradation is better, causes more reducing sugar to produce, and reduces the molecular weight of polysaccharide [11,15,19].

Studies have shown that α-glucosidase is one of the enzymes that hydrolyze polysaccharide. α-glucosidase inhibitors can effectively delay the hydrolysis and absorption of carbohydrate by inhibiting α-glucosidase at the brush edge of the small intestinal mucosa, thus improving the symptoms of hyperglycemia [22,23]. Wen et al. [24] proved that GLP found the obvious hypoglycemic activity. Research has explored that GLP and its degradation expressed the hypoglycemic effect by inhibiting α-glucosidase activity, and the polysaccharide degradation had better inhibition effect [25]. According to previous reports, the inhibitory activity of polysaccharide on α-glucosidase was related to a number of factors, such as molecular weight, monosaccharide composition, and other structures [26].

In the present study, the degradation conditions of H_2O_2-Vc, the structure of degradation products of GLP, and its inhibition effect of α-glucosidase were explored.

2. Results

2.1. *Optimized Degradation of Gracilaria Lemaneiformis Polysaccharide*

2.1.1. Results of Single Factor Experiment

To research the effect of H_2O_2-Vc concentration on degradation of GLP, the experiment was carried out under the conditions of temperature of 50 °C, reaction time of 0.5 h and H_2O_2-Vc concentration of 5, 10, 15, 20, and 25 mM, respectively. Reducing sugar content and α-glucosidase inhibition rate were taken as the screening indexes. From Figure 1a, both reducing sugar content and α-glucosidase inhibition rate were the highest when the concentration of H_2O_2-Vc concentration was 20 mM.

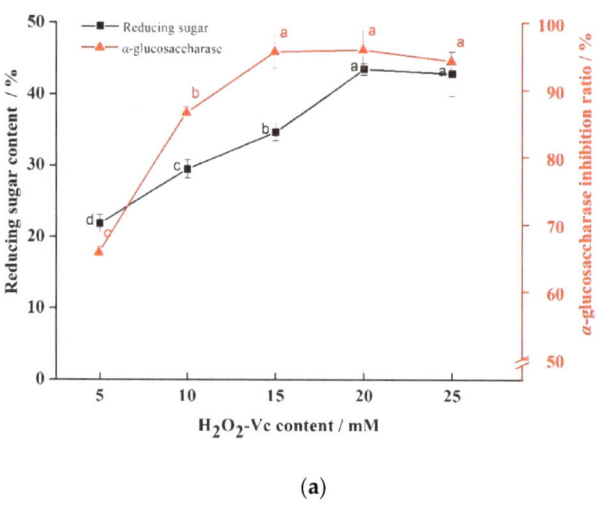

(a)

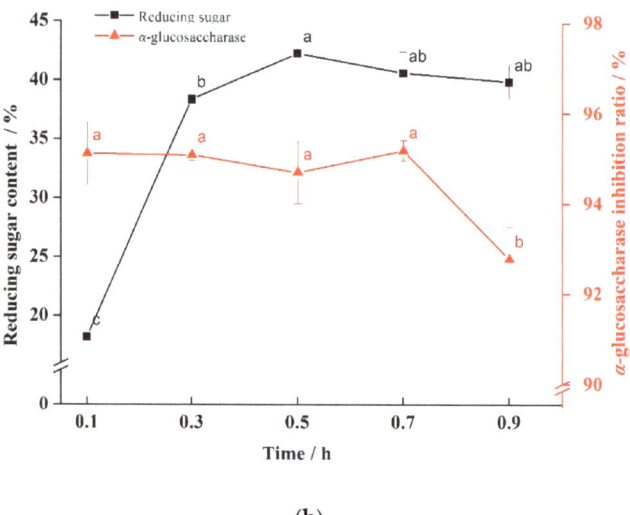

(b)

Figure 1. *Cont.*

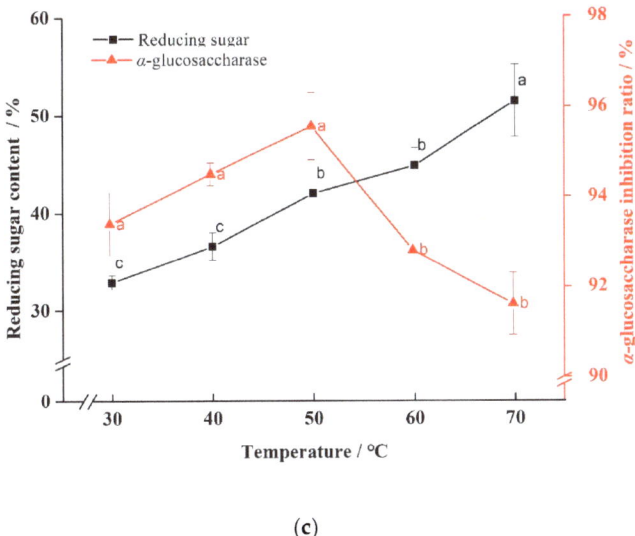

(**c**)

Figure 1. Effect of H_2O_2-Vc concentration, time, and temperature on degradation. Note: (**a**) Effect of H_2O_2-Vc concentration on degradation; (**b**) effect of time on degradation; (**c**) effect of temperature on degradation; a, b, and c represent significant differences among groups, and $p < 0.05$ indicates significant differences.

In order to study the effect of time on degradation, the concentration of H_2O_2-Vc was 20 mM (attained from Figure 1a), the temperature was 50 °C, and the time was 0.1, 0.3, 0.5, 0.7, and 0.9 h. The reducing sugar content and α-glucosidase inhibition rate were taken as indexes. The results (Figure 1b) showed that the reducing sugar content and α-glucosidase inhibition rate were the highest when the time was 0.5 h.

On the basis of the above experiments (H_2O_2-Vc concentration was 20 mM and time was 0.5 h), temperature of 30, 40, 50, 60, and 70 °C were selected to explore the influence of temperature on the degradation. The results showed that the reducing sugar content and α-glucosidase inhibition rate were higher when the temperature was 50 °C (as seen in Figure 1c).

The above results indicated that H_2O_2-Vc concentration, time, and temperature all had certain effects on degradation of GLP. The reducing sugar content and α-glucosidase inhibition rate were the best when H_2O_2-Vc was 20 mM, time was 0.5 h and temperature was 50 °C, respectively.

2.1.2. Results of Response Surface Experiment
Establishment of Regression Model

According to the single factor experiment results, H_2O_2-Vc concentration (A), time (B) and temperature (C), were selected for response surface analysis. The codes "−1", "0", and "1" severally represented the three levels of each factor (Table 1). A total of 17 experiment groups were designed, and the reducing sugar was the response value of the degradation products of GLP (Table 2). The Box–Behnken Design (BBD) principle of Design-Expert 8.0.6 was used to design and implement the corresponding surface method, and the response surface results were fitted. Table 2 presented the response surface experimental design scheme and results, and the regression equation was $Y = 40.81 - 1.35A + 0.81B + 1.98C + 0.85AB - 0.84AC - 0.5BC - 3.28A^2 - 1.87B^2 - 1.81C^2$.

Table 1. Factor level coding.

Factor	Level		
	−1	**0**	**1**
A H$_2$O$_2$-Vc concentration/mM	15	20	25
B Time/h	0.3	0.5	0.7
C Temperature/°C	40	50	60

Table 2. Experimental design and results for response surface analysis.

Code	A:H$_2$O$_2$-Vc Concentration/mM	B: Time/h	C:Temperature/°C	Y:Reducing Sugar Content/%
1	0	0	0	41.6564
2	0	0	0	40.6566
3	1	0	−1	32.9644
4	1	0	1	35.5119
5	0	1	1	39.2347
6	0	0	0	40.6399
7	−1	0	1	40.1668
8	0	0	0	41.0565
9	0	−1	−1	34.0254
10	0	−1	1	38.7351
11	−1	1	0	36.8824
12	1	1	0	36.1679
13	−1	0	−1	34.2537
14	1	−1	0	32.7301
15	0	0	0	40.0567
16	−1	−1	0	36.8499
17	0	1	−1	36.5345

Regression Model Analysis

In Table 3, F value of this model was 63.28, p value < 0.0001 (extremely significant), and the misfitting item was 0.8223 > 0.05 (insignificant). The indexes (R^2 = 0.9879 and R^2adj = 0.9722) indicated that the regression equation could accurately reflect the influence of various factors on the degradation of GLP, which can be used for the analysis and prediction of the degradation of GLP by H$_2$O$_2$-Vc. The values of A, B, C, A^2, B^2, and C^2 were all less than 0.0001, showing extremely significant difference. According to the value of F, the influence order of these three factors was C > A > B. Temperature had the greatest influence on the degradation of GLP, while time had the least influence. The p value of AB and AC were less than 0.01, while the p value of BC was greater than 0.05, indicating that the interaction between H$_2$O$_2$-Vc concentration and time was obvious, and the interaction between H$_2$O$_2$-Vc concentration and temperature was also significant, while the interaction between time and temperature was not significant.

Analysis of Model Interaction Items

Figure 2 showed the contour map and response surface map of the degradation products of GLP. The contour maps of Figure 2a,b were oval, and (c) was circular. The response surface slope of (a) and (b) were larger than (c). These results indicated that H$_2$O$_2$-Vc concentration had significant interaction with reaction time, and H$_2$O$_2$-Vc concentration had remarkable interaction with temperature, while the interaction between reaction time and temperature was not obvious, which was consistent with the results of regression model analysis.

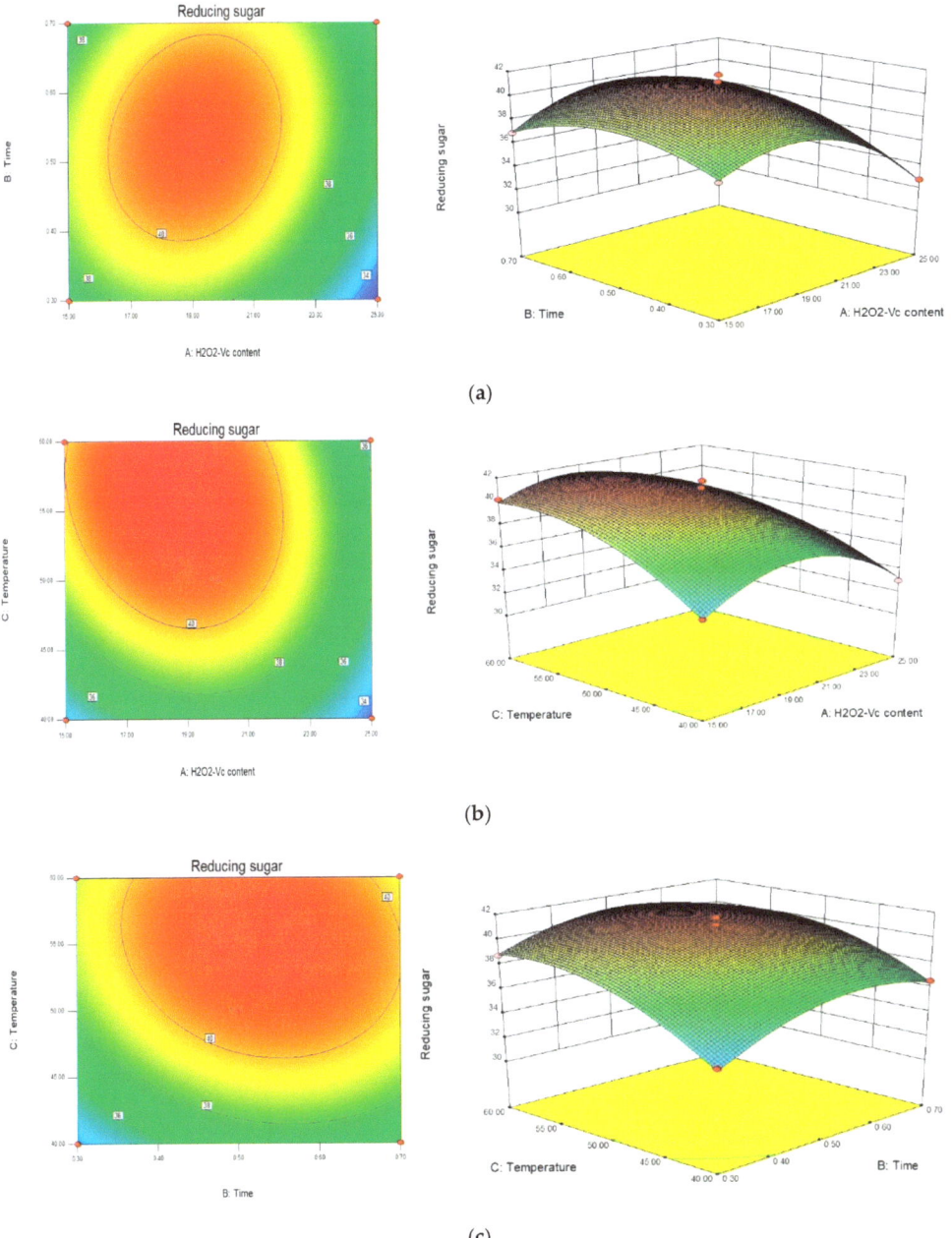

Figure 2. Response surface diagram and contour diagram of interaction of various factors on polysaccharide degradation. (**a**) The interaction between concentration and time; (**b**) The interaction between concentration and temperature; (**c**) The interaction of time and temperature.

Table 3. ANOVA of regression equation.

Source	Sun of Squares	df	Mean Square	F Value	p Value	Significance
Model	139.59	9	15.51	63.28	<0.0001	**
A-H_2O_2-Vc concentration	14.52	1	14.52	59.25	0.0001	**
B-Time	5.25	1	5.25	21.41	0.0024	**
C-Temperature	31.48	1	31.48	128.46	<0.0001	**
AB	2.90	1	2.90	11.83	0.0108	*
AC	2.83	1	2.83	11.55	0.0115	*
BC	1.01	1	1.01	4.12	0.0820	
A^2	45.35	1	45.35	185.04	<0.0001	**
B^2	14.78	1	14.78	60.31	0.0001	**
C^2	13.75	1	13.75	56.10	0.0001	**
Residual	1.72	7	0.25			
Lack of Fit	0.32	3	0.11	0.30	0.8223	
Pure Error	1.40	4	0.35			
Cor Total	141.31	16				

Note: * significant difference ($p < 0.05$); ** extremely significant difference ($p < 0.01$).

Response Surface Optimization and Validation

According to Design-Expert 8.0.6, the optimal process conditions of degradation were as follows: H_2O_2-Vc concentration was 18.64 mM, reaction time was 0.51 h, and reaction temperature was 56.03 °C. On the basis of the actual situation, the process parameters were adjusted. After adjustment, the concentration of H_2O_2-Vc was 18.7 mM, the reaction time was 0.5 h, and the reaction temperature was 56 °C. Under these conditions, the reducing sugar content of the degradation product was 45.16%. The measured value reached 41.62% (the predicted value), which proved that the process conditions of response surface optimization were accurate and reliable, and the model was suitable. The deviation between the actual measured value and the predicted value was less than 5%, indicating that the response surface optimization scheme was reliable.

2.2. The Content of Total Sugar, Reducing Sugar and Protein

In Table 4, the total sugar content of GLP, GLP-HV, GLP-H, GLP-V were 98.77%, 98.43%, 97.28%, and 97.5%, respectively, which showed no significant difference among them ($p > 0.05$). It showed us that extraction method of hot water and alcohol precipitation were more suitable for the extraction of GLP. In addition, the total sugar content of polysaccharide degradation products did not decrease. The total sugar content was only 66.68% treated by critic acid [24], which was far lower than the polysaccharide obtained by the method of water extraction and alcohol precipitation in this experiment. The total sugar content severally was 91.4% with the method of amylase-assisted extraction from Wu et al. [27]. Li et al. [4] got 59% total sugar content, illustrating that the polysaccharide obtained by acid extraction has more impurities. Moreover, the carbohydrate content was 72.06% extracted with cold water [6]. In the present experiment, the total sugar content of GLP obtained by hot water extraction was relatively high, compared with other methods, and the content did not decrease after degradation.

Table 4. The content of total sugar, reducing sugar and protein from GLP and its degradation products.

Indexes		GLP	GLP-HV	GLP-H	GLP-V
Total sugar	Content (%)	98.77 ± 5.94 a	98.43 ± 3.21 a	97.28 ± 2.63 a	97.5 ± 1.56 a
	Standard curve		y = 2.4623x + 0.0516, R^2 = 0.9939		
Reducing sugar	Content (%)	2.47 ± 0.03 c	46.92 ± 2.38 b	1.95 ± 0.15 c	50.2 ± 1.00 a
	Standard curve		y = 0.8185x − 0.0258, R^2 = 0.9999		
Protein	Content (%)	ND	ND	ND	ND
	Standard curve		y = 0.6288x + 0.5582, R^2 = 0.9902		

Note: a, b, and c represent significant differences among groups, and $p < 0.05$ indicates significant differences.

The reducing sugar of GLP was 2.47%, which enhanced the obvious degradation by H_2O_2-Vc (GLP-HV was 46.92%) or Vc (GLP-V was 50.2%). However, GLP-H was only 1.95%, significantly lower than GLP. The results proved that both H_2O_2-Vc-treated and Vc-treated promoted the production of reducing sugar, and H_2O_2-treated declined the reducing sugar content. The reducing sugar of GLP attained by Gong et al. [11] was 1.2%, lower than that of this experiment, and the content was diminished after treating with H_2O_2, which was consistent with the experimental results of this study. H_2O_2-Vc and Vc broke the glycosidic bonds, exposing more reducing sugars of polysaccharide. H_2O_2 may react with reducing groups on the sugar chain, declining the content of reducing sugar. When Vc was added, a redox reaction occurred between Vc and H_2O_2 to produce free radical, which promoted the breaking of glyosidic bonds and induced more reducing sugar. There was still a small amount of H_2O_2 that reacted with the reducing group, so the reducing sugar of GLP-HV was a little less than GLP-V.

The protein content of untreated *Gracilaria lemaneiformis* was 15.7 ± 0.0018%, detected by the Kjeldahl method. After treated by ethanol and papain, the protein of GLP was undetected with Coomassie Bright Blue method kit, which demonstrated that the protein was removed during the extraction of GLP. Liu et al. [28] detected the protein content of GLP treated by hot water was 0.98%. The protein of GLP attained by hot citric acid extraction was 1.47% [29]. Moreover, the protein content of GLP was 0.7% (enzyme extraction) [27], 1.6% (acid extraction) [4], 0.28% (extracted with cold water) [6]. From the above analysis, it can be seen that GLP obtained by other methods contain a small amount of protein, which can be removed with the method in this experiment.

2.3. Monosaccharide Composition

As exhibited in Figure 3a, the main monosaccharide components of polysaccharide and its degradation products were glucose and galactose, accompanied by a small amount of mannose, ribose, glucuronic acid, galacturonic acid, arabinose, xylose, and fucose. GLP contained 34.35% glucose and 57.37% galactose, respectively, and GLP-HV included 33.37% glucose and 59.12% galactose. H_2O_2-Vc treatment slightly increased the content of galactose, while the glucose content declined a small amount, probably because there was a little bit more free radicals to attack the glyosidic bonds linking galactose. This result was consistent with Gong et al. [11]. The monosaccharide composition of GLP extracted by this method was relatively simple, mainly consisting of glucose and galactose, compared with previous studies. The content of glucose and galactose respectively were 4.76% and 21.1% from GLP extracted by Li et al. [4]. Moreover, the level of ribose and xylose were enhanced, but rhamnose content declined after degradation.

2.4. Molecular Weight

The weight average molecular weight (Mw) of GLP was 14,78,524 Da (1478 kDa), which was higher than that of citric acid extraction (21.2 kDa and 31.5 kDa) [4,24], and it declined after degradation. In Table 5, the Mw of GLP-H and GLP-V were 1,329,838 and 1,000,630 Da, respectively, which was slightly lower than that of GLP. However, the Mw of GLP-HV was only 16,245 Da, which was much smaller than the molecular weight of GLP. It illustrated that the degradation level treated by H_2O_2-Vc was higher than alone H_2O_2 or Vc. Moreover, the value of Mw/Mn represents the molecular weight distribution, which can reflect the molecular weight distribution width and degree of polydispersity of polysaccharide. From Table 5, the Mw/Mn of GLP, GLP-HV, GLP-H, GLP-V were 144.24, 2.43, 75.96, and 47.15, respectively, which explained the GLP-HV performing the smallest distribution width, uniform distribution, and small dispersity. It was reported that the Mw of GLP was changed from 2.15×10^5 to 1.22×10^5 Da after degradation by fermentation [12], which demonstrated the degradation degree of H_2O_2-Vc was stronger than fermentation.

Table 5. The Molecular weight from GLP and its degradation products.

Molecular Weight (Da)	GLP	GLP-HV	GLP-H	GLP-V
Number average molecular weight(Mn) (Da)	10,250	6695	17,508	21,224
Weight average molecular weight(Mw) (Da)	1,478,524	16,245	1,329,838	1,000,630
Mw/Mn	144.24	2.43	75.96	47.15

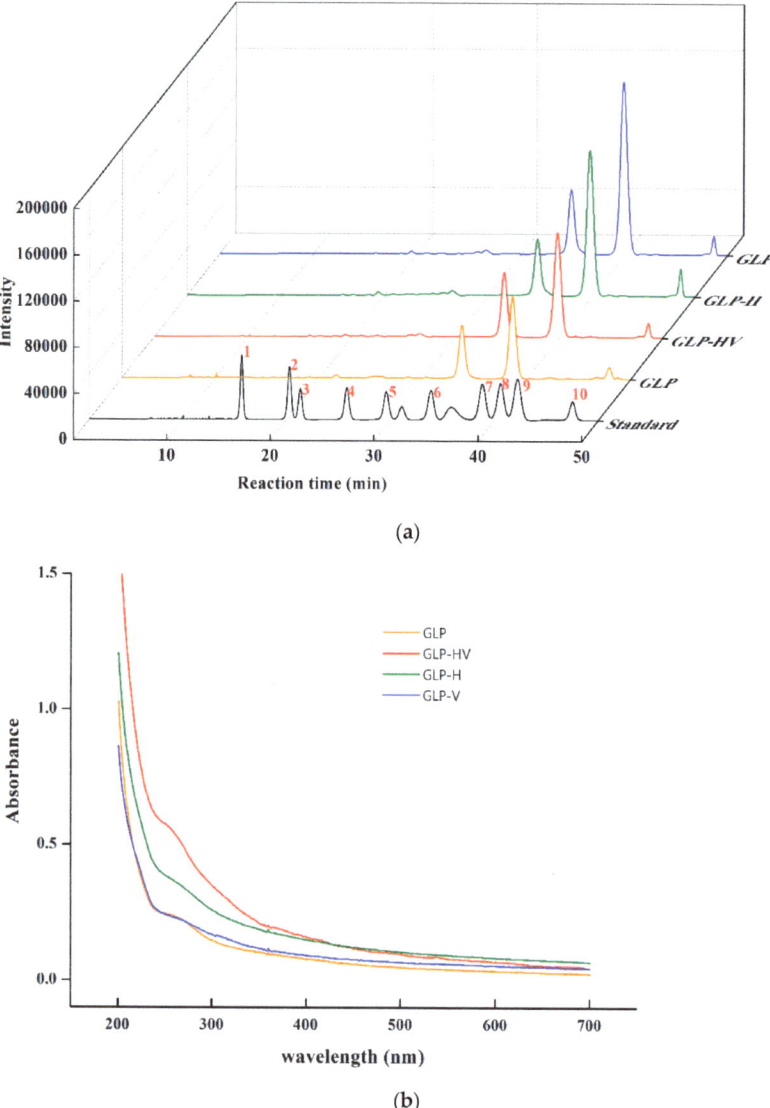

(a)

(b)

Figure 3. *Cont.*

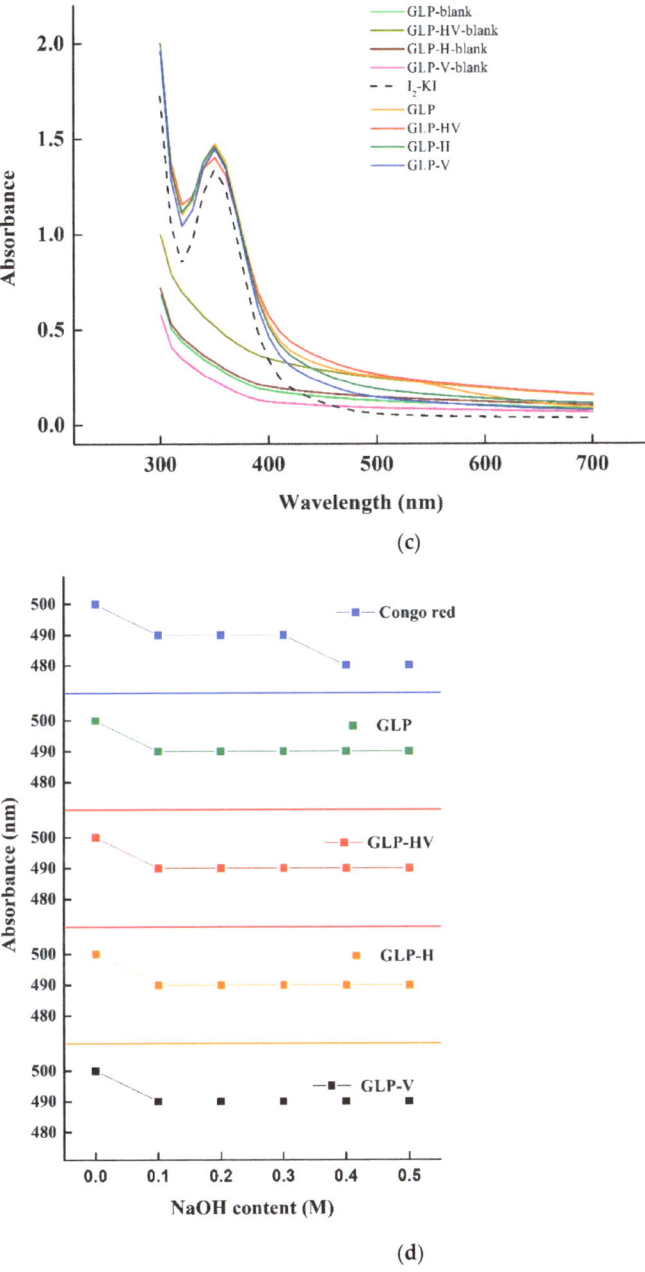

(c)

(d)

Figure 3. The monosaccharide composition, UV-visible spectroscopy, I_2-KI test, Congo red test of GLP and its degradation products. Note: (**a**) The monosaccharide composition of GLP, GLP-HV, GLP-H, GLP-V; the number of 1–10 mean as follow: 1-Mannose, 2-Ribose,3-Rhamnose, 4-Glucuronic acid, 5- Galacturonic acid, 6-Glucose, 7-Galactose, 8-Xylose,9-Arabinose,10-Fucose (**b**) The UV-visible spectroscopy analysis of GLP, GLP-HV, GLP-H, GLP-V; (**c**) The I_2-KI test of GLP, GLP-HV, GLP-H, GLP-V; (**d**) The Congo red test of GLP, GLP-HV, GLP-H, GLP-V.

2.5. UV-Visible Spectroscopy

Four polysaccharide samples were respectively scanned under UV-visible spectroscopy at 200–700 nm. As shown in Figure 3b, GLP, GLP-HV, GLP-H, GLP-V showed no absorption at 260 nm and 280 nm, indicating that there were no nucleic acid and proteins before and after the degradation of the polysaccharide, which was consistent with the determination results of protein content in Table 4.

2.6. I_2-KI Test

The blank solution of GLP, GLP-HV, GLP-H, GLP-V had no absorption peak at 300–700 nm of UV-visible spectroscopy. These four polysaccharide solutions were mixed with I_2-KI solution. After 10 min, I_2-KI had the maximum absorption peak at 350 nm, and four polysaccharides also had the maximum absorption wavelength at 350 nm when mixed with I_2-KI solution, while there was no absorption wavelength at 560 nm, indicating that the GLP, GLP-HV, GLP-H, and GLP-V contained no starch in the solution (Figure 3c). The GLP, degraded by UV-H_2O_2, also did not contain starch [11], which was consistent with the present research.

2.7. Congo Red Test

Congo red is an acidic dye soluble in water and alcohol. When it combines with the triple helix structure of polysaccharide to form a conjugate, its maximum absorption wavelength will be redshifted. However, when the concentration of NaOH increases, the complex formed by Congo red and the triple helix structure of polysaccharide will be destroyed, forming irregular curls, and the maximum absorption wavelength will first increase and then decrease [30]. From Figure 3d, GLP, GLP-HV, GLP-H, and GLP-V did not appear the phenomenon of redshifted, which were consistent with the change of pure Congo red. The results demonstrated that there was no triple helix structure in polysaccharide before and after the degradation.

2.8. Scanning Electron Microscope Analysis

The surface morphology analysis of GLP and its degradation products were explored by scanning electron microscope (SEM). The SEM images of GLP, GLP-HV, GLP-H, and GLP-V were observed in Figure 4. The SEM images at 200-fold (Figure 4a) and 1000-fold (Figure 4b) magnification indicated that the surface morphology of GLP was smooth, compact, and flaky. After the degradation with H_2O_2 and Vc, the polysaccharide structure was damaged, loose, and broken. The structure of GLP-V (treated by Vc) was damaged and became irregular (in the shapes of strips and flakes), but the surface was also smooth, compared with GLP. However, the structure of polysaccharide treated by H_2O_2 was broken, and its surface became rough and loose (GLP-H). The effect of H_2O_2-Vc degradation was more obvious, the structure was the most loose, and the damage for surface structure was the most serious, but the size of fragments was relatively uniform. The polysaccharide structure degraded by H_2O_2-Vc was more fragmented and looser. The morphologies of the polysaccharide produced by H_2O_2 degradation alone were similar to those treated by H_2O_2-Vc degradation, but the structures of the polysaccharide produced by H_2O_2-Vc were more uniform and fragmented. The probable reason was that H_2O_2 had a major effect on the structure of polysaccharide, while Vc played a supplementary role. Vc could promote H_2O_2 to generate more free radicals, breaking glyosidic bonds, so that the structure of polysaccharide became loose and broken [16].

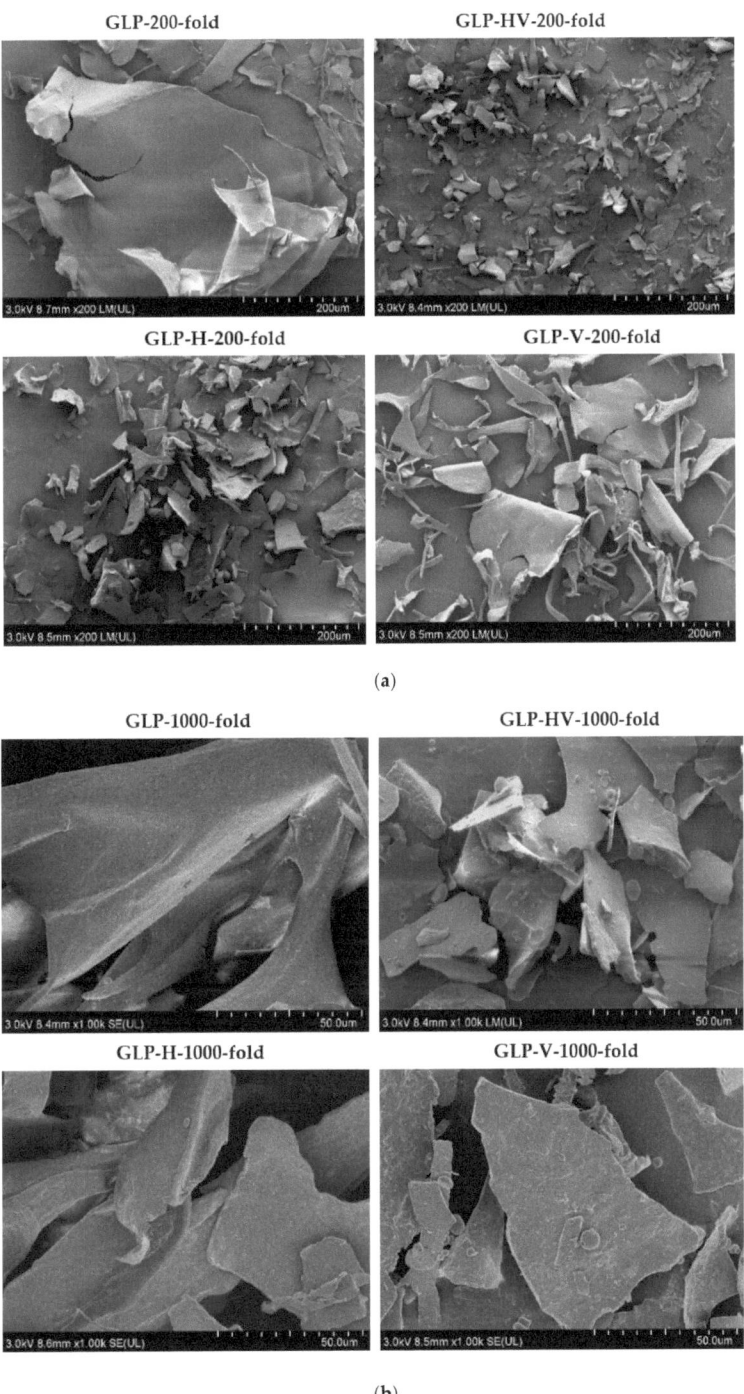

Figure 4. The surface morphology analysis of GLP and its degradation products. Note: (**a**) The surface morphology analysis of GLP, GLP-HV, GLP-H, GLP-V with the magnification of 200-fold; (**b**) The surface morphology analysis of GLP, GLP-HV, GLP-H, GLP-V with the magnification of 1000-fold.

2.9. The Inhibition Effect on α-glucosidase

α-glucosidase is a key enzyme in hydrolysis of carbohydrate which can decompose carbohydrates into glucose. The inhibition of α-glucosidase activity could reduce the production of glucose, slow down the speed of glucose to enter the blood, and then decrease postprandial blood glucose [22]. In addition, this inhibition reduces the absorption of carbohydrates by the digestive tract and intestines, stimulates insulin-dependent glucose uptake, and reduces inflammation, thereby improving the symptoms of diabetes [31]. Acarbose, an α-glucosidase inhibitor, is a complex oligosaccharide with good inhibitory effect on α-glucosidase, hence it was selected as the positive control in this experiment [26]. Figure 5 displayed that GLP and its degradation products were able to inhibit α-glucosidase activity. In particular, GLP-HV exhibited an appreciable α-glucosidase inhibition, with inhibition rate of 89.98% as the content was 5 mg/mL (Figure 5a). At the same concentration, the inhibition rates of GLP, GLP-H, and GLP-V were 52.85%, 69.53%, and 56.76%, respectively, which significantly were inferior to GLP-HV. In the figure, it was clear that the inhibition rate was dose-dependent for all samples within a certain concentration range. Liao et al. [25] attained the α-glucosidase inhibition rate of GLP degradation product, treated by 9 mM H_2O_2-Vc for 2 h, was less than 70%, which was lower than GLP-HV (89.98%) at 5 mg/mL. It pointed out that H_2O_2-Vc concentration and the reaction time of degradation played a vital effect on the hypoglycemic activity of polysaccharide. Under different degradation conditions, the molecular weight, monosaccharide composition, and other structural characteristics of the obtained polysaccharide degradation products were obviously diverse, which resulted in the difference of hypoglycemic activity in vitro. In Figure 5b, the IC_{50} value of acarbose (control), GLP, GLP-HV, GLP-H, and GLP-V were 0.053, 3.957, 0.265, 1.651, and 1.923 mg/mL, which explained the inhibition effect on α-glucosidase of these samples from high to low was acarbose > GLP-HV > GLP-H > GLP-V > GLP.

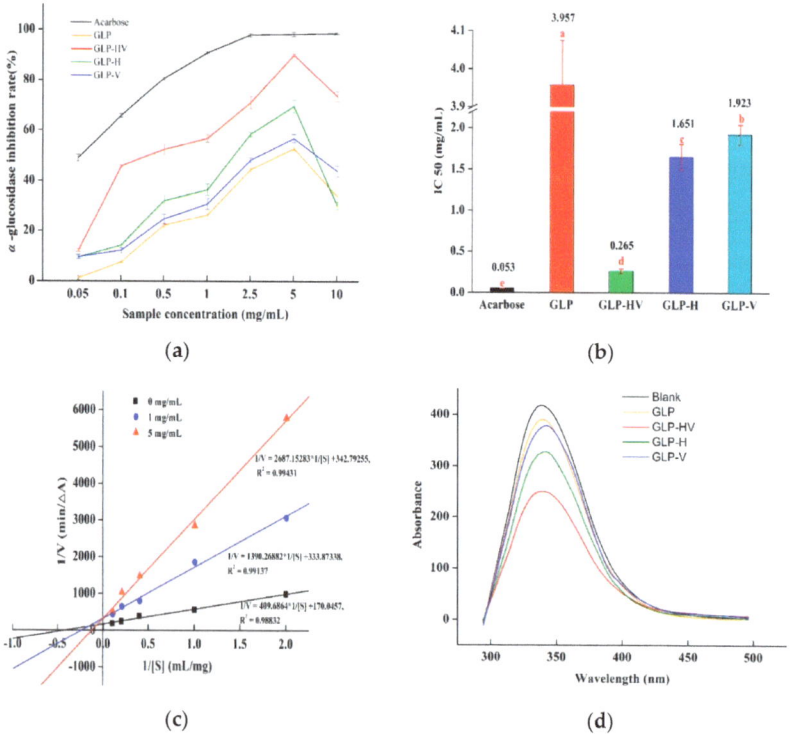

Figure 5. *Cont.*

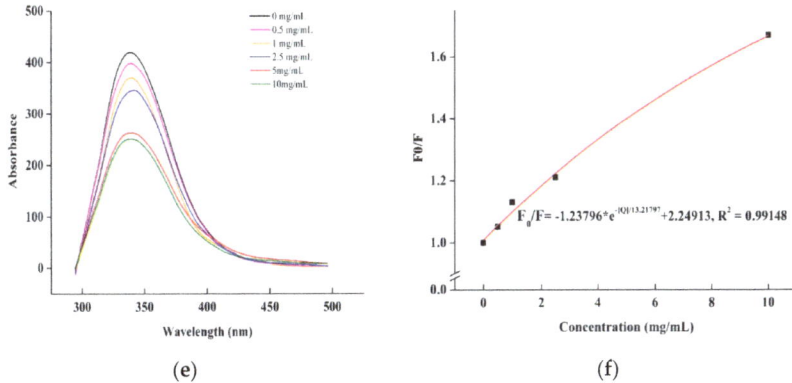

(e)   (f)

Figure 5. The inhibition effect of GLP and its degradation products on α-glucosidase. Note: (**a**) The α-glucosidase inhibition rate of GLP, GLP-HV, GLP-H, and GLP-V; (**b**) The IC_{50} value of α-glucosidase inhibition rate of GLP, GLP-HV, GLP-H, and GLP-V; (**c**) The Lineweaver–Burk curve of α-glucosidase inhibitory dynamics of GLP, GLP-HV, GLP-H, and GLP-V; (**d**) The fluorescence spectrum analysis on α-glucosidase of GLP, GLP-HV, GLP-H, and GLP-V; (**e**) The fluorescence spectrum analysis on α-glucosidase of GLP-HV; (**f**) The Stern-Volmer curve for fluorescence quenching of GLP-HV on α-glucosidase a, b, c, d and e represented significant differences among groups, and $p < 0.05$ indicates significant differences.

In Figure 5c, the Lineweaver–Burk curve of different concentrations of GLP-HV intersected in the second quadrant. From Table 6, when concentrations were 0, 1, 5 mg/mL, the *Km* values were 2.409, 4.164, and 7.839 mg/mL, and *Vmax* values were 0.005881, 0.002995, and 0.002917 mg/mL, respectively. *Km* was enhanced and *Vmax* was declined as the sample concentration increased, which were accorded with the mix of competitive and non-competitive inhibition, respectively. All of these results demonstrated that inhibition type of GLP-HV on α-glucosidase was the mix of competitive and non-competitive. The mechanism may be that samples would bind to the active sites of the enzyme, reducing the activity of the enzyme and preventing the combination of the enzyme to the substrate. On the other hand, the sample interacted with groups outside the active center of the enzyme, which had no direct inhibition effect on the enzyme, but can inhibit the release of products combined by enzyme and substrate, so as to achieve the inhibition effect. Cao et al. [32] studied the α-glucosidase inhibition effect of *Lentinus edodes* mycelia polysaccharide; the inhibition type also was mixed-type manner, which was in accordance with our results. Polysaccharides from different materials may have diverse types of α-glucosidase inhibition. Zhao et al. [33] found that the inhibition type was a competitive mode on α-glucosidase affected by polysaccharide from *Ribes nigrum* L.

Table 6. The inhibitory kinetic constant on α-glucosidase of GLP-HV.

[S] (mg/mL)	V *max* (mg/mL·min^{-1})	*Km* (mg/mL)	Inhibition Type
0	0.0059	2.409	The mix of competitive and non-competitive
1	0.0030	4.164	
5	0.0029	7.839	

Figure 5d reflected the fluorescence intensity on α-glucosidase from GLP, GLP-HV, GLP-H, and GLP-V, which confirmed that all of the samples had fluorescence quenching effect to some extent. The fluorescence intensity became weakened, and the phenomenon of red shift occurred after the addition of samples. GLP-HV performed the best impact on the fluorescence intensity, and the second was GLP-H. GLP and GLP-V exhibited the similar effect, which were a little bit worse than the first two samples. Therefore, we chose GLP-HV with series of concentrations to observe the effect on fluorescence intensity of α-glucosidase (Figure 5e). The degree of redshift was bigger and bigger as the concentration increased (the concentration from 0 to 10 mg/mL), observed by Figure 5e and the value of F (Table 6). It demonstrated that the bigger content of GLP-HV displayed the stronger combination with the luminophore groups (tryptophan, tyrosine, and phenylalanine) of α-glucosidase. It was also possible that the combination of samples with the groups of the enzyme may cause changes of the environment around the luminescent groups, thus affecting the luminescence intensity. Calculating by fluorescence quenching Stern–Volmer equation, the fluorescence parameters on α-glucosidase of GLP-HV were showed in Table 7 and Figure 5f. The quenching constant Ksv and Kq were 0.07566 L/mol and 7.566×10^6 L/mol/s, respectively. The value of Ksv was poorer than the other polysaccharide from literatures [34]. Kq was lower than 2.0×10^{10} L/mol/s [35], the maximum collision rate constant of quenchers caused by large biomolecules. On the other hand, the quenching curve between F_0/F and $[Q]$ almost showed the linear relationship. As a result, the fluorescence quenching type of GLP-HV to enzyme may be dynamic quenching, but the quenching effect was weak, according to the value of Ksv. Ka was the binding constant of GLP-HV with α-glucosidase, that could be calculated from the intercept of $\lg((F_0 - F)/F)$ versus $\lg[Q]$ curve. Such data are summarized in Table 7: Ka was 9.5082 L/mol, and the number of binding sites (n) was 0.8137 (close to 1). We noticed that the value of Ka was relatively low, and the value of n was only 1, which indicated that the binding effect of the GLP-HV to the α-glucosidase was weak and there was only one binding site.

Table 7. The fluorescence parameter on α-glucosidase of GLP-HV.

[Q] (mg/mL)	F	F_0/F	Ksv (L/mol)	Kq (L/mol/s)	Ka (L/mol)	n
0	419	1				
0.5	399	1.0518				
1	371	1.1309	0.07566	7.566×10^6	9.5082	0.8137
2.5	346	1.2107				
5	263	1.5930				
10	251	1.6690				
equation of curve	$F_0/F = -1.23796*e^{-[Q]/13.21797} + 2.24913$, $R^2 = 0.99148$				$\lg((F_0 - F)/F) = 0.8137*\lg[Q] - 0.9781$, $R^2 = 0.9788$	

According to the results of inhibition rate, IC_{50}, inhibition kinetics and fluorescence spectrum analysis, GLP-HV had a good inhibition effect on α-glucosidase in a dose-dependent manner, which was the mixed type of competitive and non-competitive. It had a certain quenching effect on fluorescence, which may be dynamic quenching. GLP-HV may have the potential to be developed as new hypoglycemic agents.

3. Discussion

The degradation degree of polysaccharide was related to H_2O_2-Vc concentration, degradation time and temperature according to single factor and response surface experiments. H_2O_2-Vc concentration in the system was very small, and the degradation time was short, which had the advantages of rapid reaction, high efficiency, and low cost. The Mw of H_2O_2 and Vc were both lower than 300 g/mol, respectively, which can be removed by dialysis without introducing impurities and interfering with the activity of polysaccharide. This method is safe and reliable that can be used in industrial production. The total sugar and protein content were not changed after degradation, indicating that H_2O_2-Vc did not introduce other impurities. In addition, the reducing content of polysaccharide was higher after degradation, and its lower Mw, exhibiting the effective degradation of H_2O_2-Vc. And the degradation effect was better than fermentation, and similar to HPT treatment (high temperature and pressure combined with Vc) from the comparison of molecular weight [12,15].

Polysaccharide degradation is attributed to the breaking of glyosidic bonds, resulting in changes in monosaccharide composition. Various degradation methods act on different glyosidic bonds, so the breakage of glyosidic bonds' location and number may be diverse, resulting in differences in the amount and content of monosaccharides exposed [11,20,21]. Xu et al. [13] found that the glucose and galactose were changed after degradation by HCl (the content of galactose was 35.9%) and enzyme (the content of galactose was 68.9%, respectively), compared with GLP (56.6%). It might be that the positions and quantities of glyosidic bonds destroyed by diverse degradation methods were different, leading to changes in monosaccharides content. However, the ratio of main monosaccharide components GLP-H (24.63% glucose and 66.39% galactose) and GLP-V (24.43% glucose and 69.64% galactose) were changed a little, compared with GLP, and exhibited the same variation. Moreover, the level of ribose and xylose enhanced, but rhamnose content declined after degradation. This phenomenon may be due to the position of glyosidic bond affected by different degradation ways. Alone, H_2O_2 or Vc treatment may break the similar position or numbers of glyosidic bond. They may cut the glyosidic bonds on both sides of galactose, promoting the produce of galactose, compared with H_2O_2-Vc treatment. The degradation of polysaccharide led to the change of monosaccharide composition, which may be the main reason for the change of glucosidase inhibition effect by polysaccharide and its production products.

The SEM results were consistent with the change of reducing sugar and molecular weight, which exhibited that H_2O_2-Vc obviously degraded the *Gracilaria lemaneiformis* polysaccharide effectively, thus could break its structure, and changed its surface morphology. Furthermore, H_2O_2-Vc treatment exhibited the better degradation effect than alone H_2O_2 or Vc treatment, might be due to the differences in the distance and degree of crosslinking between molecules. Gong et al. [11] also found that GLP presented the thick slices image with flat and smooth surface, and then changed into thin, lacerating, and rough after degradation by UV-H_2O_2. However, the polysaccharide structure was more fragmented and looser degraded by H_2O_2-Vc. Perhaps Vc reacted with H_2O_2 to produce more free radicals, which had a stronger effect on the polysaccharide molecules. The Mw of polysaccharides dreaded by H_2O_2 or Vc were only slightly less than GLP, and H_2O_2-Vc exhibited the excellent degradation effect with the minimum Mw. This finding validated the SEM result.

α-glucosidase is one of the hydrolases in the digestive tract, which is closely related to hypoglycemic activity [32]. The inhibition effect of polysaccharide on α-glucosidase can reduce the production of glucose in the blood and thus change the carbohydrate metabolism. Therefore, the inhibitory effect of polysaccharide on α-glucosidase can reflect the hypoglycemic effect in vitro. From the results of the inhibition effect of α-glucosidase, the polysaccharide treated by H_2O_2-Vc enhanced the hypoglycemic activity in vitro, compared with H_2O_2 or Vc treatment alone. GLP-HV presented higher galactose, ribose, and xylose than GLP, and lower glucose and rhamnose. Both GLP-H and GLP-V expressed similar changes with GLP-HV, but the effect were not as significant as GLP-HV. The degraded polysaccharides showed better inhibition, especially GLP-HV. It possibly was related to these changes in monosaccharide compositions. Cao et al. [32] exerted the outstanding inhibition on α-glucosidase by *Lentinus edodes* mycelia polysaccharide containing mannose, arabinose, galactose, xylose, and rhamnose. Combined with the results of molecular weight, GLP-HV had the lower Mw than GLP, GLP-H, and GLP-V. For another, the Mw of GLP-V was smaller than GLP and GLP-H, but its inhibition rate on α-glucosidase was worse than GLP-H and higher than GLP. Therefore, the good inhibition effect of GLP-HV may not only be due to the low molecular weight and monosaccharide composition, but also to the connection mode of glycoside chains, which needs to be verified by subsequent studies. Lv et al. [30] researched the backbone of WXA-1 (polysaccharide from wheat bran) was →4)-β-D-Xylp-(1→, which was substituted at O-3 positions by arabinose, glucose, and galactose residues, while the backbone of AXA-1 (polysaccharide from wheat bran) was → 4)-β-D-Xylp-(1→, which was mainly substituted at O-3 positions by arabinose. AXA-1 exhibited a stronger inhibitory effect on the activities of α-amylase and α-glucosidase compared with WXA-1. When the concentration range of GLP-HV was 0–5 mg/mL, the inhibition rate of α-glucosidase was dose-dependent, and the higher concentration played the higher inhibition rate. When the concentration was from 5 to 10 mg/mL, the inhibition rate decreased. However, fluorescence quenching effect of GLP-HV with 10 mg/mL was a little bit stronger than 5 mg/mL, which was contrary to the results of inhibition rate. The probable reason may that the inhibition type was the mix of competitive and non-competitive. GLP-HV inhibited the products of enzyme-substrate interaction rather than directly binding to the enzyme active groups. Furthermore, the strength of fluorescence quenching cannot fully represent the inhibitory effect on the enzyme. The fluorescence spectrum of α-glucosidase under this condition was due to the existence of luminescent groups such as tryptophan, tyrosine, and phenylalanine. Changes of the groups and their environment led to the changes in fluorescence intensity. The weak binding ability between GLP-HV and the luminescent group or the weak influence on the environment of the luminescent group cannot fully explain the weak inhibitory activity of the sample.

The method of hot water extraction and alcohol precipitation is a suitable extraction method for polysaccharide, with high total sugar content and without protein. H_2O_2-Vc is also an excellent degradation method, which has the advantages of high efficiency, low cost, and no by-products. Low molecular weight polysaccharide with high hypoglycemic activity could be obtained by H_2O_2-Vc degradation. Polysaccharide degradation products showed the inhibition on α-glucosidase, and GLP-HV presented the best effect in a dose-dependent manner, which was the mixed type of competitive and non-competitive. It had a certain quenching effect on fluorescence of α-glucosidase, which may be dynamic quenching. The best inhibition effect on α-glucosidase may be related to its molecular weight, monosaccharide composition and other factors.

4. Materials and Methods

4.1. Materials and Chemicals

Gracilaria lemaneiformis was purchased from Nan'ao Island (Shantou, Gguangdong, China), the Coomassie Bright Blue kit was purchased from Shanghai Biyuntian Biotechnology Co., LTD (Shanghai, China); vitamin C (Vc) and α-glucosidase were purchased from Shanghai Yuanye Biotechnology Co., LTD (Shanghai, China); P-nitrobenzene-α-d-glucoside (PNPG) was purchased from Shanghai Maclin Biochemical Technology Co., LTD (Shanghai, China).

4.2. Preparation of GLP

Gracilaria lemaneiformis was cleaned many times to remove impurities, dried in an oven at 50 °C, crushed and sifted through 40 mesh to obtain uniform powder. The powder was soaked on a shaking table (50 °C) with an ethanol volume of nine times to remove pigment, fat, and alcohol-soluble impurities. After 24 h, the filter residue was extracted and placed in a drying oven at 50 °C for drying. The GLP was extracted by hot water and precipitated by ethanol according to the previous reported methods with some modifications [11]. After 30 min of ultrasonic wall breaking, *Gracilaria lemaneiformis* was extracted with water at a ratio of 1:45 (w/v) at 90 °C for 4 h under oscillation, and then cooled to room temperature to add 1% papain and 0.5% cellulase (w/v). The mixture was incubated at 60 °C for 2 h under oscillation, and then rapidly heated in boiling water for 10 min to denature the papain and cellulase. After cooling to room temperature, the mixture was centrifuged at 8000 rpm for 15 min, and the supernatant was collected and condensed to one third of the original volume by rotary evaporation (60 °C). The concentrated solution was precipitated at 4 °C for 12 h, centrifuged for precipitation, filtered with 200 mesh gauze, and then dialyzed (7 kDa) at 4 °C for 72 h, and pure water was changed once at 4 h. After freeze-drying, GLP values were obtained.

4.3. Degradation of GLP with H_2O_2-Vc

4.3.1. Single-Factor Experiment

The degradation was adopted based on the reported method [10]. GLP was degraded by H_2O_2-Vc (mole ratio of H_2O_2 and Vc was 1:1). In brief, GLP (5 mg/mL) and H_2O_2-Vc at different concentrations (5, 10, 15, 20, and 25 mM) were added directly into the solution. Degradation times were 0.1, 0.3, 0.5, 0.7, and 0.9 h, and the temperature were maintained at 30, 40, 50, 60, and 70 °C. Reducing sugar content and α-glucosidase inhibition rate were used as screening indexes.

4.3.2. Response Surface Analysis

According to the single-factor experimental results, the response surface method was designed and implemented using the Box–Behnken Design (BBD) principle of Design-Expert 8.0.6 software, and the response surface results were fitted.

4.3.3. Preparation of Degradation Products from GLP

The polysaccharide was degraded by the optimal process obtained by the results of single-factor experiment and response surface analysis. The degradation product was neutralized (pH 7.0) with 1 M NaOH, concentrated to 1/3 volume at 60 °C using a rotary evaporator, and precipitated at 4 °C for 12 h with absolute ethanol (1:4, *v/v*). After centrifuging (8000 rpm, 15 min), the precipitation was dissolved with pure water in the magnetic blender, and then dialyzed (300 Da) at 4 °C for 48 h, and pure water was changed once at 4 h. After freeze-drying, the degradation product was obtained, named GLP-HV (*Gracilaria lemaneiformis* polysaccharide degraded by H_2O_2-Vc). Only H_2O_2 in the same concentration was used for polysaccharide, the other conditions were the same, the sample was obtained, named GLP-H (*Gracilaria lemaneiformis* polysaccharide degraded by H_2O_2). Only Vc in the same concentration was used for polysaccharide, the other conditions were the same, the sample was obtained, named GLP-V (*Gracilaria lemaneiformis* polysaccharide degraded by Vc). GLP-H and GLP-V were the controls of GLO-HV.

4.4. Analysis of Chemical Characterizatics

4.4.1. Determination of Total Sugar, Reducing Sugar and Protein Content

Total sugar, reducing sugar, and protein content were determined by phenol-sulfuric acid method with D-glucose as the standard compound, DNS (3,5-Dinitrosalicylic acid) method with D-glucose as the standard compound, and Coomassie Bright Blue kit.

4.4.2. Determination of Monosaccharide Composition

Monosaccharide composition was determined using high performance liquid chromatography (LC-20AD) according to the method reported by Kang et al. [9], with a slight modification. The analysis conducted with a drift tube temperature of 30 °C, wavelength of 250 nm, using Xtimate C18 column (4.6 mm × 250 mm, 5 μm) at 30 °C for 50 min. The monosaccharides were eluted using 0.05 M potassium dihydrogen phosphate (PH 6.7)-acetonitrile mobile phase (83:17) at a flow rate of 1 mL/min.

Derivatives of standard products: After the monosaccharide standards were dissolved in water, 250 uL 0.6 mol/L NaOH and 500 uL 0.4 mol/L PMP-methanol were added and reacted at 70 °C for 1 h. Subsequently, the solution was cooled in cold water for 10 min, 500 uL 0.3 mol/L HCl was added for neutralization, and 1 mL chloroform was added and mixed. Centrifugation was performed at 3000 r/min for 10 min. The supernatant was carefully taken and extracted three times.

Hydrolysis and derivatization of samples: appropriate amounts of samples were accurately weighed, 2 mL 2 mol/L trifluoroacetylacetone (TFA) was added and acidolized at 120 °C for 4 h. TFA was blow-dried with nitrogen and redissolved with 2 mL water. The derivatization procedure of the hydrolyzed sample solution was consistent with that of the standard.

4.4.3. Determination of Molecular Weight

Molecular weight was determined by Gel Permeation Chromatography (Shimadzu, Japan), referred to the report [36], with a slight modification. The analysis carried out on differential refractive index detector of RID-20A with a drift tube temperature of 35 °C, using TSKgel GMPWXL column for 25 min. The molecular weight was eluted using 0.1 M sodium nitrate (NaNO$_3$) and 0.06% Sodium azide (NaN$_3$) at a flow rate of 0.6 mL/min.

4.4.4. UV-Visible Spectroscopy

The method was referred to the previous research [37]. The absorption spectra of sample solutions (0.5 mg/mL) were measured using a UV-vis spectrophotometer (UV2550, Shimadzu, Japan), with the wavelength ranging from 200 to 700 nm with an interval of 1 nm.

4.4.5. I$_2$-KI Test

A polysaccharide and degradation products solution (2.0 mg/mL, 2.0 mL) was mixed with I$_2$-KI reagent (0.8 mL, containing 0.2% KI and 0.02% I$_2$, w/v) for 10 min. The absorbance was detected by a UV-vis spectrophotometer (UV2550, Japan) with the range of 300–700 nm [38].

4.4.6. Congo Red Test

Polysaccharide and degradation products solution (2 mg/L, 2.0 mL) were prepared, and 2 mL of 80 uM Congo red was added, and then 1 M NaOH was dropped to make the concentration of NaOH in different solutions vary from 0 to 0.5 mol/L. UV-vis spectrophotometer scanning (400–700 nm) was conducted to determine the maximum absorption wavelength under various concentration gradients of NaOH [33].

4.4.7. Scanning Electron Microscope Analysis (SEM)

The morphology of GLP, GLP-HV, GLP-H, and GLP-V were analyzed by SEM (SU 8010, Hitachi, Japan) [38]. These samples were dipped in a small amount of powder with conductive tape and pasted on the sample table. After spraying gold for 30–60 s, the samples were vacuumized and tested on the machine. The images were taken by SU 8010 Hitachi scanning electron microscope and the magnifications were 1000-fold and 200-flod, respectively.

4.5. The Inhibition Effect on α-Glucosidase

The inhibition effect on α-glucosidase was detected according to the previous report [26], with some modifications.

The inhibition rate: 30 μL polysaccharide and degradation products solution (0.1, 0.5, 1, 2.5, 5, 10 mg/mL), mixed with 100 μL phosphate buffer solution (PBS, 0.1 mol/L, pH 6.8,) and 30 μL α-glucoside enzyme solution (0.5 U/mL, pH 6.8, prepared by PBS) in 96-well plates, which incubated at 37 °C for 15 min. 30 μL PNPG solution (10 mmol/L, prepared by PBS) was mixed into the reaction mixture and incubated at 37 °C for 20 min. Then measured the absorbance value at 405 nm, and calculated the inhibitory activity according to the following formula:

$$\text{Inhibition rate}/\% = ((A_3 - A4) - (A_1 - A_2))/(A_3 - A4) \times 100, \qquad (1)$$

A_1: Samples and enzyme; A_2: The enzyme was replaced by PBS; A_3: Samples are replaced with pure water; A_4: Samples and enzyme were replaced with pure water and PBS, respectively.

Inhibition kinetics: The sample concentration was 0, 1, and 5 mg/mL, and the concentration of PNPG was 1, 2.5, 5, 7.5, and 10 mM, respectively. The reaction time was 20 min, and the determination was performed every 2 min. The Lineweaver–Burk curve was drawn by double reciprocal plotting method with reciprocal of substrate concentration as abscissa and reciprocal of reaction rate as ordinate, which calculated the Michaelis constant (*Km*), the maximum reaction rate (*Vmax*), according to the following formula:

$$1/v = Km/Vmax \times 1/([S]) + 1/Vmax, \tag{2}$$

V: initial reaction rate; *Vmax*: the maximum reaction rate; *[S]*: the concentration of PNPG; *Km*: the Michaelis constant.

Fluorescence spectrum analysis: The fluorescence spectrum analysis was studied according to literature [31] with some modifications. The excitation wavelength was 280 nm, the emission wavelength was 290–500 nm, and the slit width was 5 nm. 0.5 mL samples solution (5 mg/mL) and 2.5 mL α-glucosidase (5 U/mL) were taken, and the fluorescence spectrum was measured under these conditions after shaking and mixing, and the samples were replaced by PBS as blank. The samples with the best activity were prepared with concentrations of 0.1, 0.5, 1, 2.5, 5 and 10 mg/mL, and the fluorescence spectra were determined under the same conditions. The equation of Stern–Volmer was used to express the fluorescence quenching:

$$F_0/F = 1 + Ksv\,[Q] = 1 + Kq\,\tau_0\,[Q], \tag{3}$$

$$F_0/F = e^{\hat{}}(Ksv[Q]), \tag{4}$$

$$Ksv = Kq\tau_0, \tag{5}$$

$$\lg((F_0 - F)/F) = \lg Ka + n\lg[Q], \tag{6}$$

F_0: fluorescence intensity of α-glucosidase without samples; *F*: fluorescence intensity of α-glucosidase with samples; *[Q]*: the concentration of samples; τ_0: the average life of fluorescent substances without quenching agent is generally 10^{-8}; *Kq*: quenching rate constant; *Ksv*: quenching constant of Stern–Volmer. *Ka*: the binding constant between samples and α-glucosidase; n: the binding-site number.

4.6. Statistical Analysis

Data are expressed as means ± standard (SD). Duncan's multiple range test was applied to identify differences between the mean values for each group by IBM SPSS software (version 22). $p < 0.05$ was considered to represent statistical significance. The degradation experimental design and analysis was performed using Design-Expert 8.0.6. IC_{50} was calculated by IBM SPSS software 22. Figures were finished by Origin-Pro 8.5.

5. Conclusions

The optimal conditions for H_2O_2-Vc degradation were as follows: H_2O_2-Vc concentration was 18.7 mM, reaction time was 0.5 h, and reaction temperature was 56 °C. The total sugar content of GLP, GLP-HV, GLP-H and GLP-V were 98.77%, 98.43%, 97.28%, and 97.5%, respectively, and their reducing sugar were 2.47%, 46.92%, 1.95%, and 50.2%, respectively. Moreover, the Mw was reduced after degradation, and the monosaccharides were mainly glucose and galactose before and after degradation. In addition, GLP and its degradation products did not have protein, starch, and triple helix structure. The degradation method of H_2O_2-Vc is feasible, and no by-products can be produced. The SEM analysis demonstrated that H_2O_2-Vc made the structure loose and broken. All samples showed the inhibition on α-glucosidase, and GLP-HV presented the best effect in a dose-dependent manner, which was the mixed type of competitive and non-competitive. It had a certain quenching effect on fluorescence of α-glucosidase, which may be dynamic quenching. The polysaccharide degraded by H_2O_2-Vc, with low Mw, exerted the good inhibition effect on glucosidase activity.

Author Contributions: Conceptualization, X.L.; methodology, H.X.; investigation, S.C., S.Z.; resources, X.H., L.L., X.Y.; data curation, S.L.; writing—original draft preparation, X.L.; writing—review and editing, X.H., X.Y. All authors have read and agreed to the published version of the manuscript.

Funding: This work was supported by the Key-Area Research and Development Program of Guangdong Province (2020B1111030004), the National Key R&D Program of China (2019YFD0901905), the China Agriculture Research System of MOF and MARA (CARS-50), the Special Scientific Research Funds for Central Non-profit Institutes, Chinese Academy of Fishery Sciences (2020TD69), and the Central Public-interest Scientific Institution Basal Research Funds, South China Sea Fisheries Research Institute, CAFS (2021SD06).

Institutional Review Board Statement: Not applicable.

Informed Consent Statement: Not applicable.

Data Availability Statement: Data is contained within the article.

Conflicts of Interest: The authors declare no conflict of interest.

References

1. Yu, Y.-Y.; Chen, W.-D.; Liu, Y.-J.; Niu, J.; Chen, M.; Tian, L.-X. Effect of different dietary levels of Gracilaria lemaneiformis dry power on growth performance, hematological parameters and intestinal structure of juvenile Pacific white shrimp (*Litopenaeus vannamei*). *Aquaculture* **2016**, *450*, 356–362. [CrossRef]
2. Long, X.; Hu, X.; Liu, S.; Pan, C.; Chen, S.; Li, L.; Qi, B.; Yang, X. Insights on preparation, structure and activities of Gracilaria lemaneiformis polysaccharide. *Food Chem. X* **2021**, *12*, 100153. [CrossRef]
3. Fisheries Administration of Ministry of Agriculture and Rural Affairs. *China Fishery Statistical Yearbook*; China Agriculture Press: Beijing, China, 2020.
4. Li, X.; Huang, S.; Chen, X.; Xu, Q.; Ma, Y.; You, L.; Kulikouskaya, V.; Xiao, J.; Piao, J. Structural characteristic of a sulfated polysaccharide from Gracilaria Lemaneiformis and its lipid metabolism regulation effect. *Food Funct.* **2020**, *11*, 10876–10885. [CrossRef] [PubMed]
5. Sun, X.; Duan, M.; Liu, Y.; Luo, T.; Ma, N.; Song, S.; Ai, C. The beneficial effects of Gracilaria lemaneiformis polysaccharides on obesity and the gut microbiota in high fat diet-fed mice. *J. Funct. Foods* **2018**, *46*, 48–56. [CrossRef]
6. Fan, Y.; Wang, W.; Song, W.; Chen, H.; Teng, A.; Liu, A. Partial characterization and anti-tumor activity of an acidic polysaccharide from Gracilaria lemaneiformis. *Carbohydr. Polym.* **2012**, *88*, 1313–1318. [CrossRef]
7. Chen, M.-Z.; Xie, H.-G.; Yang, L.-W.; Liao, Z.-H.; Yu, J. In vitro anti-influenza virus activities of sulfated polysaccharide fractions from Gracilaria lemaneiformis. *Virol. Sin.* **2010**, *25*, 341–351. [CrossRef]
8. Wang, X.; Zhang, Z.; Zhou, H.; Sun, X.; Chen, X.; Xu, N. The anti-aging effects of Gracilaria lemaneiformis polysaccharide in Caenorhabditis elegans. *Int. J. Biol. Macromol.* **2019**, *140*, 600–604. [CrossRef]
9. Kang, Y.; Wang, Z.-J.; Xie, D.; Sun, X.; Yang, W.; Zhao, X.; Xu, N. Characterization and Potential Antitumor Activity of Polysaccharide from Gracilariopsis lemaneiformis. *Mar. Drugs* **2017**, *15*, 100. [CrossRef]
10. Chen, S.; Liu, H.; Yang, X.; Li, L.; Qi, B.; Hu, X.; Ma, H.; Li, C.; Pan, C. Degradation of sulphated polysaccharides from Grateloupia livida and antioxidant activity of the degraded components. *Int. J. Biol. Macromol.* **2020**, *156*, 660–668. [CrossRef]
11. Gong, Y.; Ma, Y.; Cheung, P.C.-K.; You, L.; Liao, L.; Pedisić, S.; Kulikouskaya, V. Structural characteristics and anti-inflammatory activity of UV/H2O2-treated algal sulfated polysaccharide from Gracilaria lemaneiformis. *Food Chem. Toxicol.* **2021**, *152*, 112157. [CrossRef]
12. Zhang, X.; Aweya, J.J.; Huang, Z.-X.; Kang, Z.-Y.; Bai, Z.-H.; Li, K.-H.; He, X.-T.; Liu, Y.; Chen, X.-Q.; Cheong, K.-L. In vitro fermentation of Gracilaria lemaneiformis sulfated polysaccharides and its agaro-oligosaccharides by human fecal inocula and its impact on microbiota. *Carbohydr. Polym.* **2020**, *234*, 115894. [CrossRef] [PubMed]
13. Xu, X.-Q.; Su, B.-M.; Xie, J.-S.; Li, R.-K.; Yang, J.; Lin, J.; Ye, X.-Y. Preparation of bioactive neoagaroligosaccharides through hydrolysis of Gracilaria lemaneiformis agar: A comparative study. *Food Chem.* **2018**, *240*, 330–337. [CrossRef] [PubMed]
14. Jin, M.; Liu, H.; Hou, Y.; Chan, Z.; Di, W.; Li, L.; Zeng, R. Preparation, characterization and alcoholic liver injury protective effects of algal oligosaccharides from Gracilaria lemaneiformis. *Food Res. Int.* **2017**, *100*, 186–195. [CrossRef] [PubMed]
15. Liu, Q.; Zhang, Y.; Shu, Z.; Liu, M.; Zeng, R.; Wang, Y.; Liu, H.; Cao, M.; Su, W.; Liu, G. Sulfated oligosaccharide of Gracilaria lemaneiformis protect against food allergic response in mice by up-regulating immunosuppression. *Carbohydr. Polym.* **2020**, *230*, 115567. [CrossRef] [PubMed]
16. Yan, S.; Pan, C.; Yang, X.; Chen, S.; Qi, B.; Huang, H. Degradation of Codium cylindricum polysaccharides by H2O2-Vc-ultrasonic and H2O2-Fe2+-ultrasonic treatment: Structural characterization and antioxidant activity. *Int. J. Biol. Macromol.* **2021**, *182*, 129–135. [CrossRef]
17. Shen, X.; Liu, Z.; Li, J.; Wu, D.; Zhu, M.; Yan, L.; Mao, G.; Ye, X.; Linhardt, R.J.; Chen, S. Development of low molecular weight heparin by H2O2/ascorbic acid with ultrasonic power and its anti-metastasis property. *Int. J. Biol. Macromol.* **2019**, *133*, 101–109. [CrossRef]
18. Shokri, Z.; Seidi, F.; Karami, S.; Li, C.; Saeb, M.R.; Xiao, H. Laccase Immobilization onto Natural Polysaccharides for Biosensing and Biodegradation. *Carbohydr. Polym.* **2021**, *262*, 117963. [CrossRef]

19. Chen, H.; Xiao, Q.; Weng, H.; Zhang, Y.; Yang, Q.; Xiao, A. Extraction of sulfated agar from Gracilaria lemaneiformis using hydrogen peroxide-assisted enzymatic method. *Carbohydr. Polym.* **2020**, *232*, 115790. [CrossRef] [PubMed]
20. Chen, X.; Li, X.; Sun-Waterhouse, D.; Zhu, B.; You, L.; Hileuskaya, K. Polysaccharides from Sargassum fusiforme after UV/H2O2 degradation effectively ameliorate dextran sulfate sodium-induced colitis. *Food Funct.* **2021**, *12*, 11747–11759. [CrossRef]
21. Li, J.; Li, S.; Liu, S.; Wei, C.; Yan, L.; Ding, T.; Linhardt, R.J.; Liu, D.; Ye, X.; Chen, S. Pectic oligosaccharides hydrolyzed from citrus canning processing water by Fenton reaction and their antiproliferation potentials. *Int. J. Biol. Macromol.* **2019**, *124*, 1025–1032. [CrossRef]
22. Nasab, S.B.; Homaei, A.; Pletschke, B.I.; Salinas-Salazar, C.; Castillo-Zacarias, C.; Parra-Saldívar, R. Marine resources effective in controlling and treating diabetes and its associated complications. *Process. Biochem.* **2020**, *92*, 313–342. [CrossRef]
23. Lim, J.; Ferruzzi, M.G.; Hamaker, B.R. Structural requirements of flavonoids for the selective inhibition of α-amylase versus α-glucosidase. *Food Chem.* **2022**, *370*, 130981. [CrossRef] [PubMed]
24. Wen, L.; Zhang, Y.; Sun-Waterhouse, D.; You, L.; Fu, X. Advantages of the polysaccharides from Gracilaria lemaneiformis over metformin in antidiabetic effects on streptozotocin-induced diabetic mice. *RSC Adv.* **2017**, *7*, 9141–9151. [CrossRef]
25. Liao, X.; Yang, L.; Chen, M.; Yu, J.; Zhang, S.; Ju, Y. The hypoglycemic effect of a polysaccharide (GLP) from Gracilaria lemaneiformis and its degradation products in diabetic mice. *Food Funct.* **2015**, *6*, 2542–2549. [CrossRef]
26. Zheng, Q.; Jia, R.-B.; Ou, Z.-R.; Li, Z.-R.; Zhao, M.; Luo, D.; Lin, L. Comparative study on the structural characterization and α-glucosidase inhibitory activity of polysaccharide fractions extracted from Sargassum fusiforme at different pH conditions. *Int. J. Biol. Macromol.* **2021**. [CrossRef] [PubMed]
27. Wu, L.; Lu, M.; Wang, S. Amylase-assisted extraction and antioxidant activity of polysaccharides from Gracilaria lemaneiformis. *3 Biotech* **2017**, *7*, 341. [CrossRef]
28. Liu, Q.-M.; Yang, Y.; Maleki, S.J.; Alcocer, M.; Xu, S.-S.; Shi, C.-L.; Cao, M.-J.; Liu, G.-M. Anti-Food Allergic Activity of Sulfated Polysaccharide from Gracilaria lemaneiformis is Dependent on Immunosuppression and Inhibition of p38 MAPK. *J. Agric. Food Chem.* **2016**, *64*, 4536–4544. [CrossRef]
29. Ren, Y.; Zheng, G.; You, L.; Wen, L.; Li, C.; Fu, X.; Zhou, L. Structural characterization and macrophage immunomodulatory activity of a polysaccharide isolated from Gracilaria lemaneiformis. *J. Funct. Foods* **2017**, *33*, 286–296. [CrossRef]
30. Lv, Q.-Q.; Cao, J.-J.; Liu, R.; Chen, H.-Q. Structural characterization, α-amylase and α-glucosidase inhibitory activities of polysaccharides from wheat bran. *Food Chem.* **2021**, *341*, 128218. [CrossRef]
31. Fu, M.; Shen, W.; Gao, W.; Namujia, L.; Yang, X.; Cao, J.; Sun, L. Essential moieties of myricetins, quercetins and catechins for binding and inhibitory activity against α-Glucosidase. *Bioorganic Chem.* **2021**, *115*, 105235. [CrossRef]
32. Cao, X.; Xia, Y.; Liu, D.; He, Y.; Mu, T.; Huo, Y.; Liu, J. Inhibitory effects of Lentinus edodes mycelia polysaccharide on α-glucosidase, glycation activity and high glucose-induced cell damage. *Carbohydr. Polym.* **2020**, *246*, 116659. [CrossRef]
33. Zhao, M.; Bai, J.; Bu, X.; Yin, Y.; Wang, L.; Yang, Y.; Xu, Y. Characterization of selenized polysaccharides from Ribes nigrum L. and its inhibitory effects on α-amylase and α-glucosidase. *Carbohydr. Polym.* **2021**, *259*, 117729. [CrossRef] [PubMed]
34. Wang, S.; Li, Y.; Huang, D.; Chen, S.; Xia, Y.; Zhu, S. The inhibitory mechanism of chlorogenic acid and its acylated derivatives on α-amylase and α-glucosidase. *Food Chem.* **2022**, *372*, 131334. [CrossRef] [PubMed]
35. Bharathi, D.; Siddlingeshwar, B.; Krishna, R.H.; Kirilova, E.M.; Divakar, D.D.; Alkheraif, A.A. Interaction of CuO and ZnO nanoparticles with 3-N-(N′-methylacetamidino) benzanthrone: A temperature dependent fluorescence quenching study. *Inorg. Chem. Commun.* **2021**, *134*, 109069. [CrossRef]
36. Zhang, S.; Hong, H.; Zhang, H.; Chen, Z. Investigation of anti-aging mechanism of multi-dimensional nanomaterials modified asphalt by FTIR, NMR and GPC. *Constr. Build. Mater.* **2021**, *305*, 124809. [CrossRef]
37. Pattanayak, S.; Chakraborty, S.; Biswas, S.; Chattopadhyay, D.; Chakraborty, M. Degradation of Methyl Parathion, a common pesticide and fluorescence quenching of Rhodamine B, a carcinogen using β-d glucan stabilized gold nanoparticles. *J. Saudi Chem. Soc.* **2018**, *22*, 937–948. [CrossRef]
38. Wang, L.; Li, L.; Gao, J.; Huang, J.; Yang, Y.; Xu, Y.; Liu, S.; Yu, W. Characterization, antioxidant and immunomodulatory effects of selenized polysaccharides from dandelion roots. *Carbohydr. Polym.* **2021**, *260*, 117796. [CrossRef]

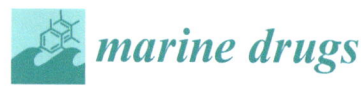

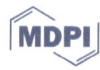

Review

Computational Approaches to Enzyme Inhibition by Marine Natural Products in the Search for New Drugs

Federico Gago

Department of Biomedical Sciences & IQM-CSIC Associate Unit, School of Medicine and Health Sciences, University of Alcalá, E-28805 Madrid, Alcalá de Henares, Spain; federico.gago@uah.es; Tel.: +34-918854514

Abstract: The exploration of biologically relevant chemical space for the discovery of small bioactive molecules present in marine organisms has led not only to important advances in certain therapeutic areas, but also to a better understanding of many life processes. The still largely untapped reservoir of countless metabolites that play biological roles in marine invertebrates and microorganisms opens new avenues and poses new challenges for research. Computational technologies provide the means to (i) organize chemical and biological information in easily searchable and hyperlinked databases and knowledgebases; (ii) carry out cheminformatic analyses on natural products; (iii) mine microbial genomes for known and cryptic biosynthetic pathways; (iv) explore global networks that connect active compounds to their targets (often including enzymes); (v) solve structures of ligands, targets, and their respective complexes using X-ray crystallography and NMR techniques, thus enabling virtual screening and structure-based drug design; and (vi) build molecular models to simulate ligand binding and understand mechanisms of action in atomic detail. Marine natural products are viewed today not only as potential drugs, but also as an invaluable source of chemical inspiration for the development of novel chemotypes to be used in chemical biology and medicinal chemistry research.

Keywords: enzyme inhibitors; databases; cheminformatics

Citation: Gago, F. Computational Approaches to Enzyme Inhibition by Marine Natural Products in the Search for New Drugs. *Mar. Drugs* **2023**, *21*, 100. https://doi.org/10.3390/md21020100

Received: 21 December 2022
Revised: 26 January 2023
Accepted: 28 January 2023
Published: 30 January 2023

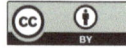

1. Overview

Both pharmacology and basic cell biology have traditionally benefited from the continuous identification and biochemical characterization of active principles obtained from natural sources. The scanty primitive chemical libraries of natural products (NPs), consisting mostly of the alkaloids and heterosides isolated from terrestrial plants that provided the foundations of modern pharmacology [1], were progressively enriched with a multitude of small- to medium-sized molecules present in numerous living creatures, both big and small, including those inhabiting seas and oceans, which together make up a huge water mass that covers >70% of Earth's total surface and hosts ~80% of all living species [2]. Nonetheless, and despite a notable renaissance in recent years [3,4], the list of marine natural products (MNPs) that have been approved or are currently found in the global marine pharmaceutical clinical pipeline (https://www.midwestern.edu/departments/marinepharmacology/clinical-pipeline, accessed on 20 December 2022) is still very limited, and only a few of these drugs actually target an enzyme.

The vastness of the largely unexplored chemical space [5] existing in marine environments poses daunting challenges in terms of (i) sample recollection, (ii) compound isolation, (iii) chemical characterization, (iv) evaluation in as many biochemical and/or biological assays as possible, preferably using validated targets and high-throughput state-of-the-art technologies [6], and (v) the identification and validation of pharmacologically relevant targets. Given the precedents of successful marine leads as a source of useful medicinal agents and biochemical probes, it can be argued that it makes sense to continue exploiting over four billion years of evolution in nature's combinatorial chemistry, often subjected to unique ecological pressures and nutrient availability, that led to selective survival advantages in the producing organisms [7]. The best studied phylogenetically diverse living beings from marine habitats include green, brown, and red algae; sponges; coelenterates (i.e., jellyfishes, corals, and sea anemones); bryozoans (i.e., invertebrates known as moss animals); the Ascidiacea class (commonly known as the ascidians, tunicates, and sea squirts); mollusks; echinoderms; phytoplankton; and innumerable bacteria and fungi. Secondary metabolites are specialized organic compounds that are not considered essential for normal growth or reproduction (under laboratory culture conditions) but instead play roles in evolution, communication (as chemical cues), and competition, or else appear to be used as chemical weaponry against prey or natural enemies in their natural environments. MNPs often feature unique scaffolds and carbocyclic skeletons, and many have been discovered following their bioassay-guided isolation, although the paucity of material usually prevents the full profiling of bioactivity [8], which is often limited to some rudimentary tests (e.g., phenotype-oriented antimicrobial or cytotoxic assays [9], and/or inhibitory activity against one enzyme or a limited set of enzymes). In this respect, it has been pointed out that micromolar activities detected in extracts should be critically analyzed because of potential artefactual assay readouts due to unspecific aggregation [10], hence the recommendation to use β-lactamase and malate dehydrogenase as counter-screening enzymes [11], among other precautionary measures.

Recent progress in understanding the genetic basis of MNP biosynthesis and the ever-increasing availability of genomic information have created unique opportunities to develop sequence-based approaches for the discovery of novel bioactive molecular entities [12]. Polyketide synthases (PKSs) and multimodular nonribosomal peptide synthetases (NRPS) stand out among the enzymes that are ultimately responsible for the highly efficient synthesis of three large subclasses of important NPs (PKs, NRPs, and PK/RP or NRP/PK hybrids) [13] through the concerted assembly of relatively simple carboxylic acid and amino acid building blocks, respectively [14,15]. Type I PKSs consist of multiple modules, with each module minimally containing three core domains: acyltransferase (AT) domain, ketosynthase (KS) domain, and thiolation (T) domain [aka acyl carrier protein (ACP) domain] [16]. These (mega)enzymes are encoded in biosynthetic gene clusters (BGCs), which have been identified for hundreds of bacterial and fungal metabolites and are highly evolved for horizontal exchange [17]. Besides, attention continues to be drawn to two facts that have significantly expanded the area of MNP research, namely (i) that some isolated MNPs are bioaccumulated in the target organism from dietary sources, e.g., algae [18]; and (ii) that a significant number of MNPs are actually produced by microbes and/or microbial interactions with the "host from whence it was isolated" [8]. The growing emphasis on the study of compounds from microbial sources (both terrestrial and marine) has been fueled by interest in (i) the central role that microorganisms play in mediating both interspecies interactions and host-microbe relationships [19]; and (ii) their natural ability to produce ribosomally synthesized and post-translationally modified peptides (RiPPs), which often contain noncanonical amino acids and structural motifs that give rise to a currently under-represented class of biologically active molecules [20,21].

Modern science (and the world at large) is overly dependent on computer and internet technologies. Computers have a long history in data management, as well as in information storage, processing, retrieval, and dissemination, and for these purposes their use has expanded enormously in recent years and has contributed to shaping the current research landscapes in bioscience and biomedicine as we know them today. The World Wide Web has become a central source of (i) information on all possible subjects that is stored and (ideally) curated in extensively hyperlinked databases; (ii) educational and research tools; and (iii) services that are intended to make life easier not only for the general public, but also for scientists, including those devoted to chemical biology, medicinal chemistry, and drug discovery. Devices ranging from pocket computers, also known as mobile or cellular phones which have superseded earlier personal digital assistants (PDA), to tablets, laptops, desktops, mainframes, and supercomputers dominate many aspects of our lives and complement human skills in numerous applications designed to utilize an ever-growing torrent of biological and chemical data in effective manners. While this is the driving force behind the increasing use of high-performance computing, machine learning and artificial intelligence for processing tons of data in a way that compensates for the inherent constraints of human cognition [22], better-informed decision making in drug discovery and development still largely relies (or so I like to believe) on the power of human judgement and life-long expertise.

The concise Guide to Pharmacology (https://www.guidetopharmacology.org/; latest release 13 October 2022, accessed on 20 December 2022) presented by the International Union of Basic and Clinical Pharmacology (IUPHAR) and the British Pharmacological Society (BPS) includes enzymes (Nature's catalysts essential to the chemistry of life) as one of the six major classes of pharmacological targets, the others being G protein-coupled receptors, ion channels, nuclear hormone receptors, catalytic receptors, and transporters (including the very large SLC superfamily of solute carriers) [23]. Over one thousand distinct human enzymes are described in the Universal Protein Knowledgebase (UniProtKB) [24], therefore representing almost half of all current human targets. Fortunately, the three-dimensional (3D) structures of many of these enzymes or closely related counterparts from other species—both in their apo forms and in complexes with ligands—have been solved and deposited in the Worldwide Protein Data Bank (wwPDB) [25], a continuously enlarging global repository established in 1971. These 3D structures facilitate the elucidation of functional mechanisms, aid in understanding the binding mode of inhibitors, and enable virtual screening (VS) and structure-based drug design (SBDD) technologies. For other enzymes of interest, we still depend on several homology modeling approaches [26], neural network-based models, such as those generated by AlphaFold [27], and artificial intelligence, which was recently employed to build the ESM Metagenomic Atlas (https://esmatlas.com/, accessed on 20 December 2022), with more than 617 million structures from all kingdoms of life [28].

Following the recommendations of the Nomenclature Committee of the International Union of Biochemistry and Molecular Biology (IUBMB, https://www.qmul.ac.uk/sbcs/iubmb/enzyme/; accessed on 20 December 2022), the wwPDB assigns Enzyme Commission (EC) numbers to protein chains in macromolecular structures according to the type of chemical reaction that they catalyze. The main classes are oxidoreductases (EC 1), transferases (EC 2), hydrolases (EC 3), lyases (EC 4), isomerases (EC 5), ligases (EC 6), and translocases (EC 7), with subclasses (with up to 4 digits) being defined on the basis of the specific donors and receptors of chemical groups that participate in the reactions and additional considerations. The main collection of functional enzyme and metabolism data is possibly BRENDA (https://www.brenda-enzymes.org/, accessed on 20 December 2022), which was established in 1987 and selected as an ELIXIR Core Data Resource [29] in 2018 [30]. In addition, the merging of MACiE (Mechanism, Annotation and Classification in Enzymes), a database of enzyme mechanisms, and CSA (Catalytic Site Atlas), a database of catalytic sites of enzymes, has resulted in the M-CSA Mechanism and Catalytic Site Atlas (http://www.ebi.ac.uk/thornton-srv/m-csa/browse/?sort=ec, accessed on 20 December 2022) [31], which consolidates a body of knowledge on enzyme structures, gene sequences, reaction mechanisms, metabolic pathways, and kinetic data that any researcher working on enzyme inhibitors should be familiar with.

Building on this introductory background information, the following sections will separately cover each of the abovementioned aspects for which specialized computer technologies have been developed in the field of enzyme inhibition by MNPs (Figure 1).

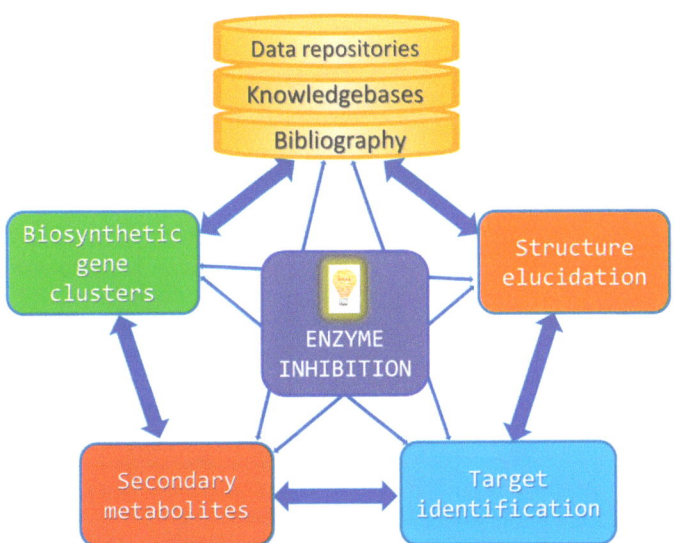

Figure 1. Simplified interrelationship diagram illustrating how the design/identification of enzyme inhibitors from marine sources can benefit from the use of computer-aided methods.

2. Bibliographical Sources and Virtual NP Databases

Chemical libraries encompassing millions of compounds include the Chemical Abstracts Service (CAS) REGISTRY database (http://www.cas.org/expertise/cascontent/registry/index.html, accessed on 20 December 2022), which is updated on a daily basis and contains >250,000 NPs out of >150 million chemical substances, PubChem (including PC-Substance, PCCompound, and PCBioAssay) [32], ChEMBL (a manually curated database of >2,300,000 bioactive molecules with drug-like properties, last update July 2022) [33], and ChemSpider (with various levels of partial to complete stereochemistry) [34]. The free-to-access resource DrugBank is a web-enabled database (https://go.drugbank.com/, accessed on 20 December 2022) that incorporates comprehensive molecular information about drugs, their mechanisms, their interactions, and their targets. First described in 2006 as a knowledgebase for drugs, drug actions, and drug targets [35], DrugBank has evolved over time in response to improvements in web standards and changing needs for drug research and development. The latest update, DrugBank 5.0 [36], was expanded to cover not only drug binding data, numerous investigational drugs, drug-drug and drug-food interactions, and SNP-associated drug effects, but also information on the influence of hundreds of drugs on metabolite levels (pharmacometabolomics), gene expression levels (pharmacotranscriptomics), and protein expression levels (pharmacoproteomics). Enzyme inhibitors (DBCAT000003) are described as "compounds or agents that combine with an enzyme in such a manner as to prevent the normal substrate-enzyme combination and the catalytic reaction".

Reviews on MNPs have been published on a regular basis in the scientific literature [37–39]. The renewed upsurge of interest in NPs, and MNPs in particular, over the last two decades has led to a rapid multiplication of databases in both the private sector and the public domain that compile general-purpose or thematic information on these naturally occurring compounds, often incorporating supplementary material published in scientific papers. A dedicated, searchable, and continuously updated database (MarinLit, https://marinlit.rsc.org/, accessed on 20 December 2022) that was established in the 1970s by Prof. John Blunt and Prof. Murray Munro (University of Canterbury, New Zealand) has been maintained by the Royal Society of Chemistry (UK) since 2014. MarinLit covers ~40,000 compounds from marine macro- and microorganisms and about the same number of references to journal articles. Among the specialized MNP databases, the Dictionary of Marine Natural Products (DMNP) [40] appeared as the first of its kind in 2008 and encompassed a subset of data from the Dictionary of Natural Products (DNP, one of several Chapman & Hall chemical dictionaries) based on the biological source of the compounds. DMNP was marketed as a book together with a CD-ROM for a desktop version, and the searchable web-based version CHEMnetBASE (https://dmnp.chemnetbase.com/, accessed on 20 December 2022) is still available (v. 31.1; updated in 2022), but only to subscribing institutions.

Virtual chemical libraries of NPs can be categorized into (i) encyclopedic and general NP databases; (ii) special subsets within fully enumerated, ultra-large scale chemical libraries specifically built to facilitate VS campaigns, e.g., ZINC [41,42]; (iii) compound collections enriched with NPs used in traditional medicines; and (iv) specialized databases focused on specific habitats, geographical regions, organisms, biological activities, or even specific NP classes. Unfortunately, many NP databases belonging to the latter two categories are rather ephemeral or rapidly become either outdated or unavailable to the scientific community [43], and the same criticism applies to many bioinformatics web services related to NPs [44]. This is most likely due to (i) a lack of funds (and/or human resources) for their sustained management and continuous upgrading, and (ii) the current overwhelming "data deluge". For these reasons, there is an urgent need for nonredundant, community-wide efforts that optimize the use of contemporary bioinformatic and chemoinformatic capabilities, as exemplified by the recently established open platform LOTUS (https://lotus.naturalproducts.net, accessed on 20 December 2022), a knowledgebase that is expected to have strong transformative potential for research on NPs and beyond [45]. In this praiseworthy initiative, data sharing within the Wikidata framework broadens interoperability and facilitates access to >750,000 referenced structure-organism pairs.

Another large and freely available NP database is Super Natural II (https://bioinf-applied.charite.de/supernatural_new/index.php; last updated: October 2022, accessed on 20 December 2022), which provides two-dimensional (2D) structures and physicochemical properties for ~326,000 molecules, as well as information about the pathways associated to their synthesis, degradation, and mechanisms of action with respect to structurally similar drugs [46]. An additional recent compilation of 400,000 non-redundant NPs was made available in 2021 [47] as the open-access COlleCtion of Open NatUral producTs (COCONUT, https://coconut.naturalproducts.net/, accessed on 20 December 2022).

One important goal of these NP databases is to facilitate a quick assessment of novelty for any newly identified compound in a natural extract. To distinguish between known and unknown compounds, it is important to have rapid and trustworthy "dereplication" methods, which rely heavily on the interpretation of molecular mass and molecular formula, as well as UV and NMR spectral data [48]. Nevertheless, the dereplication process can be problematic sometimes because (i) the present validity and accuracy of the collected information is only as good as that of the original data source; and (ii) stereochemical information on NPs is often inaccurate or incomplete. In the field of MNPs alone, it was recently reported that more than 200 structures were misassigned in the last ten years only [49]. A comparative analysis of the original and the revised structures revealed that major pitfalls still plague the structural elucidation of small molecules and, consequently, that quite a few 3D molecular structures present in databases may be inaccurate. This finding emphasizes the roles of total synthesis, X-ray crystallography, as well as chemical and biosynthetic logic, to complement spectroscopic data. Nevertheless, it is noteworthy that a much lower incidence of "impossible" structures was found in MNPs compared to NPs of plant origin.

The utilization of computer-assisted structure elucidation (CASE) programs can minimize the risk of misassignment and help identify truly novel compounds (the "unknown unknowns") [50] by generating all structures that are consistent with key data from 2D correlation spectroscopy (COSY), heteronuclear multiple bond correlation (HMBC), and 1,1-adequate sensitivity double-quantum spectroscopy (ADEQUATE) NMR experiments, and by ranking the resulting structures in order of probability. The algorithms may additionally benefit from both stereospecific NMR data and use of optimized geometries and predicted chemical shifts provided by density funtional theory (DFT) quantum mechanical calculations [51]. The absolute configuration of an MNP can be unequivocally confirmed by crystallographic analysis and, in the case of noncrystalline compounds containing a pseudo-meso core structure that results in a specific rotation ($[a]_D$) of almost zero (e.g., elatenyne), it may be necessary to absorb the compound into a porous coordination network (a "crystalline sponge") [52].

The exploration of the identities and biological activities of metabolites present in complex mixtures has benefited enormously in recent years from scalable native and functional metabolomics approaches [53]. Novel techniques, such as affinity selection mass spectrometry (MS), complemented with pulsed ultrafiltration, size exclusion chromatography, and magnetic microbead affinity selection screening, now allow the separation of non-covalent ligand-receptor complexes from other nonbinding compounds [54].

Recognizing the need for community-wide platforms to effectively share and analyze raw, processed, or identified tandem MS (MS/MS or MS^2) data of NPs, in an analogous fashion to what has been achieved in genomics and proteomics research with the GenBank® at the National Center for Biotechnology Information (NCBI) [55] and the UniProtKB [56], the open-access knowledgebase known as Global Natural Products Social Molecular Networking (GNPS, http://gnps.ucsd.edu, accessed on 20 December 2022) was presented in 2017 [57]. The spectral libraries enable unambiguous dereplication (by matching spectral features of the unknown compound(s) to curated spectral databases of reference compounds, i.e., identification of "known unknowns") [50], variable dereplication (approximate matches to spectra of related molecules), and the identification of spectra in molecular networks. Importantly, GNPS allows for the community-driven, iterative re-annotation of reference MS/MS spectra in a wiki-like fashion, and therefore it will contribute to library improvements and eventual convergence of all curated MS/MS spectra. The visualization of molecular networks in GNPS represents each spectrum as a node, and spectrum-to-spectrum alignments as edges (connections) between nodes.

3. Linking Chemical Diversity of Secondary Metabolites to Biosynthetic Gene Clusters

Secondary metabolites can be considered genetically encoded small molecules that play a variety of roles in cell biology and therefore have the potential to become chemical probes or drug leads. Their identification and characterization can benefit from a growing number of databases and genomics-based computational tools that have been compiled and hyperlinked at the Secondary Metabolite Bioinformatics Portal (SMBP (http://www.secondarymetabolites.org/, accessed on 20 December 2022) website [58]. Inherent limitations related to their low production and difficult detection, and also high rediscovery rates, can be addressed, at least in part, by searching for BGCs in genomic data and unveiling their (sometimes cryptic) metabolic potential [59]. However, the highly repetitive nature of the associated genes creates major challenges for accurate sequence assembly and analysis, hence the need for new bioinformatic tools. An example is the Natural Product Domain Seeker (NaPDoS) web service (https://npdomainseeker.sdsc.edu/napdos2/, accessed on 20 December 2022), which provides an automated method to assess the secondary metabolite biosynthetic gene diversity and novelty of strains or environments. NaPDoS analyses are based on the phylogenetic relationships of sequence tags derived from genes encoding PKS and NRPS, respectively. The sequence tags correspond to PKS-derived KS domains and NRPS-derived condensation (C) domains and are compared to an internal database of experimentally characterized biosynthetic genes, so that genes associated with uncharacterized biochemistry can be identified [60]. The latest update (NaPDoS2) greatly expands the taxonomic and functional diversity represented in the webtool database and allows larger datasets to be analyzed. Importantly, NaPDoS2 can be used to detect genes involved in the biosynthesis of specific structural classes or new biosynthetic mechanisms, and also to predict biosynthetic potential [61].

The key role of marine microbial symbionts of invertebrates in MNP biosynthesis has been increasingly recognized [62] and "genome mining" (i.e., the exploitation of genomic information for the discovery of biosynthetic pathways) [63] provides unique opportunities for (i) the identification of yet undisclosed specialized metabolites [64] and their chemical variants [63]; (ii) the genetic engineering of BGCs to obtain novel "unnatural" NPs [65]; and (iii) the heterologous expression of secondary metabolic pathways that remain silent or are poorly expressed in the absence of a specific trigger or elicitor [66]. In fact, the results of a variety of genome sequencing projects have unveiled the metabolic diversity of microorganisms (which may be overlooked under standard fermentation and detection conditions) and their tremendous biosynthetic potential. Furthermore, studies on the evolutionary history of BGCs in relation to that of the bacteria harboring them ("comparative genomics") beautifully illustrate the mechanisms by which chemical diversity is created in nature and how some NPs represent ecotype-defining traits while others appear selectively neutral [67].

Novel algorithms have been devised to systematically identify BGCs in microbial genomic sequences [12,63,68]. A network analysis of the predicted BGCs in Proteobacteria (aka Pseudomonadota, a major phylum of Gram-negative bacteria) has revealed large gene cluster families, and the experimental characterization of the most prominent one revealed two subfamilies consisting of hundreds of BGCs encoding the biochemical machinery for the synthesis of a series of remarkably conserved lipids with an aryl head group conjugated to a polyene tail (i.e., aryl polyenes) that are likely to play important roles in Gram-negative cell biology [17]. The systematic study of BGCs in Actinobacteria (actinomycetes mainly associated to sponges in marine habitats) is complicated by numerous repetitive motifs. By combining several metrics, a method for the global classification of these gene clusters into families (GCFs) has been developed, and the biosynthetic capacity of the resulting GCF network has been validated in hundreds of strains by correlating confident MS detection of known NPs with the presence or absence of their established BGCs [69].

The Minimum Information about a Biosynthetic Gene cluster (MIBiG, https://mibig.secondarymetabolites.org/, accessed on 20 December 2022) specification is a data standard that facilitates the consistent and systematic deposition and retrieval of metadata on BGCs and their molecular products [70]. MIBiG is a Genomic Standards Consortium project that builds on the Minimum Information about any Sequence (MIxS) framework to (i) identify which genes are responsible for the biosynthesis of which chemical moieties, thus systematically connecting genes and chemistry; (ii) understand the natural genetic diversity of BGCs within their environmental and ecological context; and (iii) develop an evidence-based parts registry for engineering biosynthetic pathways and gene clusters through synthetic biology. The MIBiG standard contains dedicated class-specific checklists for gene clusters encoding pathways to produce alkaloids, saccharides, terpenes, polyketides, NRPs, and RiPPs [20].

Natural antimicrobial peptides (AMPs) have been found not only in marine fish [71,72] but also in marine invertebrates [73,74] as major components of their innate host defense systems. The Antimicrobial Peptide Database (APD, https://aps.unmc.edu/, accessed on 20 December 2022), online since 2003 and last updated in June 2022 [75], defines four unified classes of AMPs on the basis of the polypeptide chain's connection patterns: (I) linear polypeptide chains (e.g., cathelicidins) [76]; (II) sidechain-linked peptides, such as disulfide-containing defensins and lantibiotics (i.e., lanthionine-containing antibiotics, e.g., microbisporicin, produced by the soil actinomycete *Microbispora corallina* [77] and mathermycin from the marine actinomycete *Marinactinospora thermotolerans* [78]); (III) polypeptide chains with side chain to backbone connection (e.g., bacterial lassos and fusaricidins); and (IV) circular peptides with a seamless backbone, i.e., N- and C-termini linked by a peptide bond (e.g., plant cyclotides and animal θ-defensins) [79]. The manually curated Database of Antimicrobial Activity and Structure of Peptides (DBAASP, http://dbaasp.org, accessed on 20 December 2022) provides detailed information (including chemical structure and activity against specific targets) on experimentally tested peptides (both natural and synthetic) that have shown antimicrobial activity as monomers, multimers, or multi-peptides [80]. The Collection of Antimicrobial Peptides (CAMP), CAMPSign, and ClassAMP are open-access resources that have been developed to advance our current understanding of AMPs, from N- and C-terminal modifications and the presence of unusual amino acids to 3D structures thorough family-specific signatures that facilitate AMP identification and classification as antibacterial, antifungal, or antiviral [81,82]. Synthetic AMPs are substantially enriched in residues with physicochemical properties known to be critical for antimicrobial activity, such as high α-helical propensity, positive charge, and hydrophobicity.

The Natural Products Atlas [83] was created as an open-access centralized knowledge-base encompassing ~25,000 microbially produced NPs using a combination of manual curation and automated data mining approaches, and was developed as a community-supported resource under findable, accessible, interoperable, and reusable (FAIR) [84] principles. It contains referenced data for molecular structure, source organism, isolation, total synthesis, and instances of structural reassignment for compounds of bacterial, fungal, and cyanobacterial origin. Its associated web interface (https://www.npatlas.org, v. 2.3.0, accessed on 20 December 2022) allows users to search by structure, substructure, and physical properties, as well as to explore the chemical space of these NPs from a variety of perspectives. The NP Atlas is integrated with other NP databases, including the MIBiG repository and the GNPS platform cited above. The NP Atlas was recently updated [19] and currently embodies (i) >32,000 compounds; (ii) a full RESTful (REST is an acronym for REpresentational State Transfer and an architectural style for distributed hypermedia systems) application programming interface (API); (iii) full taxonomic descriptions for all microbial taxa; (iv) integrated data from external resources, including CyanoMetDB (https://www.eawag.ch/en/department/uchem/projects/cyanometdb/, accessed on 20 December 2022), a comprehensive public database of secondary metabolites from cyanobacteria (aka "blue-green algae") [85]; and (v) chemical ontology terms from both ClassyFire [86] (see below) and NPClassifier (a deep-learning tool for the automated structural classification of NPs from their counted Morgan fingerprints) [87].

Finally, more than seven terabases of metagenomic data from samples collected in epipelagic and mesopelagic water locations across the globe by the *Tara* (https://fondationtaraocean.org/en/foundation/, accessed on 20 December 2022) Oceans project have been used to generate an ocean microbial reference gene catalog (http://ocean-microbiome.embl.de/companion.html, accessed on 20 December 2022) with >40 million nonredundant sequences from viruses, prokaryotes, and picoeukaryotes. Remarkably, almost three quarters of ocean microbial core functionality is shared with the human gut microbiome, and epipelagic community composition was found to be mostly driven by water temperature rather than geography or any other environmental factor [88]. A more recent analysis of 214 metagenome-assembled genomes (MAGs) recovered from the polar seawater microbiomes revealed strains that are prevalent in the polar regions while nearly undetectable in temperate seawater [89].

4. Classification and Chemoinformatic Analyses of Natural Products

The long-established Gene Ontology (GO) resource [90,91] describes our knowledge of the "universe" of biology with respect to (i) molecular functions, (ii) cellular locations, and (iii) biological processes of gene products, in terms of a dynamic, controlled vocabulary that can be applied to prokaryotes and eukaryotes, as well as to single and multicellular organisms. Along the same vein, a standardized and purely structure-based chemical ontology (ChemOnt) was recently developed to automatically assign over 77 million compounds to a taxonomy consisting of >4800 different categories by means of a computer program named ClassyFire (http://classyfire.wishartlab.com/, accessed on 20 December 2022) that is freely accessible as a web server [86]. This new taxonomy for chemical substances consists of up to 11 different levels (kingdom, superclass, class, subclass, etc.), with each of the categories defined by unambiguous, computable structural rules.

As a follow-on, the Chemical Functional Ontology (ChemFOnt), another FAIR-compliant, web-enabled resource (https://www.chemfont.ca, accessed on 20 December 2022), describes the functions and actions of >341,000 biologically important chemical substances, including primary and secondary metabolites, as well as drugs and NPs. The functional hierarchy within ChemFOnt consists of four functional "aspects" (physiological effect; disposition; process; and role), which are subdivided into twelve functional categories (health effects and organoleptic effects; sources, biological locations, and routes of exposure; environmental, natural, and industrial processes; adverse biological roles, normal biological roles, environmental roles, and industrial applications) and a total of >170,000 functional terms. At the time of publishing, ChemFOnt contained almost four million protein-chemical relationships and more than ten million chemical-functional relationships that can be adopted by other databases and software tools and be of utility not only to general chemists but also to researchers involved in genomics, metagenomics, proteomics, and metabolomics [92].

NPs are the result of nature's exploration of biologically relevant chemical space through eons of evolutionary time, hence their high diversity regarding atom connectivity and functional groups. Because they cover a broad range of sizes, 3D structures, and physicochemical properties that can be related to drug-likeness (including favorable ADME characteristics), NPs are considered not only as potential drugs, but also as an invaluable source of chemical inspiration for the development of new bioactive small molecules useful in chemical biology and medicinal chemistry research. The structural diversity of drugs was early assessed by making use of shape description methods and grouping the atoms of each drug molecule into ring, linker, framework (or scaffold) [93], and side chain [94]. A methodology that calculated the NP-likeness score—a Bayesian measure of similarity with respect to the structural space covered by NPs—proved capable of efficiently separating NPs from synthetic (i.e., man-made) molecules in a cross-validation experiment [95]. Nevertheless, rule-based procedures applied to the automated assignment of NPs to different classes, such as alkaloids, steroids, and flavonoids, have unveiled database-dependent differences in the coverage of chemical space [96]. Beyond that, several cheminformatics techniques have been used to analyze NPs and decompose them into fragments in the belief that their unique substructural features and chemical properties are likely to be optimized for protein recognition and enzyme inhibition. A recent cheminformatic analysis of the structural and physicochemical properties of NP-based drugs in comparison to top-selling brand-name synthetic drugs revealed that macrocycles occupied distinctive and relatively underpopulated regions of chemical space, while chemical probes largely overlapped with synthetic drugs [97].

Ideally, molecular diversity in drug discovery efforts should be focused on what is usually considered drug-like chemical space (aka "drug space"), which may (or may not) fully comply with Lipinski's "rule of five" [98]. A pioneering initiative to map this space made use of 72 descriptors accounting for size, lipophilicity (calculated log $P_{o/w}$), polarizability, charge, flexibility (number of nonterminal rotatable bonds), rigidity (total number of rings and rigid bonds), and hydrogen bonding abilities for a set of ~400 compounds encompassing both representative drugs ("core structures") and a number of "satellite molecules" intentionally placed outside of the drug space (i.e., possessing extreme values in one or several of the desired properties, while containing drug-like chemical fragments). By means of principal component analysis (PCA) and projections to latent structures (PLS) it was possible, after some iterations that involved the inclusion of additional randomly selected active molecules, to extract map coordinates in the form of *t*-score values and construct a chemical global positioning system (ChemGPS) [99]. The ChemGPS scores were found to describe well the latent structures extracted with PCA from a large set of compounds and appeared to be suitable for comparing multiple libraries and for keeping track of previously explored regions of chemical space. Later work (largely based on cyclooxygenase 1 and/or cyclooxygenase 2 (COX-1/2) inhibition) proposed an expansion of ChemGPS to better cover space for NPs, giving birth to ChemGPS-NP [100], which was further tuned for the improved handling of the chemical diversity encountered in NP research with a view to increasing the probability of hit identification [101]. The public ChemGPS-NP Web tool (http://chemgps.bmc.uu.se/, accessed on 20 December 2022) was then developed to allow for the exploration of NPs by navigating in a consistent 8-dimensional global map of structural characteristics built by means of PCA [102].

Following a different philosophy to chart the known chemical space explored by nature, the structural classification of natural products (SCONP) was devised to accomplish a hierarchical grouping of the scaffolds present in ~170,000 entries from the DNP by establishing parent–child relationships between them and arranging the scaffolds in a tree-like fashion [103]. Some previous processing was necessary that included structure cleansing (i.e., separation from accompanying molecules) and deglycosylation (in the case of glycosides whose active component is the aglycon part). Unfortunately, stereochemistry could not be considered in this early cheminformatic analysis so that the different possible configurations of the NP scaffolds had to be treated as being equivalent. The conversion of the resulting NP scaffolds to SMILES (simplified molecular-input line-entry system) strings [104] allowed for the comparison with those of standard synthetic molecules represented by over 10 million drug-like commercially available samples from the ZINC database [41]. This analysis revealed interesting differences not only between natural and synthetic (i.e., man-made) molecules, but also between scaffolds originating from distinct classes of organisms, i.e., plants, bacteria, and fungi. Visual comparisons of the respective structural features were effectively displayed by plotting the scaffolds according to their frequency distributions [105]. Moreover, a flexible analytics framework named Scaffold Hunter (https://scaffoldhunter.sourceforge.net/, accessed on 20 December 2022) generates and enables the visualization of virtual scaffold trees in bioactive compound collections that easily allow for the identification of new starting points for the design and synthesis of biology-oriented small molecule libraries [106]. Interestingly, a recent cluster analysis of chemical fingerprints and molecular scaffolds of >55,000 compounds reportedly isolated from marine and terrestrial microorganisms showed that three quarters of the MNPs are closely related to compounds isolated from their terrestrial counterparts [107].

The cheminformatic deconstruction of hundreds of thousands of NPs has allowed for the definition of thousands of fragment groups that represent a large portion of the chemical space defined by NPs and may guide the synthesis of "non-natural" NPs or pseudo-NPs, that is, molecules made in the lab that contain at least some of the structural features present in NPs but have not yet been found in living organisms [108]. In this regard, we must bear in mind that the prototype "antimetabolite" 6-thioguanine, which was synthesized in 1955 by Nobel Prize winners Elion and Hitchings [109], was found in 2013 to be biosynthetically produced by *Erwinia amylovora*, the bacteria responsible for fire blight pathogenesis in apple and pear trees [110]. In fact, a recent cheminformatic analysis revealed that a significant portion of biologically active synthetic compounds can be regarded as pseudo-NPs and, as such, the result of human-directed "chemical evolution" of NP structure [111]. Once again, humans imitate nature by (i) performing atom/group replacement and/or decorating with novel fragments what are thought to be privileged scaffolds for bioactivity [112–114]; or (ii) combining fragment-sized NPs and/or NP fragments to provide "hybrid NPs" [115].

Historically, the total synthesis of NPs followed by derivative synthesis ("active analogue approach" or "analogue-oriented synthesis" [116,117]) and semisynthetic procedures aimed at modifying the chemical structure of complex fermentation products have enabled a deeper understanding of structure–activity relationships (SAR). In contrast, the de novo combination of NP fragments in unique arrangements, often by virtue of innovative strategies such as "diversity-oriented synthesis" [118,119], "target-oriented and diversity-oriented organic synthesis" [120], and "synthesis-informed design" [121], has been shown to generate focused NP-like libraries containing compounds endowed with bioactivities unrelated to those of the guiding NP(s) [122–124]. Examples of successful workflows of pseudo-NP design and development are "biology-oriented synthesis" [114,125] and "pharmacophore-directed retrosynthesis" [126]. In applying the latter approach, a key first step is to elaborate a tentative pharmacophore, i.e., "an ensemble of steric and electronic features that is necessary to ensure the optimal supramolecular interactions with a specific biological target and to trigger (or block) its biological response", as defined by the International Union of Pure and Applied Chemistry (IUPAC) [127], and then devise a retrosynthetic procedure that ensures that the proposed pharmacophore is present in multiple intermediates of increasing complexity, ultimately leading to the NP. An important goal of these synthetic approaches is to find structurally simplified and optimized derivatives with lower molecular weights that can overcome commonly observed limitations, such as poor oral absorption, short half-life, and low blood–brain barrier permeability.

5. Linking NPs to Their Targets: Computational Methodologies for Building Global Networks

The popular term "druggable genome" [128] refers to the genes (or, more appropriately, gene products) that are known or predicted to interact with drugs, ideally resulting in a therapeutic benefit. Although drugs are intended to be selective (i.e., have high affinity for one single target), it is not uncommon for many molecules to bind to more than one protein, giving rise to polypharmacology and side effects. Due to the fact that many drug-target combinations are theoretically possible, the computational exploration of possible interactions can help identify potential targets.

Because the systematic identification of drug targets for NPs, regardless of their origin, using a battery of experimental binding or affinity assays, is both costly and time-consuming, a substantial amount of effort has gone into devising in silico tools that allow for the construction of global networks that connect active compounds to their cellular targets. It is expected that, by using these methods, the resulting system's pharmacology infrastructure will help to predict new drug targets for pharmacologically uncharacterized NPs and identify secondary targets (off-targets) that can aid in the rationalization of side effects of known molecules [129]. The Drug-Gene Interaction Database (DGIdb 4.0, https://www.dgidb.org/, accessed on 20 December 2022) provides information on drug-gene interactions and druggable gene products collected from publications, databases, and other web sites [130]. The latest update mostly focused on (i) the integration with crowd-sourced efforts (e.g., Wikidata) to facilitate term normalization and with the open-data web platform Drug Target Commons (https://dataverse.harvard.edu/dataverse/dtc2tdc, accessed on 20 December 2022) [131] to enable the upload of community-contributed interaction data; and (ii) export to a Network Data Exchange (NDEx) infrastructure [132] for storing, sharing and publishing biological network knowledge. The tool named substructure-drug-target network-based inference (SDTNBI) was devised to prioritize potential targets for old drugs ("drug repositioning"), failed drugs, and new chemical entities by bridging the gap between new chemical entities and known drug-target interactions (DTIs) [133]. A later modification (wSDTNBI) [134] uses weighted DTI networks, whose edge weights are correlated with binding affinities, and network-based VS, which does not rely on the receptors' 3D structures [135]. The publicly available SwissTargetPrediction web server (http://www.swisstargetprediction.ch, accessed on 20 December 2022) [136] also attempts to predict the most likely target(s) (in mice, rats, or human beings) for a SMILES-defined input molecule by using a computational method that combines different measures of similarities (both in 2D chemical structure and in 3D molecular shape) with known ligands [137]. All of these approaches, together with highly efficient receptor-based ligand docking [138], can be useful to narrow down the number of potential targets, but strict experimental confirmation and validation are needed [139,140].

The attention initially drawn [141] to certain synthetic molecules that were responsible for disproportionate percentages of hits in enzyme-based bioassays but, on closer inspection, turned out to be false actives and therefore nonprogressible hits, leading to the PAINS acronym (Pan Assay INterference compoundS) [142], was later extended to NPs [143]. As a result, some NPs have been designated as "invalid metabolic panaceas" and the concept of "residual complexity" (http://go.uic.edu/residualcomplexity, accessed on 20

December 2022) has emerged [144]. Nowadays, compounds with a PAINS chemotype can be recognized and excluded from bioassays by the judicious use of electronic substructure filters [145] and machine learning approaches [146] (e.g., Hit Dexter, https://nerdd.univie. ac.at/hitdexter3/, accessed on 20 December 2022).

Because the best link connecting NPs to their targets is arguably the experimentally determined 3D structure of the respective complexes, in the following section, I will provide some examples of MNPs and synthetic analogues that were selected on the basis of chemical novelty and submicromolar inhibition data, preferably supported by structural evidence of complex formation with pharmacologically relevant enzyme targets.

6. Selected Examples of MNPs Acting as Enzyme Inhibitors

The road from the research laboratory to the drug pipeline is long and winding. Quite often, molecules originally assayed for one biological activity end up showing promise for another unintended indication, either fortuitously or by following one of the computational approaches outlined in the previous sections.

Bengamides A and B (Figure 2) were first described as heterocyclic anthelmintics naturally present in the sponge *Jaspis cf. coriacea* [147], and later on, not only in other sponges from many biogeographic sites, but also in the terrestrial Gram-negative bacterium *Myxococcus virescens*. Decades of further research have shown that methionine aminopeptidases MetAP1 and MetAP2 (essential metalloenzymes that remove the initiator amino-terminal methionine from nascent proteins) are molecular targets for bengamides, which also display notable antiproliferative and antiangiogenic properties [148,149]. In fact, a synthetic analogue of bengamide B, LAF389, was the subject of a phase I anticancer clinical trial that, unfortunately, demonstrated no objective responses and also the occurrence of unanticipated cardiovascular events. The high-resolution 3D structures of both human MetAP1 and MetAP2 enzymes in complex with bengamide derivatives, including LAF389 (PDB entry 1QZY) [150], have been solved [151] and show these compounds bound in a manner that mimics the binding of peptide substrates, with three key hydroxyl groups on the inhibitor coordinating the di-Co(II) center in the enzyme active site. Renewed interest in bengamides is currently focused on their antibacterial activities against various drug-resistant *Mycobacterium tuberculosis* [152] and *Staphylococcus aureus* strains [153]. Incidentally, the mycotoxin fumagillin, first isolated from *Aspergillus fumigatus* and originally studied also as an antiangiogenic agent and human MetAP2 inhibitor [154], has been widely used for more than 60 years in apiculture to control nosema disease in honey bees effectively [155] because the microsporidian *Nosema apis* lacks MetAP1 and targeting MetAP2 suppresses infection.

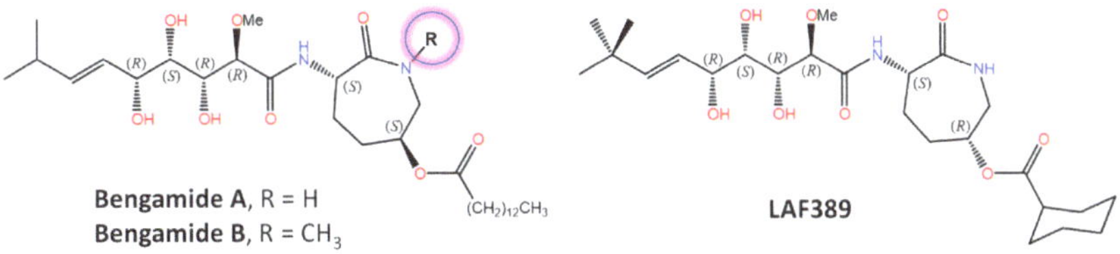

Bengamide A, R = H
Bengamide B, R = CH₃
$(CH_2)_{12}CH_3$

LAF389

Figure 2. Chemical structures of naturally occurring bengamides A and B, which appear to be encoded by a mixed PKS/NRPS BGC, and the synthetic analogue LAF389.

Another showcase example is provided by gracilin A (Figure 3), a nor-diterpene metabolite originally isolated from the Mediterranean sponge *Spongionella gracilis* [156], that was initially reported as a potent phospholipase A_2 (PLA$_2$) inhibitor [157] and later shown to mimic the immunosuppressive effects of cyclosporin A through interaction with cyclophilin A (CypA) [158]. In a recent pharmacophore-directed retrosynthesis application, a theoretically derived pharmacophore of gracilin A was chosen as an early synthetic target. Then, sequential increases in the complexity of this minimal structure enabled SAR profiling and the identification of structurally less complex derivatives of gracilin A that displayed selectivity for mitochondrial CypD over CypA inhibition as well as significant neuroprotective and/or immunosuppressive activities [126].

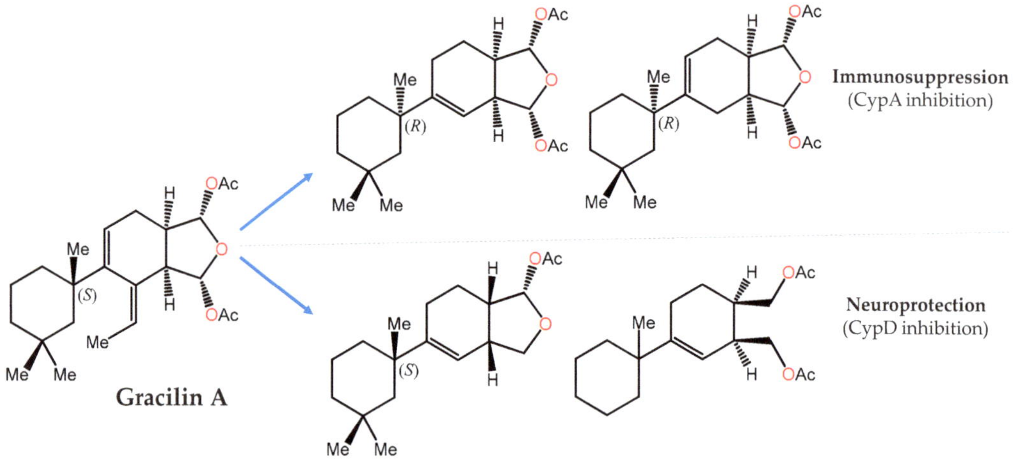

Figure 3. Pharmacophore-directed chemical modifications of gracillin A leading to novel compounds with distinct pharmacodynamic profiles by selective CypA vs. CypD inhibition [126].

The sesterterpenoids [159] are metabolites first isolated from marine sponges of the *Thorectidae* family, which includes the genera *Cacospongia*, *Fasciospongia*, *Luffariella*, and *Thorecta*, that often contain biologically active butenolide and hydroxybutenolide groups in their structures [160]. The anti-inflammatory activity of manoalide and luffolide (Figure 4a) was related to the inactivation of secretory PLA$_2$, whereas for cacospongionolide F this biological effect was shown to involve the inhibition of the nuclear factor-κB (NF-κB) pathway as well [161]. In contrast, the related dysidiolide (Figure 4b) from the Caribbean sponge *Dysidea etherea* de Laubenfels (Dysideidae family) was the first known natural inhibitor of the cyclin-dependent kinase (CDK)-activating phosphatases cdc25A and cdc25B, with IC$_{50}$ values in the micromolar range [162]. Later on, dysidiolide and distinctly decorated analogues prepared from *ent*-halimic acid following a classical "active analogue approach" were shown to cause stage-specific arrest of proliferating cancer cells, but again at low micromolar concentrations [163]. Because cdc25A was found to be present in the same protein structure similarity cluster (PSSC) [164] as 11β-hydroxysteroid dehydrogenase type 1 (11βHSD1, an enzyme that catalyzes the conversion of cortisone to cortisol), the SCONP-guided [103] selection of the 1,2,3,4,4*a*,5,6,7-octahydronaphthalene scaffold present in dysidiolide led to a focused compound library (Figure 4b) that showed the submicromolar inhibition of 11βHSD1 and selectivity over 11βHSD2 [165].

The bisulfide bromotyrosine- and oxime-containing derivatives psammaplin A and bisaprasin (Figure 5) were originally characterized as nanomolar inhibitors of histone deacetylases and DNA methyltransferase enzymes [166,167], but it is known today that they are used by marine sponges, such as *Pseudoceratina purpurea* and *Aplysinella rhax*, in their chemical communication [168] and quorum sensing [169] systems to prevent biofilm formation and attenuate virulence factor expression by pathogenic microorganisms.

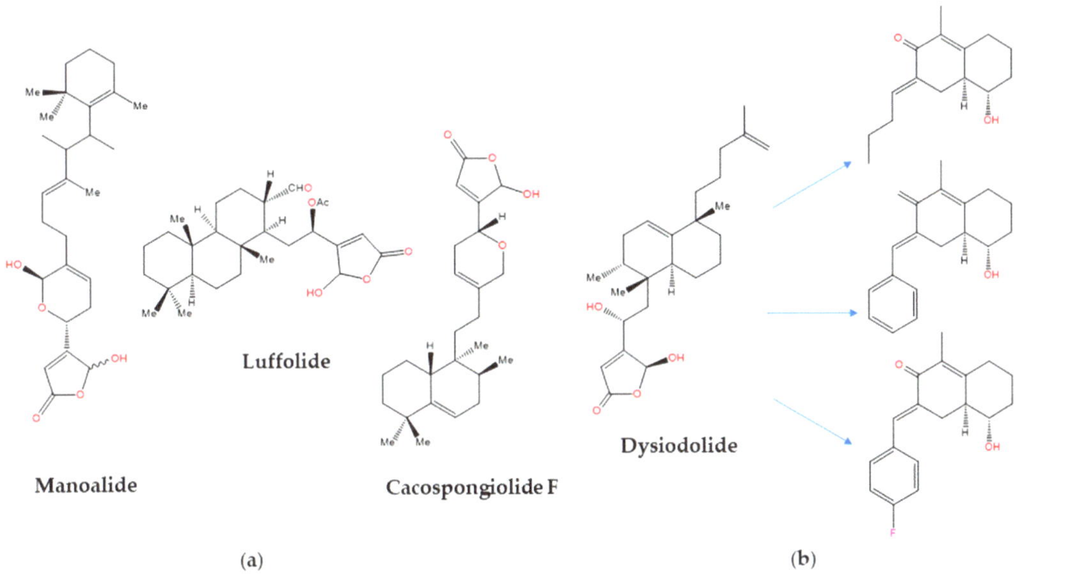

Figure 4. Examples of MNPs containing hydroxybutenolide moiety. (**a**) PLA$_2$-inhibiting sesterterpenoids of marine origin; (**b**) SCONP-guided [103] evolution from dysidiolide to a focused library of submicromolar inhibitors of 11βHSD1 that showed some selectivity over 11βHSD2 [165].

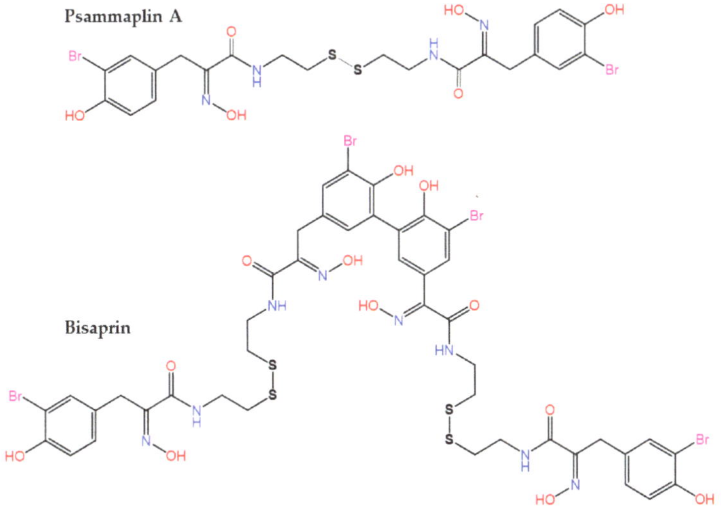

Figure 5. Structures of psammaplin A and its biphenylic dimer bisaprasin.

A number of MNPs are potent inhibitors of proteases, an important drug target class in human diseases that is integrated in MEROPS (http://www.ebi.ac.uk/merops/, accessed on 20 December 2022), a database of proteolytic enzymes, their substrates and inhibitors [170]. Gallinamide A (Figure 6), a metabolite of the marine cyanobacterium *Schizothrix* sp. that originally displayed modest antimalarial activity, was subsequently reisolated and characterized as a potent and irreversible inhibitor of the human cysteine protease cathepsin L (k_i = 9000 ± 260 M^{-1} s^{-1}), with 8- to 320-fold greater selectivity over the closely related cathepsins V or B [171]. Docking-guided modifications to improve the binding affinity resulted in notably enhanced potency against cathepsin L ($K_i = 0.0937 \pm 0.01$ nM and $k_{inact}/K_i = 8{,}730{,}000$). Gallinamide and its analogs also displayed the potent inhibition of the highly homologous cruzain, an essential *Trypanosoma cruzi* cysteine protease, as well as cytotoxic activity on intracellular *T. cruzi* amastigotes [172]. Importantly, the biochemical data indicated that inhibitor potency was driven by the rate of formation of the reversible enzyme:inhibitor complex, rather than by the rate of covalent modification. The resolution of the 3D co-crystal structure of the complex formed between cruzain and gallinamide A later confirmed the proposed binding pose and revealed the expected covalent bond formed between the drug's Michael acceptor enamide and the active site Cys25 thiol (PDB entry 7JUJ) [173].

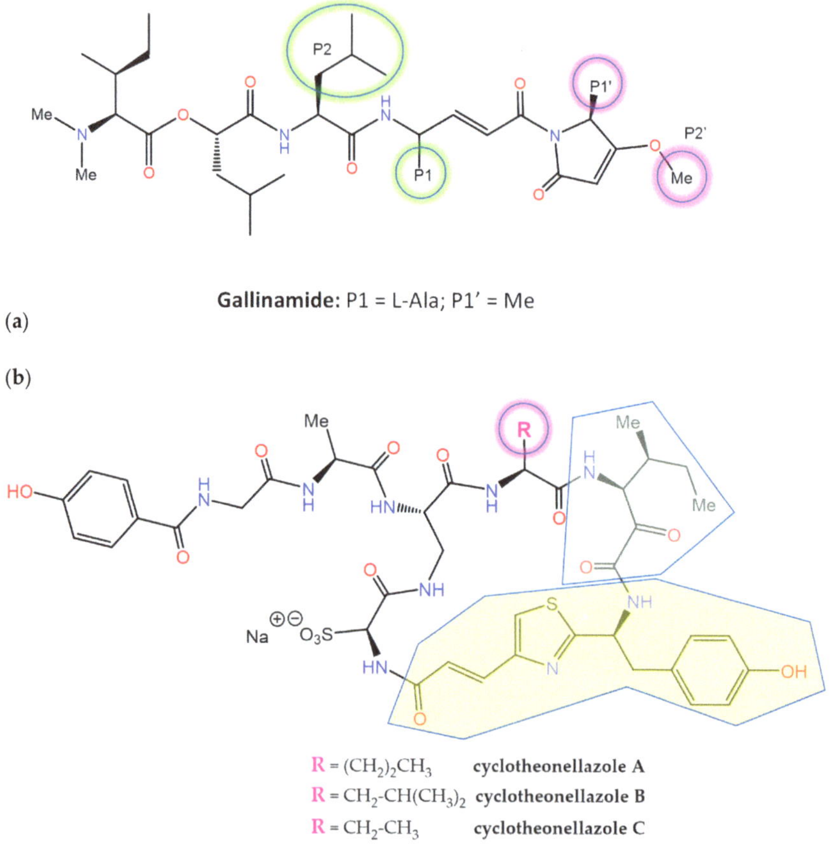

Gallinamide: P1 = L-Ala; P1' = Me

(a)

(b)

R = (CH₂)₂CH₃   **cyclotheonellazole A**
R = CH₂-CH(CH₃)₂   **cyclotheonellazole B**
R = CH₂-CH₃   **cyclotheonellazole C**

Figure 6. Chemical structures of protease inhibitors (**a**) gallinamide and (**b**) cyclotheonellazoles A–C. The 4-propenoyl-2-tyrosylthiazole (Ptt) and 3-amino-4-methyl-2-oxohexanoic acid (Amoha) subunits in the cyclotheonellazoles are highlighted in yellow and green, respectively.

The in vitro antiplasmodial activity of an extract of the sponge *Theonella aff. swinhoei* collected in Madagascar was ascribed, in part, to the previously known actin-binding metabolite swinholide A [174]. Further work disclosed the presence of three unusual cyclic peptides, cyclotheonellazoles A–C (Figure 6), containing six nonproteinogenic amino acids out of the eight composing units (of which the most novel were 4-propenoyl-2-tyrosylthiazole and 3-amino-4-methyl-2-oxohexanoic acid). These macrocyclic peptides are thought to be produced by hybrid PKS-NRPS enzymes from symbiotic bacteria and were found not to be active against *Plasmodium*, but instead displayed the nanomolar and sub-nanomolar inhibition of chymotrypsin and elastase, respectively [175]. This latter enzyme has been considered an important target to prevent acute lung injury/acute respiratory distress syndrome (ALI/ARDS) in COVID-19 patients, and the inhibition of its activity by cyclotheonellazole A has been recently shown to reduce lung edema and pathological deterioration in an ALI mouse model, comparing favorably with the clinically approved elastase inhibitor sivelestat [176].

The (Ahp)-containing cyclodepsipeptide family of cyanobacterial NPs biosynthesized by NRPS is noteworthy for the ability of many of its members (Figure 7) to inhibit several serine proteases, most notably human neutrophil elastase and kallikreins [177], by virtue of mimicking the natural substrates. The 3-amino-6-hydroxy-2-piperidone (Ahp) unit serves as the general pharmacophore, whereas the adjacent (Z)-2-amino-2-butenoic acid confers selectivity for elastase [178]. The depsipeptide molassamide was purified and characterized from cyanobacterial assemblages of *Dichothrix utahensis* as a new analogue of the cytostatic depsipeptide dolastatin 13 (originally isolated from the sea hare *Dolabella auricularia*) [179] that inhibited elastase and chymotrypsin at submicromolar concentrations, but not trypsin [180]. The analysis of the X-ray crystal structure of porcine elastase in complex with lyngbyastatin 7 (PDB code 4GVU) and SAR studies resulted in the synthesis of symplostatin 5, whose activity was comparable to that of sivelestat in short-term assays and more sustained in longer-term assays [181]. Complex fractionation guided by MS^2 metabolomics (molecular networking) [182], together with HPLC, NMR, and chiral chromatography, allowed for the identification of tutuilamides A and B from *Schizothrix* sp., along with tutuilamide C from a *Coleofasciculus* sp. These novel structures (Figure 7), which are also potent elastase inhibitors, bind reversibly to this enzyme, as shown in the co-crystal structure of tutuilamide A in complex with porcine elastase (PDB code 6TH7), despite the fact that they feature an unusual vinyl chloride-containing residue. An additional hydrogen bond relative to lyngbyastatin 7 has been proposed as the element responsible for its enhanced inhibitory potency [183]. More recently, yet another family of new Ahp-cyclodepsipeptides, the rivulariapeptolides, with nanomolar potency as serine protease inhibitors, was identified from an environmental cyanobacteria community using a scalable, bioactivity-focused, native metabolomics approach [184].

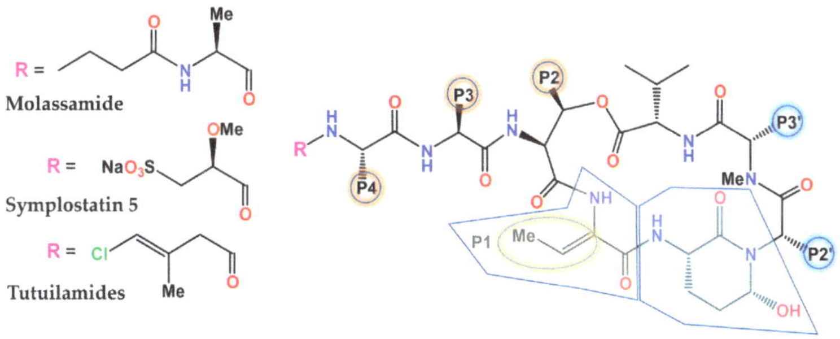

Figure 7. General structure of selected Ahp-cyclodepsipeptides. The 3-amino-6-hydroxy-2-piperidone (Ahp) and (Z)-2-amino-2-butenoic acid (Abu) subunits are highlighted in blue and green, respectively. The nature of the **P** substituents varies among family members and synthetic analogues.

The human proteasome, a multicatalytic enzyme complex that is responsible for the regulated non-lysosomal degradation of cellular proteins, gained notorious pharmacological relevance when the synthetic boron-containing bortezomib (originally developed by ProScript to treat muscle weakness and muscle loss associated with AIDS, as well as muscular dystrophy) was approved in 2003 by the FDA as Velcade® (co-developed by Millennium/Takeda and Janssen-Cilag) for the treatment of relapsed/refractory multiple myeloma (MM) and mantle cell lymphoma. Carfilzomib (Figure 8), an α',β'-epoxyketone-containing analog of the NP epoximicin—first identified in an Indian soil actinomycete strain [185]—was also approved in 2012 as Kyprolis® (Onyx Pharmaceuticals) for clinical use in MM patients, in combination with lenalidomide and dexamethasone. Marizomib (aka salinosporamide A) is a structurally and pharmacologically unique MNP that contains a β-lactone-γ-lactam (Figure 8) and is produced by the marine actinomycete *Salinispora tropica*. Marizomib not only inhibits the chymotrypsin-like activity of the proteasome (via a novel mechanism involving the acylation of the O^γ in the N-terminal catalytic Thr residue followed by the displacement of chloride) but also those of the caspase-like and trypsin-like subunits [186]. In addition to its "pan-proteasome" pharmacodynamic activity, marizomib crosses the blood-brain barrier, and for these reasons it has been extensively studied, first preclinically [187], and then in phase I–III clinical trials, both alone and in combination. Many other MNP scaffolds continue serving as inspiration for the design and synthesis of potent 20S human proteasome inhibitors, including carmaphycins A and B (Figure 8) from a marine cyanobacterium *Symploca* species and fellutamide B, originally isolated from *Penicillium fellutanium*, a fungus found in the gastrointestinal tract of the marine fish *Apogon endekataenia* [188]. In the development of potent covalent inhibitors of the proteasome, ligand docking and binding energy calculations have highlighted the importance of the optimization of the prior noncovalent binding mode, through conformational restraints, in a pose close to that found in the transition state [189].

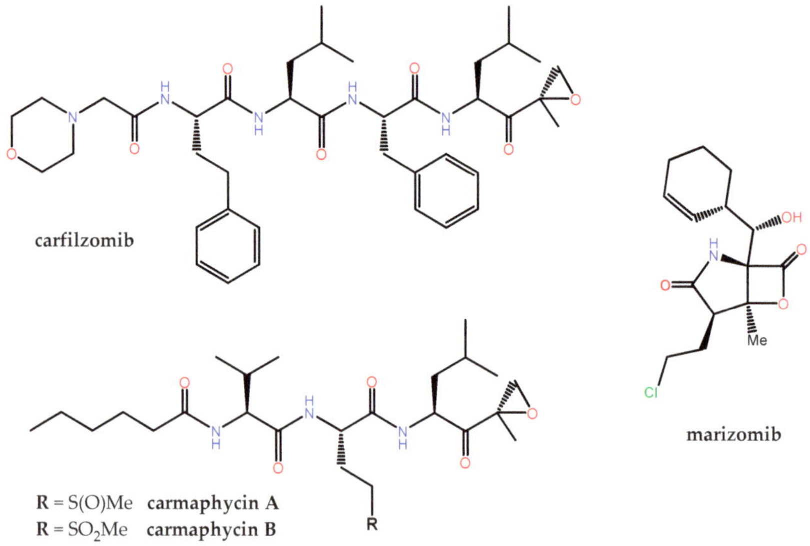

Figure 8. Chemical structure of selected proteasome inhibitors: carfilzomib (clinically approved), marizomib (in clinical trials), and carmaphycins A and B (investigational).

Protein kinases are validated drug targets because (i) kinase deregulation plays an essential role in many disease states, and (ii) many inhibitors have already shown therapeutic benefit (almost one hundred are currently approved for clinical use). This bioactivity is of broad scope and has been reported for various MNPs obtained from different sources, including bacteria and cyanobacteria, fungi, algae, soft corals, sponges, and animals [6,190]. Of note, a significant number of them were originally isolated from terrestrial sources and subsequently found in marine organisms too, and vice versa. For example, the pan-kinase inhibitor staurosporine (a pentacyclic indolo(2,3-*a*)carbazole first discovered in 1977 from the bacterium *Streptomyces staurosporeus*) was one of the early tools used to probe the cellular effects of blocking the ATP-binding pocket in different protein kinases. In 2002, 11-hydroxystaurosporine (Figure 9) was reported to be present in an ascidian *Eudistoma* species collected in Micronesia and to be a more potent inhibitor of protein kinase C than staurosporine itself [191]. Another early potent pan-kinase inhibitor is (*Z*)-hymenialdisine, which owes its name to *Hymeniacidon aldis*, the sponge where it was originally found.

These and many other MNPs inspired synthetic work on analogues and novel scaffolds that paved the ground for the discovery of imatinib (Gleevec®), a landmark drug that has (i) significantly improved the outcomes of patients with chronic myelogenous leukemia by inhibiting the oncogenic BCR–ABL tyrosine kinase; (ii) shown remarkable clinical efficacy in the treatment of other malignancies; (iii) helped establish the concept of "targeted therapy" in the field of cancer research; (iv) fostered the concept of "precision medicine", i.e., tailor the chemotherapeutic treatment to the unique genetic changes in an individual's cancer cells; and (v) fuel the extremely rich and rewarding research on protein kinase inhibitors [192].

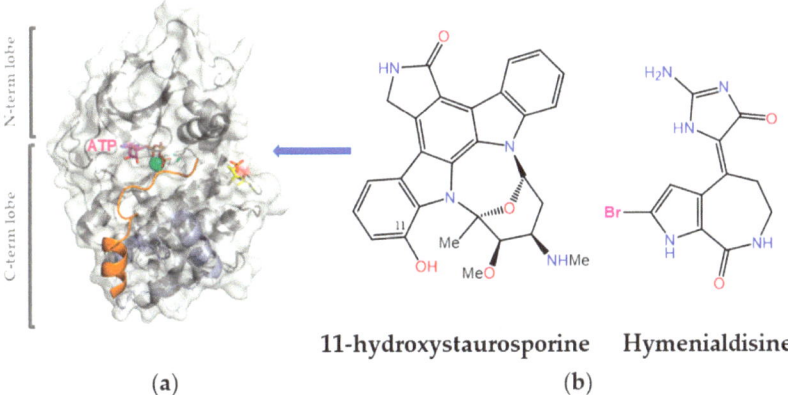

11-hydroxystaurosporine   Hymenialdisine

(a)   (b)

Figure 9. Early small-molecule protein kinase inhibitors of marine origin. (**a**) A representative protein kinase structure (PDB code 3FJQ) showing a bound peptide inhibitor (orange) and an ATP molecule (purple) plus two Mn^{2+} ions (green spheres) in the crevice that separates the N- and C-terminal lobes. The C-terminal lobe (bottom) contains the activation sites (T196 and phosphorylated T198 in yellow) and substrate-binding site (residues 230–260 in light blue). (**b**) Chemical structures of two early pan-kinase inhibitors.

A top priority in the development of novel protein kinase inhibitors is to understand selectivity so that the tendency of one given drug to bind to other unintended kinases (off-targets) can be suppressed or attenuated. To this end, kinome-wide inhibitory selectivity profiling is necessary because small assay panels cannot provide a robust measure of selectivity [193]. Binding site similarity searches, as performed in the KinomeFEATURE (https://simtk.org/projects/kdb, accessed on 20 December 2022) [194] and KID [195] databases, along with machine learning models that map the activity profile of inhibitors across the entire human kinome [196], as exemplified by Drug Discovery Maps [197], can be of help not only to gain insight into the structural basis of kinase cross-inhibition, but also to predict the binding affinities of novel kinase inhibitors.

Cortistatin A (Figure 10a) was isolated as an antiangiogenic steroidal alkaloid from the marine sponge *Corticium simplex* and should not be confused with the somatostatin-like cortistatin neuropeptides. It consists of a 9(10→19)-*abeo*-androstane and isoquinoline skeleton and was originally shown to inhibit the proliferation of human umbilical vein endothelial cells at nanomolar concentrations [198]. It was later found that this MNP selectively inhibits the mediator-associated cyclin-dependent kinase CDK8 and disproportionately induces the upregulation of superenhancer-associated genes in acute myeloid leukemia cell lines [199]. The crystal structure of the ternary complex of CDK8 bound to cyclin C and cortistatin A (PDB code 4CRL) revealed exquisite shape complementarity between this alkaloid and the ATP-binding pocket of CDK8 (Figure 10b), with the crucial isoquinoline [200] making essential hydrogen bonding interactions with the peptide backbone.

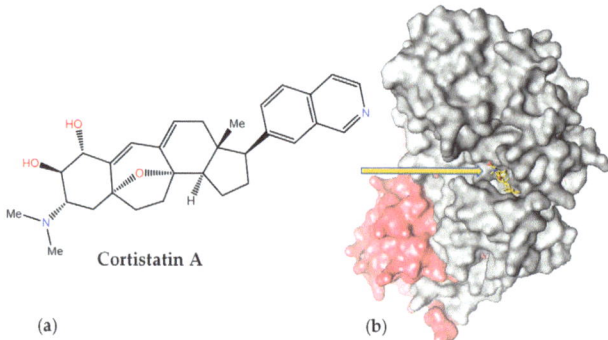

(a)

(b)

Figure 10. Inhibition of mediator-associated cyclin-dependent kinase CDK8 by cortistatin A. (**a**) Chemical structure of cortistatin A. (**b**) Schematic view of the complex between cyclin C (pink) and CDK8 (grey) showing cortistatin A (yellow sticks) bound inside the ATP-binding pocket of CDK8 (PDB code 4CRL).

The last example in this review is provided by sphaerimicin A (Figure 11), a complex macrocyclic uridine nucleoside derivative isolated from *Sphaerisporangium* sp. SANK60911 using a genome mining approach focused on the enzyme uridine-5′-aldehyde transaldolase [201]. Even though this is a terrestrial actinomycete, it is closely related to other marine species [202] that contain similar BGCs, hence its inclusion in this section. Sphaeromicin A exhibits nanomolar inhibitory activity on bacterial MraY, an integral membrane enzyme that catalyzes the transfer of phospho-*N*-acetylmuramyl pentapeptide from UDP-*N*-acetylmuramyl pentapeptide (Park's nucleotide) to the phospholipid undecaprenyl phosphate during the lipid cycle of peptidoglycan biosynthesis. In an elegant example of molecular design assisted by theoretical conformational analysis and NMR data, the simplified analogues with defined stereochemistry SPM-1 and SPM-2 were synthesized [203]. The fact that SPM-1 turned out to be 54-fold more potent than SPM-2 against MraY from *Aquifex aeolicus* (MraY$_{AA}$) revealed the importance of the conformationally restrained macrocycle for target binding, an aspect that was clarified even further when the 3D structure of the MraY$_{AA}$:SPM-1 complex was solved by X-ray crystallography. Therefore structure-based optimization is now feasible in order to develop MraY inhibitors with the potential of becoming novel antibiotics against drug-resistant bacteria.

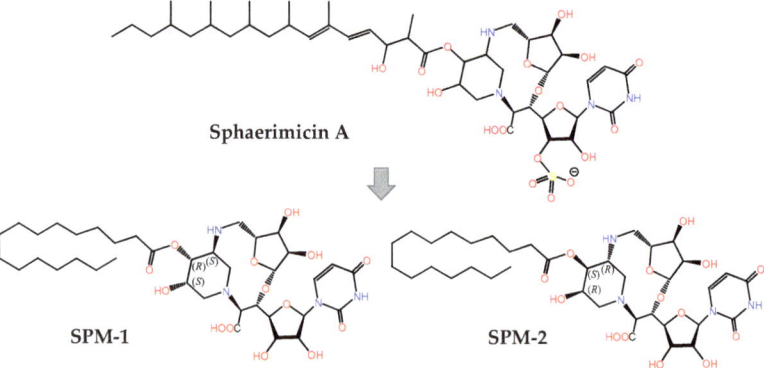

Figure 11. Chemical structures of the naturally occurring sphaerimicin A (containing the undetermined stereogenic centers circled in grey) and synthetic simplified analogues SPM-1 and SPM-2 with defined stereochemistry, which is critical for inhibitory potency. The X-ray crystal structure of the MraY:SPM-1 complex has recently been determined (PDB code 8CXR) [203].

7. Conclusions and Outlook

Computational methodologies play indispensable roles in the exploration of the vast chemical space covered by MNPs by helping, among many other tasks, to (i) elucidate their chemical composition and 3D structure; (ii) store, process, curate, and organize huge amounts of information related to source organisms, biosynthesis, and bioactivity; and (iii) connect biological activities with both molecular scaffolds and target binding sites [204]. The limits of biologically relevant chemical space for enzyme inhibitors are defined by the specific binding interactions taking place between small- and medium-sized molecules (e.g., terpenoids, alkaloids, polyketides, non-ribosomal peptides, and RiPPs) [20] and a number of selected orthosteric and allosteric pockets in macromolecular catalysts that have evolved over billions of years [205].

Some of the molecular entities recently found in marine microbiota can easily defy and outperform a chemist's imagination and ingenuity, and also be endowed with unexpected, and even unprecedented, bioactivities that may inspire more synthetic creativity. A historical example is the clinically used cytarabine (aka cytosine arabinoside or arabinosyl cytosine, Ara-C), a synthetic pyrimidine nucleoside that was developed in the imitation of spongothymidine, a nucleoside originally isolated from the Caribbean sponge *Tethya crypta*. Many other analogues, however, did not follow the same fate and, in fact, the potential of MNPs as therapeutic agents for human diseases has been realized only in a few cases, which attests to the enormous difficulties of progressing many of these compounds through the drug pipeline with the final goal of demonstrating an acceptable benefit-risk balance in clinical trials and thereafter. We must be confident that the new generations of cross-disciplinary trained scientists working in community-wide networks (e.g., Ocean Medicines, https://cordis.europa.eu/project/id/690944, accessed on 20 December 2022) will overcome existing hurdles to find valuable new medicines inspired by, or based on, MNPs.

It seems clear that the integration of information from various sources, including high-throughput phenotypic screening and BGC engineering, using computational methods has revolutionized NP research and can speed up the process of discovering new biologically active molecules from marine and terrestrial sources. A major bottleneck in these efforts is to identify the macromolecular target that is responsible for the observed (or assigned) mechanism of action, a problem that is usually aggravated when dealing with complex mixtures of MNPs. The recent success in the functional characterization of several NPs and the identification of bioactive metabolites upon integrating results from untargeted metabolomics, high-content image analysis of perturbation-treated cells, and gene expression signatures [206] on a data-driven multi-platform raises the hope for the accelerated discovery of novel pharmacologically active MNPs in the near future.

Funding: This research was funded by the Spanish MICINN (Project PID2019-104070RB-C22).

Data Availability Statement: Data sharing is not applicable.

Acknowledgments: I am grateful to Xavier Avilés (Universidad de Barcelona, Spain) for his kind invitation to contribute to this special issue, and to Schrodinger LLC for the provision of the educational version of PyMOL v. 1.7.4.5 (2022) that was used for 3D figure composition.

Conflicts of Interest: The author declares no conflict of interest.

References

1. Funayama, S.; Cordell, G.A. *Alkaloids: A Treasury of Poisons and Medicines*; Elsevier: Amsterdam, The Netherlands, 2014.
2. Mora, C.; Tittensor, D.P.; Adl, S.; Simpson, A.G.; Worm, B. How many species are there on Earth and in the ocean? *PLoS Biol.* **2011**, *9*, e1001127. [CrossRef] [PubMed]
3. Mayer, A.M.; Glaser, K.B.; Cuevas, C.; Jacobs, R.S.; Kem, W.; Little, R.D.; McIntosh, J.M.; Newman, D.J.; Potts, B.C.; Shuster, D.E. The odyssey of marine pharmaceuticals: A current pipeline perspective. *Trends Pharmacol. Sci.* **2010**, *31*, 255–265. [CrossRef] [PubMed]
4. Glaser, K.B.; Mayer, A.M. A renaissance in marine pharmacology: From preclinical curiosity to clinical reality. *Biochem. Pharmacol.* **2009**, *78*, 440–448. [CrossRef] [PubMed]

5. Reymond, J.L. The chemical space project. *Acc. Chem. Res.* **2015**, *48*, 722–730. [CrossRef] [PubMed]
6. Bharate, S.B.; Sawant, S.D.; Singh, P.P.; Vishwakarma, R.A. Kinase inhibitors of marine origin. *Chem. Rev.* **2013**, *113*, 6761–6815. [CrossRef] [PubMed]
7. Newman, D.J.; Cragg, G.M.; Battershill, C.N. Therapeutic agents from the sea: Biodiversity, chemo-evolutionary insight and advances to the end of Darwin's 200th year. *Diving Hyperb. Med.* **2009**, *39*, 216–225.
8. Newman, D.J.; Cragg, G.M. Natural products as sources of new drugs over the nearly four decades from 01/1981 to 09/2019. *J. Nat. Prod.* **2020**, *83*, 770–803. [CrossRef]
9. Nakao, Y.; Fusetani, N. Enzyme Inhibitors from Marine Invertebrates. In *Handbook of Marine Natural Products*; Fattorusso, E., Gerwick, W.H., Taglialatela-Scafati, O., Eds.; Springer Science+Business Media B.V.: Dordrecht, The Netherlands, 2012; pp. 1145–1229.
10. Duan, D.; Doak, A.K.; Nedyalkova, L.; Shoichet, B.K. Colloidal aggregation and the in vitro activity of traditional Chinese medicines. *ACS Chem. Biol.* **2015**, *10*, 978–988. [CrossRef]
11. Seidler, J.; McGovern, S.L.; Doman, T.N.; Shoichet, B.K. Identification and prediction of promiscuous aggregating inhibitors among known drugs. *J. Med. Chem.* **2003**, *46*, 4477–4486. [CrossRef]
12. Blin, K.; Shaw, S.; Kloosterman, A.M.; Charlop-Powers, Z.; van Wezel, G.P.; Medema, M.H.; Weber, T. antiSMASH 6.0: Improving cluster detection and comparison capabilities. *Nucleic Acids Res.* **2021**, *49*, W29–W35. [CrossRef]
13. Weissman, K.J. The structural biology of biosynthetic megaenzymes. *Nat. Chem. Biol.* **2015**, *11*, 660–670. [CrossRef]
14. Fischbach, M.A.; Walsh, C.T. Biochemistry. Directing biosynthesis. *Science* **2006**, *314*, 603–605. [CrossRef] [PubMed]
15. Jurjens, G.; Kirschning, A.; Candito, D.A. Lessons from the synthetic chemist nature. *Nat. Prod. Rep.* **2015**, *32*, 723–737. [CrossRef] [PubMed]
16. Sherman, D.H.; Rath, C.M.; Mortison, J.; Scaglione, J.B.; Kittendorf, J.D. Biosynthetic Principles in Marine Natural Product Systems. In *Handbook of Marine Natural Products*; Fattorusso, E., Gerwick, W.H., Taglialatela-Scafati, O., Eds.; Springer Nature Switzerland AG: Dordrecht, The Netherlands, 2012; pp. 947–976.
17. Cimermancic, P.; Medema, M.H.; Claesen, J.; Kurita, K.; Wieland Brown, L.C.; Mavrommatis, K.; Pati, A.; Godfrey, P.A.; Koehrsen, M.; Clardy, J.; et al. Insights into secondary metabolism from a global analysis of prokaryotic biosynthetic gene clusters. *Cell* **2014**, *158*, 412–421. [CrossRef]
18. Harizani, M.; Ioannou, E.; Roussis, V. The *Laurencia* paradox: An endless source of chemodiversity. *Prog. Chem. Org. Nat. Prod.* **2016**, *102*, 91–252. [CrossRef]
19. van Santen, J.A.; Poynton, E.F.; Iskakova, D.; McMann, E.; Alsup, T.A.; Clark, T.N.; Fergusson, C.H.; Fewer, D.P.; Hughes, A.H.; McCadden, C.A.; et al. The Natural Products Atlas 2.0: A database of microbially-derived natural products. *Nucleic Acids Res.* **2022**, *50*, D1317–D1323. [CrossRef] [PubMed]
20. Arnison, P.G.; Bibb, M.J.; Bierbaum, G.; Bowers, A.A.; Bugni, T.S.; Bulaj, G.; Camarero, J.A.; Campopiano, D.J.; Challis, G.L.; Clardy, J.; et al. Ribosomally synthesized and post-translationally modified peptide natural products: Overview and recommendations for a universal nomenclature. *Nat. Prod. Rep.* **2013**, *30*, 108–160. [CrossRef] [PubMed]
21. Dang, T.; Sussmuth, R.D. Bioactive peptide natural products as lead structures for medicinal use. *Acc. Chem. Res.* **2017**, *50*, 1566–1576. [CrossRef]
22. Korteling, J.E.; van de Boer-Visschedijk, G.C.; Blankendaal, R.A.M.; Boonekamp, R.C.; Eikelboom, A.R. Human-versus Artificial Intelligence. *Front. Artif. Intell.* **2021**, *4*, 622364. [CrossRef]
23. Alexander, S.P.H.; Fabbro, D.; Kelly, E.; Mathie, A.; Peters, J.A.; Veale, E.L.; Armstrong, J.F.; Faccenda, E.; Harding, S.D.; Pawson, A.J.; et al. The concise guide to pharmacology 2019/20: Enzymes. *Br. J. Pharmacol.* **2019**, *176* (Suppl. S1), S297–S396. [CrossRef]
24. UniProt, C. UniProt: The universal protein knowledgebase in 2021. *Nucleic Acids Res.* **2021**, *49*, D480–D489. [CrossRef]
25. Burley, S.K.; Berman, H.M.; Kleywegt, G.J.; Markley, J.L.; Nakamura, H.; Velankar, S. Protein Data Bank (PDB): The single global macromolecular structure archive. *Methods Mol. Biol.* **2017**, *1607*, 627–641. [CrossRef] [PubMed]
26. Hameduh, T.; Haddad, Y.; Adam, V.; Heger, Z. Homology modeling in the time of collective and artificial intelligence. *Comput. Struct. Biotechnol. J.* **2020**, *18*, 3494–3506. [CrossRef] [PubMed]
27. Jumper, J.; Evans, R.; Pritzel, A.; Green, T.; Figurnov, M.; Ronneberger, O.; Tunyasuvunakool, K.; Bates, R.; Zidek, A.; Potapenko, A.; et al. Highly accurate protein structure prediction with AlphaFold. *Nature* **2021**, *596*, 583–589. [CrossRef]
28. Lin, Z.; Akin, H.; Rao, R.; Hie, B.; Zhu, Z.; Lu, W.; Smetanin, N.; Verkuil, R.; Kabeli, O.; Shmueli, Y.; et al. Evolutionary-scale prediction of atomic level protein structure with a language model. *bioRxiv* **2022**. [CrossRef]
29. Drysdale, R.; Cook, C.E.; Petryszak, R.; Baillie-Gerritsen, V.; Barlow, M.; Gasteiger, E.; Gruhl, F.; Haas, J.; Lanfear, J.; Lopez, R.; et al. The ELIXIR Core Data Resources: Fundamental infrastructure for the life sciences. *Bioinformatics* **2020**, *36*, 2636–2642. [CrossRef]
30. Chang, A.; Jeske, L.; Ulbrich, S.; Hofmann, J.; Koblitz, J.; Schomburg, I.; Neumann-Schaal, M.; Jahn, D.; Schomburg, D. BRENDA, the ELIXIR core data resource in 2021: New developments and updates. *Nucleic Acids Res.* **2021**, *49*, D498–D508. [CrossRef]
31. Ribeiro, A.J.M.; Holliday, G.L.; Furnham, N.; Tyzack, J.D.; Ferris, K.; Thornton, J.M. Mechanism and Catalytic Site Atlas (M-CSA): A database of enzyme reaction mechanisms and active sites. *Nucleic Acids Res.* **2018**, *46*, D618–D623. [CrossRef]
32. Kim, S.; Chen, J.; Cheng, T.; Gindulyte, A.; He, J.; He, S.; Li, Q.; Shoemaker, B.A.; Thiessen, P.A.; Yu, B.; et al. PubChem in 2021: New data content and improved web interfaces. *Nucleic Acids Res.* **2021**, *49*, D1388–D1395. [CrossRef]
33. Mendez, D.; Gaulton, A.; Bento, A.P.; Chambers, J.; De Veij, M.; Felix, E.; Magarinos, M.P.; Mosquera, J.F.; Mutowo, P.; Nowotka, M.; et al. ChEMBL: Towards direct deposition of bioassay data. *Nucleic Acids Res.* **2019**, *47*, D930–D940. [CrossRef]

34. Pence, H.E.; Williams, A. Chemspider: An online chemical information resource. *J. Chem. Educ.* **2010**, *87*, 1123–1124. [CrossRef]
35. Wishart, D.S.; Knox, C.; Guo, A.C.; Shrivastava, S.; Hassanali, M.; Stothard, P.; Chang, Z.; Woolsey, J. DrugBank: A comprehensive resource for in silico drug discovery and exploration. *Nucleic Acids Res.* **2006**, *34*, D668–D672. [CrossRef] [PubMed]
36. Wishart, D.S.; Feunang, Y.D.; Guo, A.C.; Lo, E.J.; Marcu, A.; Grant, J.R.; Sajed, T.; Johnson, D.; Li, C.; Sayeeda, Z.; et al. DrugBank 5.0: A major update to the DrugBank database for 2018. *Nucleic Acids Res.* **2018**, *46*, D1074–D1082. [CrossRef] [PubMed]
37. Faulkner, D.J. Marine natural products. *Nat. Prod. Rep.* **2002**, *19*, 1R–49R. [CrossRef]
38. Blunt, J.W.; Carroll, A.R.; Copp, B.R.; Davis, R.A.; Keyzers, R.A.; Prinsep, M.R. Marine natural products. *Nat. Prod. Rep.* **2018**, *35*, 8–53. [CrossRef] [PubMed]
39. Carroll, A.R.; Copp, B.R.; Davis, R.A.; Keyzers, R.A.; Prinsep, M.R. Marine natural products. *Nat. Prod. Rep.* **2022**, *39*, 1122–1171. [CrossRef]
40. Blunt, J.; Munro, M.H.G. *Dictionary of Marine Natural Products, with CD-ROM*; Chapman & Hall/CRC: Boca Raton, FA, USA, 2008.
41. Sterling, T.; Irwin, J.J. ZINC 15—Ligand discovery for everyone. *J. Chem. Inf. Model.* **2015**, *55*, 2324–2337. [CrossRef]
42. Irwin, J.J.; Tang, K.G.; Young, J.; Dandarchuluun, C.; Wong, B.R.; Khurelbaatar, M.; Moroz, Y.S.; Mayfield, J.; Sayle, R.A. ZINC20-A free ultralarge-scale chemical database for ligand discovery. *J. Chem. Inf. Model.* **2020**, *60*, 6065–6073. [CrossRef]
43. Sorokina, M.; Steinbeck, C. Review on natural products databases: Where to find data in 2020. *J. Cheminform.* **2020**, *12*, 20. [CrossRef]
44. Kern, F.; Fehlmann, T.; Keller, A. On the lifetime of bioinformatics web services. *Nucleic Acids Res.* **2020**, *48*, 12523–12533. [CrossRef]
45. Rutz, A.; Sorokina, M.; Galgonek, J.; Mietchen, D.; Willighagen, E.; Gaudry, A.; Graham, J.G.; Stephan, R.; Page, R.; Vondrasek, J.; et al. The LOTUS initiative for open knowledge management in natural products research. *Elife* **2022**, *11*, e70780. [CrossRef] [PubMed]
46. Banerjee, P.; Erehman, J.; Gohlke, B.O.; Wilhelm, T.; Preissner, R.; Dunkel, M. Super Natural II–a database of natural products. *Nucleic Acids Res.* **2015**, *43*, D935–D939. [CrossRef] [PubMed]
47. Sorokina, M.; Merseburger, P.; Rajan, K.; Yirik, M.A.; Steinbeck, C. COCONUT online: Collection of Open Natural Products database. *J. Cheminform.* **2021**, *13*, 2. [CrossRef] [PubMed]
48. Blunt, J.; Munro, M.; Upjohn, M. The Role of Databases in Marine Natural Products Research. In *Handbook of Marine Natural Products*; Fattorusso, E., Gerwick, W.H., Taglialatela-Scafati, O., Eds.; Springer Science+Business Media B.V.: Dordrecht, The Netherlands, 2012; pp. 389–421.
49. Shen, S.M.; Appendino, G.; Guo, Y.W. Pitfalls in the structural elucidation of small molecules. A critical analysis of a decade of structural misassignments of marine natural products. *Nat. Prod. Rep.* **2022**, *39*, 1803–1832. [CrossRef]
50. Wishart, D.S. Computational strategies for metabolite identification in metabolomics. *Bioanalysis* **2009**, *1*, 1579–1596. [CrossRef]
51. Burns, D.C.; Mazzola, E.P.; Reynolds, W.F. The role of computer-assisted structure elucidation (CASE) programs in the structure elucidation of complex natural products. *Nat. Prod. Rep.* **2019**, *36*, 919–933. [CrossRef]
52. Urban, S.; Brkljaca, R.; Hoshino, M.; Lee, S.; Fujita, M. Determination of the absolute configuration of the pseudo-symmetric natural product elatenyne by the crystalline sponge method. *Angew. Chem. Int. Ed. Engl.* **2016**, *55*, 2678–2682. [CrossRef]
53. Rinschen, M.M.; Ivanisevic, J.; Giera, M.; Siuzdak, G. Identification of bioactive metabolites using activity metabolomics. *Nat. Rev. Mol. Cell Biol.* **2019**, *20*, 353–367. [CrossRef]
54. Muchiri, R.N.; van Breemen, R.B. Affinity selection-mass spectrometry for the discovery of pharmacologically active compounds from combinatorial libraries and natural products. *J. Mass Spectrom.* **2021**, *56*, e4647. [CrossRef]
55. Benson, D.A.; Cavanaugh, M.; Clark, K.; Karsch-Mizrachi, I.; Lipman, D.J.; Ostell, J.; Sayers, E.W. GenBank. *Nucleic Acids Res.* **2013**, *41*, D36–D42. [CrossRef]
56. Magrane, M.; UniProt, C. UniProt Knowledgebase: A hub of integrated protein data. *Database* **2011**, *2011*, bar009. [CrossRef] [PubMed]
57. Wang, M.; Carver, J.J.; Phelan, V.V.; Sanchez, L.M.; Garg, N.; Peng, Y.; Nguyen, D.D.; Watrous, J.; Kapono, C.A.; Luzzatto-Knaan, T.; et al. Sharing and community curation of mass spectrometry data with Global Natural Products Social Molecular Networking. *Nat. Biotechnol.* **2016**, *34*, 828–837. [CrossRef] [PubMed]
58. Weber, T.; Kim, H.U. The secondary metabolite bioinformatics portal: Computational tools to facilitate synthetic biology of secondary metabolite production. *Synth. Syst. Biotechnol.* **2016**, *1*, 69–79. [CrossRef]
59. Scherlach, K.; Hertweck, C. Mining and unearthing hidden biosynthetic potential. *Nat. Commun.* **2021**, *12*, 3864. [CrossRef] [PubMed]
60. Ziemert, N.; Podell, S.; Penn, K.; Badger, J.H.; Allen, E.; Jensen, P.R. The natural product domain seeker NaPDoS: A phylogeny based bioinformatic tool to classify secondary metabolite gene diversity. *PLoS ONE* **2012**, *7*, e34064. [CrossRef]
61. Klau, L.J.; Podell, S.; Creamer, K.E.; Demko, A.M.; Singh, H.W.; Allen, E.E.; Moore, B.S.; Ziemert, N.; Letzel, A.C.; Jensen, P.R. The Natural Product Domain Seeker version 2 (NaPDoS2) webtool relates ketosynthase phylogeny to biosynthetic function. *J. Biol. Chem.* **2022**, *298*, 102480. [CrossRef]
62. Albarano, L.; Esposito, R.; Ruocco, N.; Costantini, M. Genome mining as new challenge in natural products discovery. *Mar. Drugs* **2020**, *18*, 199. [CrossRef]
63. Medema, M.H.; Fischbach, M.A. Computational approaches to natural product discovery. *Nat. Chem. Biol.* **2015**, *11*, 639–648. [CrossRef]

64. Winter, J.M.; Behnken, S.; Hertweck, C. Genomics-inspired discovery of natural products. *Curr. Opin. Chem. Biol.* **2011**, *15*, 22–31. [CrossRef]
65. Lane, A.L.; Moore, B.S. A sea of biosynthesis: Marine natural products meet the molecular age. *Nat. Prod. Rep.* **2011**, *28*, 411–428. [CrossRef]
66. Bonet, B.; Teufel, R.; Crusemann, M.; Ziemert, N.; Moore, B.S. Direct capture and heterologous expression of *Salinispora* natural product genes for the biosynthesis of enterocin. *J. Nat. Prod.* **2015**, *78*, 539–542. [CrossRef] [PubMed]
67. Jensen, P.R. Natural products and the gene cluster revolution. *Trends Microbiol.* **2016**, *24*, 968–977. [CrossRef] [PubMed]
68. Medema, M.H. The year 2020 in natural product bioinformatics: An overview of the latest tools and databases. *Nat. Prod. Rep.* **2021**, *38*, 301–306. [CrossRef] [PubMed]
69. Doroghazi, J.R.; Albright, J.C.; Goering, A.W.; Ju, K.S.; Haines, R.R.; Tchalukov, K.A.; Labeda, D.P.; Kelleher, N.L.; Metcalf, W.W. A roadmap for natural product discovery based on large-scale genomics and metabolomics. *Nat. Chem. Biol.* **2014**, *10*, 963–968. [CrossRef] [PubMed]
70. Medema, M.H.; Kottmann, R.; Yilmaz, P.; Cummings, M.; Biggins, J.B.; Blin, K.; de Bruijn, I.; Chooi, Y.H.; Claesen, J.; Coates, R.C.; et al. Minimum information about a biosynthetic gene cluster. *Nat. Chem. Biol.* **2015**, *11*, 625–631. [CrossRef] [PubMed]
71. Masso-Silva, J.A.; Diamond, G. Antimicrobial peptides from fish. *Pharmaceuticals* **2014**, *7*, 265–310. [CrossRef] [PubMed]
72. Barroso, C.; Carvalho, P.; Goncalves, J.F.M.; Rodrigues, P.N.S.; Neves, J.V. Antimicrobial peptides: Identification of two b-defensins in a teleost fish, the european sea bass (*Dicentrarchus labrax*). *Pharmaceuticals* **2021**, *14*, 566. [CrossRef]
73. Tincu, J.A.; Taylor, S.W. Antimicrobial peptides from marine invertebrates. *Antimicrob. Agents Chemother.* **2004**, *48*, 3645–3654. [CrossRef]
74. Sychev, S.V.; Sukhanov, S.V.; Panteleev, P.V.; Shenkarev, Z.O.; Ovchinnikova, T.V. Marine antimicrobial peptide arenicin adopts a monomeric twisted beta-hairpin structure and forms low conductivity pores in zwitterionic lipid bilayers. *Pept. Sci.* **2017**, *110*, e23093. [CrossRef]
75. Wang, G.; Li, X.; Wang, Z. APD3: The antimicrobial peptide database as a tool for research and education. *Nucleic Acids Res.* **2016**, *44*, D1087–D1093. [CrossRef] [PubMed]
76. Broekman, D.C.; Zenz, A.; Gudmundsdottir, B.K.; Lohner, K.; Maier, V.H.; Gudmundsson, G.H. Functional characterization of codCath, the mature cathelicidin antimicrobial peptide from Atlantic cod (*Gadus morhua*). *Peptides* **2011**, *32*, 2044–2051. [CrossRef] [PubMed]
77. Castiglione, F.; Lazzarini, A.; Carrano, L.; Corti, E.; Ciciliato, I.; Gastaldo, L.; Candiani, P.; Losi, D.; Marinelli, F.; Selva, E.; et al. Determining the structure and mode of action of microbisporicin, a potent lantibiotic active against multiresistant pathogens. *Chem. Biol.* **2008**, *15*, 22–31. [CrossRef] [PubMed]
78. Chen, E.; Chen, Q.; Chen, S.; Xu, B.; Ju, J.; Wang, H. Mathermycin, a lantibiotic from the marine actinomycete *Marinactinospora thermotolerans* SCSIO 00652. *Appl. Environ. Microbiol.* **2017**, *83*, e00926-17. [CrossRef] [PubMed]
79. Wang, G. The antimicrobial peptide database provides a platform for decoding the design principles of naturally occurring antimicrobial peptides. *Protein Sci.* **2020**, *29*, 8–18. [CrossRef]
80. Pirtskhalava, M.; Amstrong, A.A.; Grigolava, M.; Chubinidze, M.; Alimbarashvili, E.; Vishnepolsky, B.; Gabrielian, A.; Rosenthal, A.; Hurt, D.E.; Tartakovsky, M. DBAASP v3: Database of antimicrobial/cytotoxic activity and structure of peptides as a resource for development of new therapeutics. *Nucleic Acids Res.* **2021**, *49*, D288–D297. [CrossRef]
81. Waghu, F.H.; Idicula-Thomas, S. Collection of antimicrobial peptides database and its derivatives: Applications and beyond. *Protein Sci.* **2020**, *29*, 36–42. [CrossRef]
82. Gawde, U.; Chakraborty, S.; Waghu, F.H.; Barai, R.S.; Khanderkar, A.; Indraguru, R.; Shirsat, T.; Idicula-Thomas, S. CAMPR4: A database of natural and synthetic antimicrobial peptides. *Nucleic Acids Res.* **2022**, *51*, D377–D383. [CrossRef]
83. van Santen, J.A.; Jacob, G.; Singh, A.L.; Aniebok, V.; Balunas, M.J.; Bunsko, D.; Neto, F.C.; Castano-Espriu, L.; Chang, C.; Clark, T.N.; et al. The Natural Products Atlas: An open access knowledge base for microbial natural products discovery. *ACS Cent. Sci.* **2019**, *5*, 1824–1833. [CrossRef]
84. Wilkinson, M.D.; Dumontier, M.; Aalbersberg, I.J.; Appleton, G.; Axton, M.; Baak, A.; Blomberg, N.; Boiten, J.W.; da Silva Santos, L.B.; Bourne, P.E.; et al. The FAIR Guiding Principles for scientific data management and stewardship. *Sci. Data* **2016**, *3*, 160018. [CrossRef]
85. Jones, M.R.; Pinto, E.; Torres, M.A.; Dorr, F.; Mazur-Marzec, H.; Szubert, K.; Tartaglione, L.; Dell'Aversano, C.; Miles, C.O.; Beach, D.G.; et al. CyanoMetDB, a comprehensive public database of secondary metabolites from cyanobacteria. *Water Res.* **2021**, *196*, 117017. [CrossRef]
86. Djoumbou Feunang, Y.; Eisner, R.; Knox, C.; Chepelev, L.; Hastings, J.; Owen, G.; Fahy, E.; Steinbeck, C.; Subramanian, S.; Bolton, E.; et al. ClassyFire: Automated chemical classification with a comprehensive, computable taxonomy. *J. Cheminform.* **2016**, *8*, 61. [CrossRef]
87. Kim, H.W.; Wang, M.; Leber, C.A.; Nothias, L.F.; Reher, R.; Kang, K.B.; van der Hooft, J.J.J.; Dorrestein, P.C.; Gerwick, W.H.; Cottrell, G.W. NPClassifier: A deep neural network-based structural classification tool for natural products. *J. Nat. Prod.* **2021**, *84*, 2795–2807. [CrossRef]
88. Sunagawa, S.; Coelho, L.P.; Chaffron, S.; Kultima, J.R.; Labadie, K.; Salazar, G.; Djahanschiri, B.; Zeller, G.; Mende, D.R.; Alberti, A.; et al. Ocean plankton. Structure and function of the global ocean microbiome. *Science* **2015**, *348*, 1261359. [CrossRef]

89. Cao, S.; Zhang, W.; Ding, W.; Wang, M.; Fan, S.; Yang, B.; McMinn, A.; Wang, M.; Xie, B.B.; Qin, Q.L.; et al. Structure and function of the Arctic and Antarctic marine microbiota as revealed by metagenomics. *Microbiome* **2020**, *8*, 47. [CrossRef]

90. Ashburner, M.; Ball, C.A.; Blake, J.A.; Botstein, D.; Butler, H.; Cherry, J.M.; Davis, A.P.; Dolinski, K.; Dwight, S.S.; Eppig, J.T.; et al. Gene ontology: Tool for the unification of biology. The Gene Ontology Consortium. *Nat. Genet.* **2000**, *25*, 25–29. [CrossRef]

91. Gene Ontology, C. The Gene Ontology resource: Enriching a GOld mine. *Nucleic Acids Res.* **2021**, *49*, D325–D334. [CrossRef]

92. Wishart, D.S.; Girod, S.; Peters, H.; Oler, E.; Jovel, J.; Budinski, Z.; Milford, R.; Lui, V.W.; Sayeeda, Z.; Mah, R.; et al. ChemFOnt: The chemical functional ontology resource. *Nucleic Acids Res.* **2022**, *51*, D1220–D1229. [CrossRef]

93. Bemis, G.W.; Murcko, M.A. The properties of known drugs. 1. Molecular frameworks. *J. Med. Chem.* **1996**, *39*, 2887–2893. [CrossRef]

94. Bemis, G.W.; Murcko, M.A. Properties of known drugs. 2. Side chains. *J. Med. Chem.* **1999**, *42*, 5095–5099. [CrossRef]

95. Ertl, P.; Roggo, S.; Schuffenhauer, A. Natural product-likeness score and its application for prioritization of compound libraries. *J. Chem. Inf. Model.* **2008**, *48*, 68–74. [CrossRef]

96. Chen, Y.; García de Lomana, M.; Friedrich, N.O.; Kirchmair, J. Characterization of the chemical space of known and readily obtainable natural products. *J. Chem. Inf. Model.* **2018**, *58*, 1518–1532. [CrossRef]

97. Stone, S.; Newman, D.J.; Colletti, S.L.; Tan, D.S. Cheminformatic analysis of natural product-based drugs and chemical probes. *Nat. Prod. Rep.* **2022**, *39*, 20–32. [CrossRef]

98. Zhang, M.Q.; Wilkinson, B. Drug discovery beyond the 'rule-of-five'. *Curr. Opin. Biotechnol.* **2007**, *18*, 478–488. [CrossRef]

99. Oprea, T.I.; Gottfries, J. Chemography: The art of navigating in chemical space. *J. Comb. Chem.* **2001**, *3*, 157–166. [CrossRef]

100. Larsson, J.; Gottfries, J.; Bohlin, L.; Backlund, A. Expanding the ChemGPS chemical space with natural products. *J. Nat. Prod.* **2005**, *68*, 985–991. [CrossRef]

101. Larsson, J.; Gottfries, J.; Muresan, S.; Backlund, A. ChemGPS-NP: Tuned for navigation in biologically relevant chemical space. *J. Nat. Prod.* **2007**, *70*, 789–794. [CrossRef]

102. Rosén, J.; Lövgren, A.; Kogej, T.; Muresan, S.; Gottfries, J.; Backlund, A. ChemGPS-NP(Web): Chemical space navigation online. *J. Comput. Aided Mol. Des.* **2009**, *23*, 253–259. [CrossRef]

103. Koch, M.A.; Schuffenhauer, A.; Scheck, M.; Wetzel, S.; Casaulta, M.; Odermatt, A.; Ertl, P.; Waldmann, H. Charting biologically relevant chemical space: A structural classification of natural products (SCONP). *Proc. Natl. Acad. Sci. USA* **2005**, *102*, 17272–17277. [CrossRef]

104. Weininger, D. SMILES, a chemical language and information system. 1. Introduction to methodology and encoding rules. *J. Chem. Inf. Model.* **1988**, *28*, 31–36. [CrossRef]

105. Ertl, P.; Schuhmann, T. Cheminformatics analysis of natural product scaffolds: Comparison of scaffolds produced by animals, plants, fungi and bacteria. *Mol. Inform.* **2020**, *39*, e2000017. [CrossRef]

106. Schafer, T.; Kriege, N.; Humbeck, L.; Klein, K.; Koch, O.; Mutzel, P. Scaffold Hunter: A comprehensive visual analytics framework for drug discovery. *J. Cheminform.* **2017**, *9*, 28. [CrossRef]

107. Voser, T.M.; Campbell, M.D.; Carroll, A.R. How different are marine microbial natural products compared to their terrestrial counterparts? *Nat. Prod. Rep.* **2022**, *39*, 7–19. [CrossRef]

108. Over, B.; Wetzel, S.; Grutter, C.; Nakai, Y.; Renner, S.; Rauh, D.; Waldmann, H. Natural-product-derived fragments for fragment-based ligand discovery. *Nat. Chem.* **2013**, *5*, 21–28. [CrossRef]

109. Elion, G.B.; Hitchings, G.H. The synthesis of 6-thioguanine. *J. Am. Chem. Soc.* **2002**, *77*, 1676. [CrossRef]

110. Coyne, S.; Chizzali, C.; Khalil, M.N.; Litomska, A.; Richter, K.; Beerhues, L.; Hertweck, C. Biosynthesis of the antimetabolite 6-thioguanine in *Erwinia amylovora* plays a key role in fire blight pathogenesis. *Angew. Chem. Int. Ed. Engl.* **2013**, *52*, 10564–10568. [CrossRef]

111. Grigalunas, M.; Brakmann, S.; Waldmann, H. Chemical evolution of natural product structure. *J. Am. Chem. Soc.* **2022**, *144*, 3314–3329. [CrossRef]

112. Müller, G. Medicinal chemistry of target family-directed masterkeys. *Drug Discov. Today* **2003**, *8*, 681–691. [CrossRef]

113. Bon, R.S.; Waldmann, H. Bioactivity-guided navigation of chemical space. *Acc. Chem. Res.* **2010**, *43*, 1103–1114. [CrossRef]

114. Wetzel, S.; Bon, R.S.; Kumar, K.; Waldmann, H. Biology-oriented synthesis. *Angew. Chem. Int. Ed. Engl.* **2011**, *50*, 10800–10826. [CrossRef]

115. Rodrigues, T.; Reker, D.; Schneider, P.; Schneider, G. Counting on natural products for drug design. *Nat. Chem.* **2016**, *8*, 531–541. [CrossRef]

116. Seiple, I.B.; Zhang, Z.; Jakubec, P.; Langlois-Mercier, A.; Wright, P.M.; Hog, D.T.; Yabu, K.; Allu, S.R.; Fukuzaki, T.; Carlsen, P.N.; et al. A platform for the discovery of new macrolide antibiotics. *Nature* **2016**, *533*, 338–345. [CrossRef] [PubMed]

117. Könst, Z.A.; Szklarski, A.R.; Pellegrino, S.; Michalak, S.E.; Meyer, M.; Zanette, C.; Cencic, R.; Nam, S.; Voora, V.K.; Horne, D.A.; et al. Synthesis facilitates an understanding of the structural basis for translation inhibition by the lissoclimides. *Nat. Chem.* **2017**, *9*, 1140–1149. [CrossRef]

118. Tan, D.S.; Foley, M.A.; Shair, M.D.; Schreiber, S.L. Stereoselective synthesis of over two million compounds having structural features both reminiscent of natural products and compatible with miniaturized cell-based assays. *J. Am. Chem. Soc.* **1998**, *120*, 8565–8566. [CrossRef]

119. Galloway, W.R.J.D.; Isidro-Llobet, A.; Spring, D.R. Diversity-oriented synthesis as a tool for the discovery of novel biologically active small molecules. *Nat. Commun.* **2010**, *1*, 80. [CrossRef]

120. Schreiber, S.L. Target-oriented and diversity-oriented organic synthesis in drug discovery. *Science* **2000**, *287*, 1964–1969. [CrossRef]
121. Wender, P.A. Toward the ideal synthesis and molecular function through synthesis-informed design. *Nat. Prod. Rep.* **2014**, *31*, 433–440. [CrossRef] [PubMed]
122. Cremosnik, G.S.; Liu, J.; Waldmann, H. Guided by evolution: From biology oriented synthesis to pseudo natural products. *Nat. Prod. Rep.* **2020**, *37*, 1497–1510. [CrossRef] [PubMed]
123. Karageorgis, G.; Foley, D.J.; Laraia, L.; Waldmann, H. Principle and design of pseudo-natural products. *Nat. Chem.* **2020**, *12*, 227–235. [CrossRef]
124. Karageorgis, G.; Foley, D.J.; Laraia, L.; Brakmann, S.; Waldmann, H. Pseudo natural products-chemical evolution of natural product structure. *Angew. Chem. Int. Ed. Engl.* **2021**, *60*, 15705–15723. [CrossRef]
125. van Hattum, H.; Waldmann, H. Biology-oriented synthesis: Harnessing the power of evolution. *J. Am. Chem. Soc.* **2014**, *136*, 11853–11859. [CrossRef]
126. Abbasov, M.E.; Alvariño, R.; Chaheine, C.M.; Alonso, E.; Sánchez, J.A.; Conner, M.L.; Alfonso, A.; Jaspars, M.; Botana, L.M.; Romo, D. Simplified immunosuppressive and neuroprotective agents based on gracilin A. *Nat. Chem.* **2019**, *11*, 342–350. [CrossRef] [PubMed]
127. Wermuth, C.G.; Ganellin, C.R.; Lindberg, P.; Mitscher, L.A. Glossary of terms used in medicinal chemistry (IUPAC Recommendations 1998). *Pure Appl. Chem.* **1998**, *70*, 1129–1143. [CrossRef]
128. Hopkins, A.L.; Groom, C.R. The druggable genome. *Nat. Rev. Drug Discov.* **2002**, *1*, 727–730. [CrossRef] [PubMed]
129. Fang, J.; Wu, Z.; Cai, C.; Wang, Q.; Tang, Y.; Cheng, F. Quantitative and systems pharmacology. 1. In silico prediction of drug-target interactions of natural products enables new targeted cancer therapy. *J. Chem. Inf. Model.* **2017**, *57*, 2657–2671. [CrossRef] [PubMed]
130. Freshour, S.L.; Kiwala, S.; Cotto, K.C.; Coffman, A.C.; McMichael, J.F.; Song, J.J.; Griffith, M.; Griffith, O.L.; Wagner, A.H. Integration of the Drug-Gene Interaction Database (DGIdb 4.0) with open crowdsource efforts. *Nucleic Acids Res.* **2021**, *49*, D1144–D1151. [CrossRef]
131. Tang, J.; Tanoli, Z.U.; Ravikumar, B.; Alam, Z.; Rebane, A.; Vaha-Koskela, M.; Peddinti, G.; van Adrichem, A.J.; Wakkinen, J.; Jaiswal, A.; et al. Drug Target Commons: A community effort to build a consensus knowledge base for drug-target interactions. *Cell Chem. Biol.* **2018**, *25*, 224–229.e2. [CrossRef]
132. Pillich, R.T.; Chen, J.; Churas, C.; Liu, S.; Ono, K.; Otasek, D.; Pratt, D. NDEx: Accessing network models and streamlining network biology workflows. *Curr. Protoc.* **2021**, *1*, e258. [CrossRef]
133. Wu, Z.; Cheng, F.; Li, J.; Li, W.; Liu, G.; Tang, Y. SDTNBI: An integrated network and chemoinformatics tool for systematic prediction of drug-target interactions and drug repositioning. *Brief. Bioinform.* **2017**, *18*, 333–347. [CrossRef]
134. Wu, Z.; Ma, H.; Liu, Z.; Zheng, L.; Yu, Z.; Cao, S.; Fang, W.; Wu, L.; Li, W.; Liu, G.; et al. wSDTNBI: A novel network-based inference method for virtual screening. *Chem. Sci.* **2022**, *13*, 1060–1079. [CrossRef]
135. Wu, Z.; Li, W.; Liu, G.; Tang, Y. Network-based methods for prediction of drug-target interactions. *Front. Pharmacol.* **2018**, *9*, 1134. [CrossRef]
136. Gfeller, D.; Michielin, O.; Zoete, V. Shaping the interaction landscape of bioactive molecules. *Bioinformatics* **2013**, *29*, 3073–3079. [CrossRef] [PubMed]
137. Gfeller, D.; Grosdidier, A.; Wirth, M.; Daina, A.; Michielin, O.; Zoete, V. SwissTargetPrediction: A web server for target prediction of bioactive small molecules. *Nucleic Acids Res.* **2014**, *42*, W32–W38. [CrossRef] [PubMed]
138. Gentile, F.; Yaacoub, J.C.; Gleave, J.; Fernandez, M.; Ton, A.T.; Ban, F.; Stern, A.; Cherkasov, A. Artificial intelligence-enabled virtual screening of ultra-large chemical libraries with deep docking. *Nat. Protoc.* **2022**, *17*, 672–697. [CrossRef] [PubMed]
139. Keiser, M.J.; Setola, V.; Irwin, J.J.; Laggner, C.; Abbas, A.I.; Hufeisen, S.J.; Jensen, N.H.; Kuijer, M.B.; Matos, R.C.; Tran, T.B.; et al. Predicting new molecular targets for known drugs. *Nature* **2009**, *462*, 175–181. [CrossRef] [PubMed]
140. Lounkine, E.; Keiser, M.J.; Whitebread, S.; Mikhailov, D.; Hamon, J.; Jenkins, J.L.; Lavan, P.; Weber, E.; Doak, A.K.; Cote, S.; et al. Large-scale prediction and testing of drug activity on side-effect targets. *Nature* **2012**, *486*, 361–367. [CrossRef]
141. McGovern, S.L.; Caselli, E.; Grigorieff, N.; Shoichet, B.K. A common mechanism underlying promiscuous inhibitors from virtual and high-throughput screening. *J. Med. Chem.* **2002**, *45*, 1712–1722. [CrossRef]
142. Baell, J.B.; Holloway, G.A. New substructure filters for removal of pan assay interference compounds (PAINS) from screening libraries and for their exclusion in bioassays. *J. Med. Chem.* **2010**, *53*, 2719–2740. [CrossRef]
143. Baell, J.B. Feeling Nature's PAINS: Natural products, natural product drugs, and pan assay interference compounds (PAINS). *J. Nat. Prod.* **2016**, *79*, 616–628. [CrossRef]
144. Bisson, J.; McAlpine, J.B.; Friesen, J.B.; Chen, S.N.; Graham, J.; Pauli, G.F. Can invalid bioactives undermine natural product-based drug discovery? *J. Med. Chem.* **2016**, *59*, 1671–1690. [CrossRef]
145. Baell, J.B.; Nissink, J.W.M. Seven year itch: Pan-assay interference compounds (PAINS) in 2017-utility and limitations. *ACS Chem. Biol.* **2018**, *13*, 36–44. [CrossRef]
146. Stork, C.; Chen, Y.; Sicho, M.; Kirchmair, J. Hit Dexter 2.0: Machine-learning models for the prediction of frequent hitters. *J. Chem. Inf. Model.* **2019**, *59*, 1030–1043. [CrossRef] [PubMed]
147. Quiñoà, E.; Adamczeski, M.; Crews, P.; Bakus, G.J. Bengamides, heterocyclic anthelmintics from a Jaspidae marine sponge. *J. Org. Chem.* **1986**, *51*, 4494–4497. [CrossRef]
148. Wang, Y.Q.; Miao, Z.H. Marine-derived angiogenesis inhibitors for cancer therapy. *Mar. Drugs* **2013**, *11*, 903–933. [CrossRef]

149. White, K.N.; Tenney, K.; Crews, P. The bengamides: A mini-review of natural sources, analogues, biological properties, biosynthetic origins, and future prospects. *J. Nat. Prod.* **2017**, *80*, 740–755. [CrossRef]

150. Towbin, H.; Bair, K.W.; DeCaprio, J.A.; Eck, M.J.; Kim, S.; Kinder, F.R.; Morollo, A.; Mueller, D.R.; Schindler, P.; Song, H.K.; et al. Proteomics-based target identification: Bengamides as a new class of methionine aminopeptidase inhibitors. *J. Biol. Chem.* **2003**, *278*, 52964–52971. [CrossRef]

151. Xu, W.; Lu, J.P.; Ye, Q.Z. Structural analysis of bengamide derivatives as inhibitors of methionine aminopeptidases. *J. Med. Chem.* **2012**, *55*, 8021–8027. [CrossRef] [PubMed]

152. Lu, J.P.; Yuan, X.H.; Yuan, H.; Wang, W.L.; Wan, B.; Franzblau, S.G.; Ye, Q.Z. Inhibition of *Mycobacterium tuberculosis* methionine aminopeptidases by bengamide derivatives. *ChemMedChem* **2011**, *6*, 1041–1048. [CrossRef] [PubMed]

153. Porras-Alcalá, C.; Moya-Utrera, F.; García-Castro, M.; Sánchez-Ruiz, A.; López-Romero, J.M.; Pino-González, M.S.; Díaz-Morilla, A.; Kitamura, S.; Wolan, D.W.; Prados, J.; et al. The development of the bengamides as new antibiotics against drug-resistant bacteria. *Mar. Drugs* **2022**, *20*, 373. [CrossRef]

154. Liu, S.; Widom, J.; Kemp, C.W.; Crews, C.M.; Clardy, J. Structure of human methionine aminopeptidase-2 complexed with fumagillin. *Science* **1998**, *282*, 1324–1327. [CrossRef]

155. Bailey, L. Effect of fumagillin upon *Nosema apis* (Zander). *Nature* **1953**, *171*, 212–213. [CrossRef]

156. Rateb, M.E.; Houssen, W.E.; Schumacher, M.; Harrison, W.T.; Diederich, R.; Ebel, R.; Jaspars, M. Bioactive diterpene derivatives from the marine sponge *Spongionella* sp. *J. Nat. Prod.* **2009**, *72*, 1471–1476. [CrossRef] [PubMed]

157. Potts, B.C.; Faulkner, D.J.; Jacobs, R.S. Phospholipase A_2 inhibitors from marine organisms. *J. Nat. Prod.* **1992**, *55*, 1701–1717. [CrossRef] [PubMed]

158. Sánchez, J.A.; Alfonso, A.; Leirós, M.; Alonso, E.; Rateb, M.E.; Jaspars, M.; Houssen, W.E.; Ebel, R.; Tabudravu, J.; Botana, L.M. Identification of *Spongionella* compounds as cyclosporine A mimics. *Pharmacol. Res.* **2016**, *107*, 407–414. [CrossRef]

159. Li, K.; Gustafson, K.R. Sesterterpenoids: Chemistry, biology, and biosynthesis. *Nat. Prod. Rep.* **2021**, *38*, 1251–1281. [CrossRef] [PubMed]

160. Ebada, S.S.; Lin, W.; Proksch, P. Bioactive sesterterpenes and triterpenes from marine sponges: Occurrence and pharmacological significance. *Mar. Drugs* **2010**, *8*, 313–346. [CrossRef] [PubMed]

161. Posadas, I.; De Rosa, S.; Terencio, M.C.; Paya, M.; Alcaraz, M.J. Cacospongionolide B suppresses the expression of inflammatory enzymes and tumour necrosis factor-alpha by inhibiting nuclear factor-kappa B activation. *Br. J. Pharmacol.* **2003**, *138*, 1571–1579. [CrossRef]

162. Gunasekera, S.P.; McCarthy, P.J.; Kelly-Borges, M.; Lobkovsky, E.; Clardy, J. Dysidiolide: A novel protein phosphatase inhibitor from the Caribbean sponge *Dysidea etheria* de Laubenfels. *J. Am. Chem. Soc.* **1996**, *118*, 8759–8760. [CrossRef]

163. Marcos, I.S.; Escola, M.A.; Moro, R.F.; Basabe, P.; Diez, D.; Sanz, F.; Mollinedo, F.; de la Iglesia-Vicente, J.; Sierra, B.G.; Urones, J.G. Synthesis of novel antitumoural analogues of dysidiolide from *ent*-halimic acid. *Bioorg. Med. Chem.* **2007**, *15*, 5719–5737. [CrossRef]

164. Dekker, F.J.; Koch, M.A.; Waldmann, H. Protein structure similarity clustering (PSSC) and natural product structure as inspiration sources for drug development and chemical genomics. *Curr. Opin. Chem. Biol.* **2005**, *9*, 232–239. [CrossRef]

165. Koch, M.A.; Wittenberg, L.O.; Basu, S.; Jeyaraj, D.A.; Gourzoulidou, E.; Reinecke, K.; Odermatt, A.; Waldmann, H. Compound library development guided by protein structure similarity clustering and natural product structure. *Proc. Natl. Acad. Sci. USA* **2004**, *101*, 16721–16726. [CrossRef]

166. Pina, I.C.; Gautschi, J.T.; Wang, G.Y.; Sanders, M.L.; Schmitz, F.J.; France, D.; Cornell-Kennon, S.; Sambucetti, L.C.; Remiszewski, S.W.; Perez, L.B.; et al. Psammaplins from the sponge *Pseudoceratina purpurea*: Inhibition of both histone deacetylase and DNA methyltransferase. *J. Org. Chem.* **2003**, *68*, 3866–3873. [CrossRef] [PubMed]

167. Kim, D.H.; Shin, J.; Kwon, H.J. Psammaplin A is a natural prodrug that inhibits class I histone deacetylase. *Exp. Mol. Med.* **2007**, *39*, 47–55. [CrossRef] [PubMed]

168. El-Sayed, A.M. The Pherobase: Database of Pheromones and Semiochemicals; 2022. Available online: https://pherolist.org/ (accessed on 20 December 2022).

169. Oluwabusola, E.T.; Katermeran, N.P.; Poh, W.H.; Goh, T.M.B.; Tan, L.T.; Diyaolu, O.; Tabudravu, J.; Ebel, R.; Rice, S.A.; Jaspars, M. Inhibition of the quorum sensing system, elastase production and biofilm formation in *Pseudomonas aeruginosa* by psammaplin A and bisaprasin. *Molecules* **2022**, *27*, 1721. [CrossRef]

170. Rawlings, N.D.; Barrett, A.J.; Thomas, P.D.; Huang, X.; Bateman, A.; Finn, R.D. The MEROPS database of proteolytic enzymes, their substrates and inhibitors in 2017 and a comparison with peptidases in the PANTHER database. *Nucleic Acids Res.* **2018**, *46*, D624–D632. [CrossRef] [PubMed]

171. Miller, B.; Friedman, A.J.; Choi, H.; Hogan, J.; McCammon, J.A.; Hook, V.; Gerwick, W.H. The marine cyanobacterial metabolite gallinamide A is a potent and selective inhibitor of human cathepsin L. *J. Nat. Prod.* **2014**, *77*, 92–99. [CrossRef] [PubMed]

172. Boudreau, P.D.; Miller, B.W.; McCall, L.I.; Almaliti, J.; Reher, R.; Hirata, K.; Le, T.; Siqueira-Neto, J.L.; Hook, V.; Gerwick, W.H. Design of gallinamide a analogs as potent inhibitors of the cysteine proteases human cathepsin l and *Trypanosoma cruzi* cruzain. *J. Med. Chem.* **2019**, *62*, 9026–9044. [CrossRef]

173. Barbosa Da Silva, E.; Sharma, V.; Hernandez-Alvarez, L.; Tang, A.H.; Stoye, A.; O'Donoghue, A.J.; Gerwick, W.H.; Payne, R.J.; McKerrow, J.H.; Podust, L.M. Intramolecular interactions enhance the potency of gallinamide A analogues against *Trypanosoma cruzi*. *J. Med. Chem.* **2022**, *65*, 4255–4269. [CrossRef]

174. Klenchin, V.A.; King, R.; Tanaka, J.; Marriott, G.; Rayment, I. Structural basis of swinholide A binding to actin. *Chem. Biol.* **2005**, *12*, 287–291. [CrossRef]
175. Issac, M.; Aknin, M.; Gauvin-Bialecki, A.; De Voogd, N.; Ledoux, A.; Frederich, M.; Kashman, Y.; Carmeli, S. Cyclotheonellazoles A–C, potent protease inhibitors from the marine sponge *Theonella aff. swinhoei*. *J. Nat. Prod.* **2017**, *80*, 1110–1116. [CrossRef]
176. Cui, Y.; Zhang, M.; Xu, H.; Zhang, T.; Zhang, S.; Zhao, X.; Jiang, P.; Li, J.; Ye, B.; Sun, Y.; et al. Elastase inhibitor cyclotheonellazole A: Total synthesis and in vivo biological evaluation for acute lung injury. *J. Med. Chem.* **2022**, *65*, 2971–2987. [CrossRef]
177. Köcher, S.; Resch, S.; Kessenbrock, T.; Schrapp, L.; Ehrmann, M.; Kaiser, M. From dolastatin 13 to cyanopeptolins, micropeptins, and lyngbyastatins: The chemical biology of Ahp-cyclodepsipeptides. *Nat. Prod. Rep.* **2020**, *37*, 163–174. [CrossRef] [PubMed]
178. Chen, Q.Y.; Luo, D.; Seabra, G.M.; Luesch, H. Ahp-Cyclodepsipeptides as tunable inhibitors of human neutrophil elastase and kallikrein 7: Total synthesis of tutuilamide A, serine protease selectivity profile and comparison with lyngbyastatin 7. *Bioorg. Med. Chem.* **2020**, *28*, 115756. [CrossRef] [PubMed]
179. Pettit, G.R.; Kamano, Y.; Herald, C.L.; Dufresne, C.; Cerny, R.L.; Herald, D.L.; Schmidt, J.M.; Kizu, H. Antineoplastic agent. 174. Isolation and structure of the cytostatic depsipeptide dolastatin 13 from the sea hare *Dolabella auricularia*. *J. Am. Chem. Soc.* **1989**, *111*, 5015–5017. [CrossRef]
180. Gunasekera, S.P.; Miller, M.W.; Kwan, J.C.; Luesch, H.; Paul, V.J. Molassamide, a depsipeptide serine protease inhibitor from the marine cyanobacterium *Dichothrix utahensis*. *J. Nat. Prod.* **2010**, *73*, 459–462. [CrossRef] [PubMed]
181. Salvador, L.A.; Taori, K.; Biggs, J.S.; Jakoncic, J.; Ostrov, D.A.; Paul, V.J.; Luesch, H. Potent elastase inhibitors from cyanobacteria: Structural basis and mechanisms mediating cytoprotective and anti-inflammatory effects in bronchial epithelial cells. *J. Med. Chem.* **2013**, *56*, 1276–1290. [CrossRef]
182. Yu, M.; Dolios, G.; Petrick, L. Reproducible untargeted metabolomics workflow for exhaustive MS2 data acquisition of MS1 features. *J. Cheminform.* **2022**, *14*, 6. [CrossRef]
183. Keller, L.; Canuto, K.M.; Liu, C.; Suzuki, B.M.; Almaliti, J.; Sikandar, A.; Naman, C.B.; Glukhov, E.; Luo, D.; Duggan, B.M.; et al. Tutuilamides A–C: Vinyl-chloride-containing cyclodepsipeptides from marine cyanobacteria with potent elastase inhibitory properties. *ACS Chem. Biol.* **2020**, *15*, 751–757. [CrossRef]
184. Reher, R.; Aron, A.T.; Fajtova, P.; Stincone, P.; Wagner, B.; Perez-Lorente, A.I.; Liu, C.; Shalom, I.Y.B.; Bittremieux, W.; Wang, M.; et al. Native metabolomics identifies the rivulariapeptolide family of protease inhibitors. *Nat. Commun.* **2022**, *13*, 4619. [CrossRef]
185. Hanada, M.; Sugawara, K.; Kaneta, K.; Toda, S.; Nishiyama, Y.; Tomita, K.; Yamamoto, H.; Konishi, M.; Oki, T. Epoxomicin, a new antitumor agent of microbial origin. *J. Antibiot.* **1992**, *45*, 1746–1752. [CrossRef]
186. Levin, N.; Spencer, A.; Harrison, S.J.; Chauhan, D.; Burrows, F.J.; Anderson, K.C.; Reich, S.D.; Richardson, P.G.; Trikha, M. Marizomib irreversibly inhibits proteasome to overcome compensatory hyperactivation in multiple myeloma and solid tumour patients. *Br. J. Haematol.* **2016**, *174*, 711–720. [CrossRef]
187. Potts, B.C.; Albitar, M.X.; Anderson, K.C.; Baritaki, S.; Berkers, C.; Bonavida, B.; Chandra, J.; Chauhan, D.; Cusack, J.C., Jr.; Fenical, W.; et al. Marizomib, a proteasome inhibitor for all seasons: Preclinical profile and a framework for clinical trials. *Curr. Cancer Drug Targets* **2011**, *11*, 254–284. [CrossRef] [PubMed]
188. Hubbell, G.E.; Tepe, J.J. Natural product scaffolds as inspiration for the design and synthesis of 20S human proteasome inhibitors. *RSC Chem. Biol.* **2020**, *1*, 305–332. [CrossRef] [PubMed]
189. Kawamura, S.; Unno, Y.; Tanaka, M.; Sasaki, T.; Yamano, A.; Hirokawa, T.; Kameda, T.; Asai, A.; Arisawa, M.; Shuto, S. Investigation of the noncovalent binding mode of covalent proteasome inhibitors around the transition state by combined use of cyclopropylic strain-based conformational restriction and computational modeling. *J. Med. Chem.* **2013**, *56*, 5829–5842. [CrossRef] [PubMed]
190. Li, T.; Wang, N.; Zhang, T.; Zhang, B.; Sajeevan, T.P.; Joseph, V.; Armstrong, L.; He, S.; Yan, X.; Naman, C.B. A systematic review of recently reported marine derived natural product kinase inhibitors. *Mar. Drugs* **2019**, *17*, 493. [CrossRef] [PubMed]
191. Kinnel, R.B.; Scheuer, P.J. 11-Hydroxystaurosporine: A highly cytotoxic, powerful protein kinase C inhibitor from a tunicate. *J. Org. Chem.* **1992**, *57*, 6327–6329. [CrossRef]
192. Cohen, P.; Cross, D.; Janne, P.A. Kinase drug discovery 20 years after imatinib: Progress and future directions. *Nat. Rev. Drug Discov.* **2021**, *20*, 551–569. [CrossRef]
193. Karaman, M.W.; Herrgard, S.; Treiber, D.K.; Gallant, P.; Atteridge, C.E.; Campbell, B.T.; Chan, K.W.; Ciceri, P.; Davis, M.I.; Edeen, P.T.; et al. A quantitative analysis of kinase inhibitor selectivity. *Nat. Biotechnol.* **2008**, *26*, 127–132. [CrossRef]
194. Lo, Y.C.; Liu, T.; Morrissey, K.M.; Kakiuchi-Kiyota, S.; Johnson, A.R.; Broccatelli, F.; Zhong, Y.; Joshi, A.; Altman, R.B. Computational analysis of kinase inhibitor selectivity using structural knowledge. *Bioinformatics* **2019**, *35*, 235–242. [CrossRef]
195. Dai, X.; Xu, Y.; Qiu, H.; Qian, X.; Lin, M.; Luo, L.; Zhao, Y.; Huang, D.; Zhang, Y.; Chen, Y.; et al. KID: A kinase-focused interaction database and its application in the construction of kinase-focused molecule databases. *J. Chem. Inf. Model.* **2022**, *62*, 6022–6034. [CrossRef]
196. Manning, G.; Whyte, D.B.; Martinez, R.; Hunter, T.; Sudarsanam, S. The protein kinase complement of the human genome. *Science* **2002**, *298*, 1912–1934. [CrossRef]
197. Janssen, A.P.A.; Grimm, S.H.; Wijdeven, R.H.M.; Lenselink, E.B.; Neefjes, J.; van Boeckel, C.A.A.; van Westen, G.J.P.; van der Stelt, M. Drug discovery maps, a machine learning model that visualizes and predicts kinome-inhibitor interaction landscapes. *J. Chem. Inf. Model.* **2019**, *59*, 1221–1229. [CrossRef]

198. Aoki, S.; Watanabe, Y.; Sanagawa, M.; Setiawan, A.; Kotoku, N.; Kobayashi, M. Cortistatins A, B, C, and D, anti-angiogenic steroidal alkaloids, from the marine sponge *Corticium simplex*. *J. Am. Chem. Soc.* **2006**, *128*, 3148–3149. [CrossRef] [PubMed]
199. Pelish, H.E.; Liau, B.B.; Nitulescu, II; Tangpeerachaikul, A.; Poss, Z.C.; Da Silva, D.H.; Caruso, B.T.; Arefolov, A.; Fadeyi, O.; Christie, A.L.; et al. Mediator kinase inhibition further activates super-enhancer-associated genes in AML. *Nature* **2015**, *526*, 273–276. [CrossRef] [PubMed]
200. Aoki, S.; Watanabe, Y.; Tanabe, D.; Arai, M.; Suna, H.; Miyamoto, K.; Tsujibo, H.; Tsujikawa, K.; Yamamoto, H.; Kobayashi, M. Structure-activity relationship and biological property of cortistatins, anti-angiogenic spongean steroidal alkaloids. *Bioorg. Med. Chem.* **2007**, *15*, 6758–6762. [CrossRef]
201. Funabashi, M.; Baba, S.; Takatsu, T.; Kizuka, M.; Ohata, Y.; Tanaka, M.; Nonaka, K.; Spork, A.P.; Ducho, C.; Chen, W.C.; et al. Structure-based gene targeting discovery of sphaerimicin, a bacterial translocase I inhibitor. *Angew. Chem. Int. Ed. Engl.* **2013**, *52*, 11607–11611. [CrossRef] [PubMed]
202. Li, L.; Gui, Y.H.; Xu, Q.H.; Lin, H.W.; Lu, Y.H. *Spongiactinospora rosea* gen. nov., sp. nov., a new member of the family Streptosporangiaceae. *Int. J. Syst. Evol. Microbiol.* **2019**, *69*, 427–433. [CrossRef] [PubMed]
203. Nakaya, T.; Yabe, M.; Mashalidis, E.H.; Sato, T.; Yamamoto, K.; Hikiji, Y.; Katsuyama, A.; Shinohara, M.; Minato, Y.; Takahashi, S.; et al. Synthesis of macrocyclic nucleoside antibacterials and their interactions with MraY. *Nat. Commun.* **2022**, *13*, 7575. [CrossRef]
204. Pereira, R.B.; Evdokimov, N.M.; Lefranc, F.; Valentao, P.; Kornienko, A.; Pereira, D.M.; Andrade, P.B.; Gomes, N.G.M. Marine-derived anticancer agents: Clinical benefits, innovative mechanisms, and new targets. *Mar. Drugs* **2019**, *17*, 329. [CrossRef]
205. Lipinski, C.; Hopkins, A. Navigating chemical space for biology and medicine. *Nature* **2004**, *432*, 855–861. [CrossRef]
206. Hight, S.K.; Clark, T.N.; Kurita, K.L.; McMillan, E.A.; Bray, W.; Shaikh, A.F.; Khadilkar, A.; Haeckl, F.P.J.; Carnevale-Neto, F.; La, S.; et al. High-throughput functional annotation of natural products by integrated activity profiling. *Proc. Natl. Acad. Sci. USA* **2022**, *119*, e2208458119. [CrossRef]

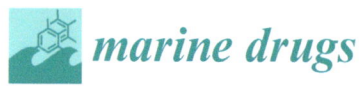

Article

Isolation and Characterization of NpCI, a New Metallocarboxypeptidase Inhibitor from the Marine Snail *Nerita peloronta* with Anti-*Plasmodium falciparum* Activity

Aymara Cabrera-Muñoz [1], Yusvel Sierra-Gómez [1], Giovanni Covaleda-Cortés [2], Mey L. Reytor [1], Yamile González-González [1], José M. Bautista [3], Francesc Xavier Avilés [2,*] and Maday Alonso-del-Rivero [1,*]

[1] Centro de Estudio de Proteínas, Facultad de Biología, Universidad de la Habana, La Habana 10400, Cuba
[2] Institut de Biotecnologia i de Biomedicina and Departament de Bioquímica, Universitat Autònoma de Barcelona, 08193 Bellaterra, Spain
[3] Departamento de Bioquímica y Biología Molecular, Facultad de Veterinaria, Universidad Complutense de Madrid, Ciudad Universitaria, 28040 Madrid, Spain
* Correspondence: FrancescXavier.Aviles@uab.cat (F.X.A.); maday@fbio.uh.cu (M.A.-d.-R.)

Abstract: Metallocarboxypeptidases are zinc-dependent peptide-hydrolysing enzymes involved in several important physiological and pathological processes. They have been a target of growing interest in the search for natural or synthetic compound binders with biomedical and drug discovery purposes, i.e., with potential as antimicrobials or antiparasitics. Given that marine resources are an extraordinary source of bioactive molecules, we screened marine invertebrates for new inhibitory compounds with such capabilities. In this work, we report the isolation and molecular and functional characterization of NpCI, a novel strong metallocarboxypeptidase inhibitor from the marine snail *Nerita peloronta*. NpCI was purified until homogeneity using a combination of affinity chromatography and RP-HPLC. It appeared as a 5921.557 Da protein with 53 residues and six disulphide-linked cysteines, displaying a high sequence similarity with NvCI, a carboxypeptidase inhibitor isolated from *Nerita versicolor*, a mollusc of the same genus. The purified inhibitor was determined to be a slow- and tight-binding inhibitor of bovine CPA (Ki = 1.1×10^{-8} mol/L) and porcine CPB (Ki = 8.15×10^{-8} mol/L) and was not able to inhibit proteases from other mechanistic classes. Importantly, this inhibitor showed antiplasmodial activity against *Plasmodium falciparum* in an in vitro culture (IC$_{50}$ = 5.5 µmol/L), reducing parasitaemia mainly by inhibiting the later stages of the parasite's intraerythrocytic cycle whilst having no cytotoxic effects on human fibroblasts. Interestingly, initial attempts with other related proteinaceous carboxypeptidase inhibitors also displayed similar antiplasmodial effects. Coincidentally, in recent years, a metallocarboxypeptidase named PfNna1, which is expressed in the schizont phase during the late intraerythrocytic stage of the parasite's life cycle, has been described. Given that NpCI showed a specific parasiticidal effect on *P. falciparum*, eliciting pyknotic/dead parasites, our results suggest that this and related inhibitors could be promising starting agents or lead compounds for antimalarial drug discovery strategies.

Keywords: metallocarboxipeptidases; carboxypeptidase inhibitor; slow- and tight-binding inhibitor; marine invertebrate; *Plasmodium falciparum*; antimalarial

Citation: Cabrera-Muñoz, A.; Sierra-Gómez, Y.; Covaleda-Cortés, G.; Reytor, M.L.; González-González, Y.; Bautista, J.M.; Avilés, F.X.; Alonso-del-Rivero, M. Isolation and Characterization of NpCI, a New Metallocarboxypeptidase Inhibitor from the Marine Snail *Nerita peloronta* with Anti-*Plasmodium falciparum* Activity. *Mar. Drugs* **2023**, *21*, 94. https://doi.org/10.3390/md21020094

Academic Editor: Bill J. Baker

Received: 29 November 2022
Revised: 24 January 2023
Accepted: 25 January 2023
Published: 28 January 2023

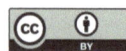
1. Introduction

Metallocarboxypeptidases (MCPs) are zinc-dependent peptide-hydrolysing enzymes involved in important physiological and pathological processes [1–3]. Due to the important functions of these enzymes, their proteolytic activity is controlled in many instances. One of the most efficient control mechanisms is protease inhibitors of natural origins, either organic or proteinaceous [3].

In contrast to the wide variety of reported proteinaceous inhibitors of endopeptidases, only a few natural inhibitors of metallocarboxypeptidases have been described to date [4].

Several inhibitors have been isolated from plants, including tomato metallocarboxypeptidase inhibitor (TMCI) and potato carboxypeptidase inhibitor (PCI) [5,6]; invertebrates, such as tick carboxypeptidase inhibitor (TCI) and *Haemaphysalis longicornis* carboxypeptidase inhibitor (HTCI) [7,8], leech carboxypeptidase inhibitor (LCI) [9], *Ascaris suum* carboxypeptidase inhibitor (ACI) from the intestinal parasite *Ascaris suum* [10], *Nerita versicolor* carboxypeptidase inhibitor (NvCI) from the marine mollusc *Nerita versicolor* [11,12], and *Sabellastarte magnifica* carboxypeptidase inhibitor (SmCI) from the marine annelid *Sabellastarte magnifica* [13]; and mammals, including latexin from humans and rats [14,15]. All of these are classified as tight-binding inhibitors against the cognate enzymes. These inhibitors have demonstrated potential in the treatment of several diseases in which carboxypeptidases are involved. For example, PCI and TCI, inhibitors of the TAFI (*thrombin-activatable fibrinolysis inhibitor*) metallocarboxypeptidase, have been used as fibrinolytic agents to treat massive pulmonary embolism [16,17] and acute thrombotic events [18]. In addition, human latexin has exhibited potential as a tumour suppressor [19,20].

On the other hand, the potential of strong inhibitors of metallocarboxypeptidases (PCI, LCI, benzyl succinate) to inhibit the growth of *Plasmodium falciparum* in culture has also been proposed [21]. This property has been related to the occurrence of a unique gene coding for an Nna1-like carboxypeptidase in *P. falciparum* [22,23] belonging to the cytosolic carboxypeptidase subfamily (CCPs and M14C). In addition, it has been shown that these enzymes participate in α-tubulin processing, an important mechanism in the dynamics of microtubules during cell division in parasites [23–25]. Therefore, its inhibition could produce a negative effect on parasite development [21]. These findings point to this enzyme as a potentially attractive target to treat parasitic infections. It is worth noting that several unsuccessful attempts have been made to isolate or recombinantly produce the enzyme in an active state.

Due to the importance of this enzyme and the absence of inhibitors targeting it or its subfamily of metallocarboxypeptidases, the availability of new and specific inhibitors could contribute to the design of novel antimalarials as well as to advances in enzyme–inhibitor structure–function knowledge. In this regard, a clear inhibitory activity was recently detected against the related model enzymes of bovine carboxypeptidase A (bCPA) and porcine carboxypeptidases B (pCPB) in an aqueous extract from the marine mollusc *Nerita peloronta* [26]. In addition, extracts from other marine invertebrates, in particular from three ascidians, were reported to inhibit the growth of *P. falciparum* in vitro [27]. These results suggest that *N. peloronta* extract could be a potential and attractive source of carboxypeptidase inhibitors with antimalarial activity. Taking these elements into account, in this work, we set out to identify, purify, and molecularly and functionally characterize a carboxypeptidase inhibitor from the marine mollusc *N. peloronta* (NpCI) as well as test its ability to arrest the growth of *P. falciparum*, which was shown to be successful.

2. Results

2.1. Purification of NpCI

The inhibitor NpCI was purified until homogeneity from the mollusc extract treated with 2.5% TCA. The TCA-treated extract showed a total inhibitory activity of 45.15 U and specific activity of 0.3 U/mg towards bCPA. A chromatogram depicting the purification using a CPA–ethyloxy–*Sepharose* CL–6B matrix is displayed in Figure 1a. The elution of bound proteins, achieved by increasing the pH to 12.0, was observed in a single protein small peak, in which the inhibitory activity was concentrated. This chromatography allowed us to recover 80% of the inhibitor applied and obtain a 13-fold purification grade. The active fractions were pooled and applied to an RP-HPLC chromatography C8 column, giving rise to a main symmetric peak with CPA inhibitory activity (Figure 1b). Overall, a purification grade of 103-fold was achieved, with a yield of 78.6%.

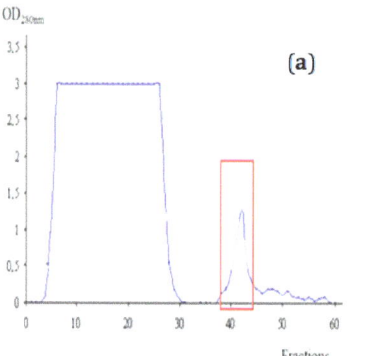
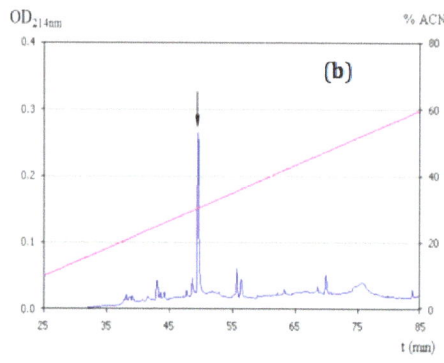

Figure 1. Purification of NpCI from *Nerita peloronta* clarified extract. (**a**) CPA affinity chromatography: column—7.0 × 1.0 cm; linear flow rate—17.0 cm/h. (**b**) RP-HPLC in C8 column with a linear gradient between H_2O-TFA 0.1% and acetonitrile (ACN)-TFA 0.1% (*v/v*) in the 10–60% range: linear flow rate—377 cm/h. The blue line represents absorbance at 280 nm (**a**) or 214 nm (**b**).

A summary of the purification procedure is shown in Table 1.

Table 1. NpCI purification and summary.

Step	[Prots] (mg/mL)	Inhibitory Activity (Ut)	Specific Activity (U/mg)	Yield (%)	Purification (Times)
TCA-clarified extract	3.010	0.903	0.300	100	1
Affinity chromatography	0.183	0.724	3.956	80.2	13
RP-HPLC	0.023	0.710	30.87	78. 6	103

2.2. Molecular Characterization of NpCI

A mass spectrometry analysis allowed for the complete molecular characterization of purified NpCI in terms of its molecular mass, number of free and linked cysteines, and full-length amino acid sequence. The ESI-MS spectra obtained for native NpCI showed signals for the multicharged ions of the inhibitor (Figure 2). Signals A5 and A4 corresponded to ions with five and four positive charges, respectively, which allowed for the derivation of the mass of native NpCI as 5925.84 Da, calculated as the average from the signals of the different ions. This value is in agreement with the major signal obtained in the analysis of the active fractions from affinity chromatography. It should be noted that this value was refined afterwards with a precisely tuned and calibrated mass spectrometer to exact mass values of 5921.557 Da and 5927.604 Da for the native and reduced forms, respectively.

In addition, the mass spectrometry analysis of a reduced and carbamidomethylated sample showed an increase of 350.1 Da in the molecular mass of the inhibitor versus the unmodified inhibitor (Figure 3). This fits with the presence of six disulphide-linked Cys residues in the protein, confirmed in the native and reduced forms through analysis with Ellman's reagent.

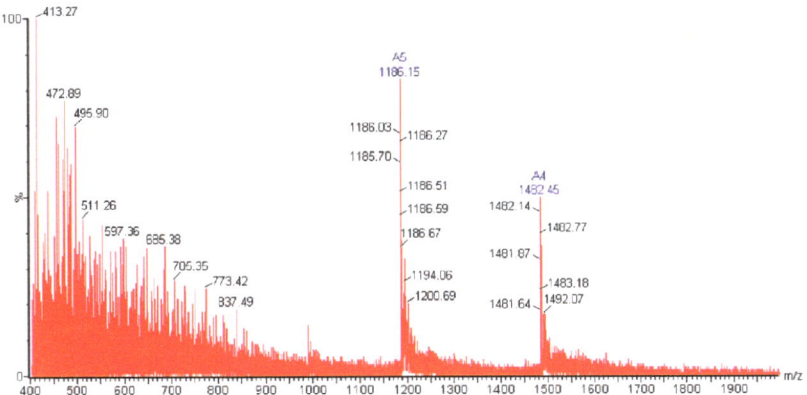

Figure 2. ESI-MS intact mass spectrum analysis from the RP-HPLC NpCI fraction.

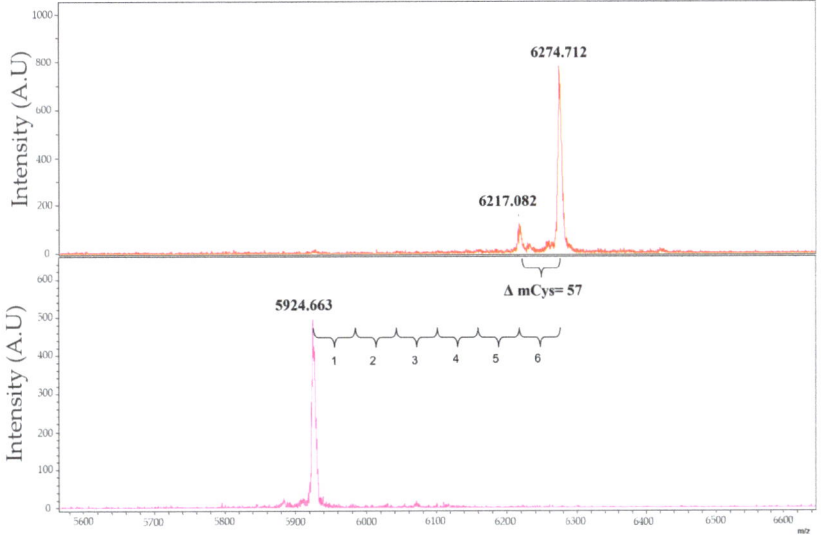

Figure 3. MALDI-TOF mass spectrum of NpCI in the carbamidomethylated and native forms (top and bottom panels, respectively). Samples were treated with 2,5-dihydroxyacetonephosphate (DHAP) as matrix.

Subsequently, the protein sequence of NpCI was derived via the combined analysis of its N-terminal sequencing by automated Edman degradation and the generation of peptides with different proteases, followed by RP-HPLC purification and LC.ESI-MS/MS analysis, which were carried out on both the isolated peptides and the mixtures. The use of trypsin and Glu-C proteinases produced various sets of peptides. The MS/MS analyses of their sequences gave rise to a full coverage of the NpCI sequence, from residues 1 to 53, as shown in Figure 4. This sequence was finally validated through high resolution/high accuracy MALDI.MS analysis using a properly calibrated Bruker timsTOF fleX mass spectrometer, with exact masses of 5921.557 Da ($\pm$0.002Da) and 5927.604 Da ($\pm$0.002 Da) for the native and reduced forms (mono-charged species), respectively. These data fit exactly with the additive masses of the NpCI residues within its putative (now derived) full sequence, as well as with the state of its six cysteine residues in their disulphide-linked forms.

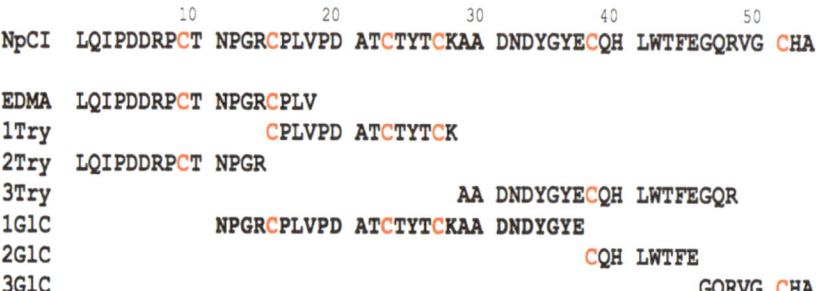

```
               10          20          30          40          50
NpCI   LQIPDDRPCT  NPGRCPLVPD  ATCTYTCKAA  DNDYGYECQH  LWTFEGQRVG  CHA

EDMA   LQIPDDRPCT  NPGRCPLV
1Try               CPLVPD  ATCTYTCK
2Try   LQIPDDRPCT  NPGR
3Try                                AA  DNDYGYECQH  LWTFEGQR
1GlC               NPGRCPLVPD  ATCTYTCKAA  DNDYGYE
2GlC                                        CQH  LWTFE
3GlC                                                       GQRVG  CHA
```

Figure 4. Partial sequences and assembly of NpCI, derived using different experimental approaches. The N-terminus sequence was derived via automated Edman degradation (EDMA) and extended through the LC.ESI-MS/MS sequencing of tryptic peptides (1+2+3 Try) and Glu-C (1+2+3Gl C)-selected endoproteinase-cleaved peptides, as shown in the figure. Cysteine residues are displayed in red. The derived putative 53-residue full protein sequence of NpCI (shown at the top) was validated by fitting its mass with the exact mass of native and intact NpCI derived through a high resolution/high accuracy analysis using MALDI-TOF MS.

As shown in the comparative alignment in Figure 5, the derived full sequence was highly similar to that of NvCI, a carboxypeptidase inhibitor from the marine snail *N. versicolor* of the same genus, which was previously sequenced and characterized by one of our groups [12]. Differences were detected at residues 1–3, 10, 34, 41, and 52—that is, 7 residues of 53 (86.8% of homology)—most of them corresponding to conservative substitutions. The maintenance of the six cysteine residue positions in the two homologous inhibitors, most likely keeping the same disulphide pattern detected in NvCI, is noteworthy.

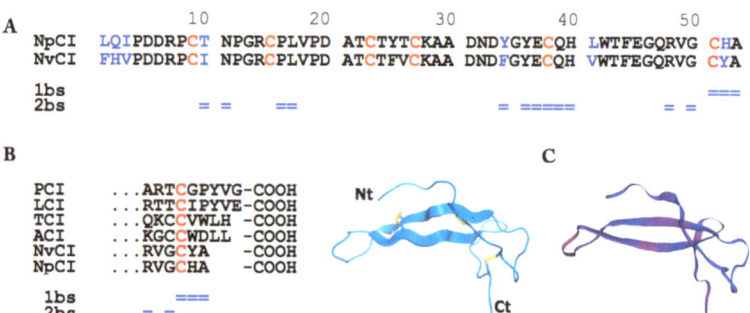

Figure 5. NpCI sequence and conformational analysis. (**A**) NpCI and NvCI sequence alignment. Cysteine residues are highlighted in red, substitutions in blue. The primary and secondary binding sites (1bs and 2bs, respectively) of NvCI to M14 metallocarboxypeptidases [11] are indicated (= sign). (**B**) The boundary between the compact central region and the short C-terminal tail is detected at the last cysteine (in red), as shown by the sequence alignment of the C-tails of NpCI and other proteinaceous carboxypeptidase inhibitors: PCI—the inhibitor from potato [5]; LCI—from leeches [9]; TCI—from ticks [7]; ACI—from *Ascaris suum* [8]; NvCI—from *Nerita versicolor* [11]. (**C**) Cartoon-like representation (left) of the conformation of NvCI from its crystal structure [11] and modelled folding of NpCI (right) displaying a central compact region, a long N-tail, and a short C-tail. Disulphide bonds, represented in yellow for NvCI (left), are most likely the same in NpCI.

A comparison of the C-terminal tail of NpCI with that of other described carboxypeptidase inhibitors is shown in Figure 5b. Low similarities were detected among the inhibitors (with the exception of the NpCI/NvCI pair) regarding both the conservation of residues and tail sizes, which ranged from two to five residues. This merits discussion given that it is an important region including the primary and part of the secondary binding site [11].

Furthermore, conformational modelling using *Swiss-Model* [28] and the two available crystal structures (of protein complexes) containing NvCI, used as high-homology templates [11,29], showed that modelled NpCI was characterized by a central compact region (two antiparallel β strands), a long N-tail, and a short C-tail (Figure 5c). The obtained model was compatible with the same disulphide bond pairings as NvCI.

2.3. Kinetic Characterization of NpCI

For an in-depth characterization of the inhibition of bCPA and porcine carboxypeptidase B (pCPB) by NpCI, the minimum time required for the establishment of the enzyme–inhibitor equilibrium was determined. The incubation of the enzymes and the inhibitor, at a fixed concentration, for 3, 5, 10, 12, and 30 min before the assay showed that there were statistically significant differences in inhibition between 3 and 10 min. However, after a 10 min incubation, the inhibitory activity did not change significatively, indicating that this was a sufficient time for the establishment of the enzyme–inhibitor equilibrium; it was therefore selected for the following experiments. These results allowed us to qualify NpCI as a slow-binding inhibitor of bCPA and pCPB.

Using the 10 min incubation time, the inhibition constants (K_i) of NpCI against bCPA and pCPB were determined. The experiments were performed under conditions where $E_0/Ki \leq 10$ and $[S_0] = 1K_M$. The fitting of the Morrison equation [30] to the experimental data allowed for the calculation of the K_{iap} values of 5.5×10^{-9} mol/L and 8.15×10^{-8} mol/L for the inhibition of bCPA and pCPB, respectively. In both cases, concave curves for the v_i/v_0 vs. $[I_0]$ plots were obtained, indicating the reversibility of the inhibition (Figure 6a,b). The derived K_i values allowed us to confirm that NpCI is a tight-binding inhibitor of bCPA and pCPB under these experimental conditions.

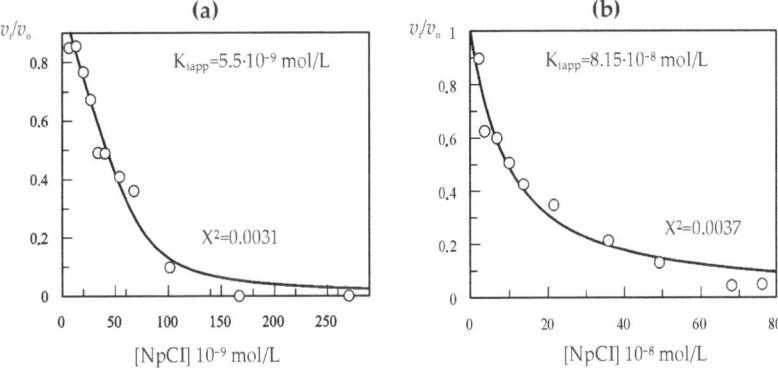

Figure 6. Kinetic characterization of NpCI. (**a**) K_i value determination against bCPA. (**b**) K_i value determination against pCPB. The fitting of the Morrison equation to the experimental data is displayed, generated using the Grafit program.

To evaluate the effect of substrate concentration on the inhibitory activity of NpCI, a kinetic analysis was performed with substrate concentrations equivalent to 0.5, 1, and 1.5 K_M. The increase in substrate concentration in the assay did not produce a statistically significant decrease in inhibitory activity against pCPB. However, a decrease was observed in the bCPA case when the substrate concentration was increased. This result suggests that the substrate can displace NpCI from the active site of the enzyme, which is a characteristic behaviour of competitive inhibitors (data not shown). Based on this behaviour, the K_i value of NpCI against bCPA was recalculated considering the substrate concentration and the equation described by Bieth [31] for competitive inhibitors, obtaining a value equal to 1.1×10^{-8} mol/L.

After the inhibition of bCPA and pCPB by NpCI, its capability to inhibit serine and cysteine proteases was evaluated. Accordingly, it was determined that NpCI was unable to inhibit porcine pancreatic elastase, bovine pancreatic trypsin, and chymotrypsin, as well as subtilisin A from *Bacillus licheniformis* and papain from *Carica papaya*, with an $[I_0]/[E_0]$ rate higher than 200, indicating a narrow specificity of NpCI for metallocarboxypeptidases.

2.4. Inhibitory Effect of Purified NpCI on P. falciparum Growth

Considering that Plasmodium spp. Contain a rather unique cytoplasmic carboxypeptidase [22,23] and having observed inhibitory activity by similar metallocarboxypeptidase inhibitors against this parasite [21], we aimed to evaluate the direct effect of the purified form of NpCI against *P. falciparum* Dd2 (a chloroquine-resistant strain), since in previous assays (not shown) the crude extract of *N. peloronta* was shown to result in the growth delay of *P. falciparum* Dd2 in vitro. In addition, the effect of the inhibitor against the chloroquine-sensitive *P. falciparum* 3D7 strain was also evaluated.

The purified form of NpCI showed antiplasmodial activity in a dose-dependent manner. Increasing the inhibitor concentration clearly reduced parasite growth (Figure 7a). An IC_{50} value of 5.5 μmol/L was obtained for the NpCI fraction against *P. falciparum* Dd2. The chloroquine control used in parallel resulted in IC_{50} values for both *P. falciparum* strains tested Dd2 and 3D7 within the expected range (0.175 and 0.016 μmol/L, respectively), validating the inhibition assay.

The effect of the inhibitor on the intraerythrocytic stages of *P. falciparum* Dd2's life cycle was also assessed using microscopy (Figure 7b). For this purpose, the levels of parasitaemia and the forms corresponding to the different life cycle stages, as well as pyknotic parasites, were analysed by microscopy and quantified at different inhibitor concentrations (Figures S1 and 7b). In the absence of NpCI, *P. falciparum* Dd2 showed the highest levels of parasitaemia (12–14%) with parasites in all stages, mainly rings and trophozoites that had completed the cycle at 48 h from ring-synchronized cultures. However, with NpCI, the cycle was significantly delayed, observed as a decrease in parasitaemia and the abundant presence of schizonts even at concentrations below the IC_{50} value. Furthermore, the abundant presence of pyknotic forms demonstrated the parasiticidal effect of NpCI on the parasite. In fact, the highest concentration tested (88 μmol/L) was completely lethal to the *P. falciparum* Dd2 culture, as only pyknotic forms were observed therein (Figure 7b). These results suggest that the inhibition of growth by NpCI occurs mainly during parasite development towards maturation to merozoite, prior to schizont rupture.

Finally, it was investigated whether the inhibitory effect of NpCI on *P. falciparum* Dd2 was maintained in other non-chloroquine-resistant strains. A comparison between the 3D7 and Dd2 strains (Figure 7c) showed similar inhibitory strength at the concentrations tested, suggesting that its effect may be transferable to other strains of *P. falciparum* through similar mechanisms of delayed maturation.

The above observations suggest the need to evaluate the cytotoxic effect of NpCI on human cells. Importantly, it was determined that NpCI did not significantly affect human fibroblast cell viability (Figure 7d). Even at the highest concentration tested (six times the IC_{50} value obtained for *P. falciparum* Dd2), the percentage of cell lethality was always lower than 25%; thus, NpCI can be considered as non-toxic to this cell line.

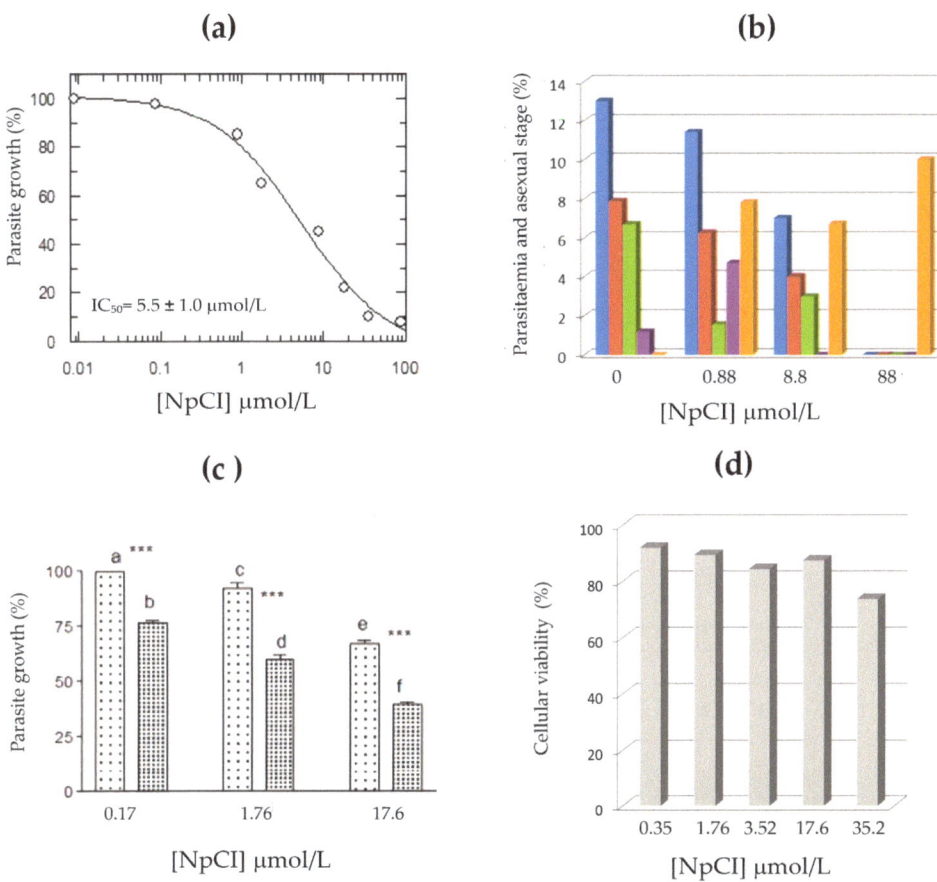

Figure 7. In vitro activity of NpCI in *P. falciparum* and human cells. (**a**) Representative curve of the dose–response effect of NpCI on *P. falciparum* Dd2. Parasites were grown in erythrocyte cultures at 1% initial parasitaemia and incubated with different concentrations of inhibitor. The DNA content was determined at 48 h by microfluorimetry. (**b**) Effect of NpCI on the life cycle of *P. falciparum* Dd2. The presence of different stages of the parasite was observed in culture. Bars indicate percentages of total parasitaemia (dark blue), ring stage (red), trophozoite stage (green), schizont stage (violet), and pyknotic bodies (orange). Data were obtained from the microscopic observation of Wright's-stained smears from cultures treated for 48 h with different concentrations of NpCI. Percentages were calculated from counts of at least 1000 erythrocytes. (**c**) Comparison of the in vitro inhibitory activity of NpCI for two strains of *P. falciparum*, 3D7 (left) and Dd2 (right), at identical NpCI concentrations. Letters indicate differences for $p \leq 0.001$, according to post-ANOVA Tukey–Kramer test. (**d**) Cell viability of human fibroblast culture (1BR3G) during 24 h treatment at different NpCI concentrations. For each condition, the percentage of viable cells was determined and plotted.

3. Discussion

Metallocarboxypeptidases (MCPs) are zinc-dependent enzymes that hydrolyse the C-terminal residue(s) of peptides and proteins. Their activity is tightly regulated due to the important processes in which they are involved. Several MCPs have been linked to chronic human diseases, such as cancer, fibrinolysis, and inflammation, as well as infectious diseases. Consequently, MCPs and their inhibitors have attracted considerable medical interest as potential drug targets [2,3,32–34].

Marine species constitute an extraordinary source of bioactive molecules, and a number of these molecules have been tested as antimalarials [35], including protease inhibitors [36]. Many protease inhibitors isolated from marine invertebrates are active against serine proteases and, to a lesser extent, cysteine proteases, although inhibitors from other mechanistic classes have also been isolated. Regarding carboxypeptidase inhibitors, only two of proteinaceous character have been previously described in marine invertebrates, one of which belongs to the phylum Mollusca [11–13]. Therefore, the latter is still an unexplored field.

As mentioned earlier, previous studies have reported the capacity of both proteinaceous and organic (synthetic) inhibitors of metallocarboxypeptidases to inhibit the growth of *P. falciparum* in culture, indicating antimalarial potential [21]. This effect could be related to the occurrence and role of a unique gene in *P. falciparum* coding for an M14C metallocarboxypeptidase, a subfamily of enzymes involved in tubulin processing, which is an essential process in cell development [23–25]. Increasing evidence for such compounds and their capabilities has therefore gained interest in the development of antimalarials. In our case, we aimed to characterize one of these inhibitors, NpCI, isolated from marine snail *N. peloronta* specimens collected on the Cuban Atlantic coast. For NpCI purification, a combination of TCA and affinity chromatography using CPA–ethyloxy–*Sepharose* as a matrix was employed. A highly purified form was produced using this method. The final refinement of purification, when required (as for protein sequencing), was accomplished using C8 RP-HPLC.

The mass spectrometry analysis of the purified inhibitor revealed that native NpCI had an average molecular mass of 5925.84 Da, as well as masses of 5921.557 Da and 5927.604 Da for the monoisotopic major forms of the native and reduced forms, respectively. These figures fit exactly with those derived from the deduced protein sequence through the application of the peptide/protein calculator on the Expasy server [28] and are in the mass range of most MCP proteinaceous inhibitors described to date. Only SmCI, from the marine worm *S. magnifica*, and latexin, from mammals, have molecular masses higher than 10 kDa (19.7 kDa and 26 kDa, respectively) [5,6,8–10,13,14]. The molecular mass obtained here is in agreement with that reported for NvCI, the only carboxypeptidase inhibitor isolated from molluscs until now [11]. Both inhibitors have 86.7% homology.

The amino acid sequence of NpCI, obtained via the combined analysis of its N-terminal sequence using automated Edman degradation and the generation of peptides with distinct proteases, followed by HPLC purification and/or LC.ESI-MS/MS analysis, showed that the protein consisted of 53 residues with a theoretical mass of 5927.61 Da. This result is in accordance with the molecular mass determined using MS, if it is considered that the six Cys residues form disulphide bonds. A list of the peptides generated and sequenced is shown in Table S1 in the Supplementary Materials. The protein has a high percentage of hydrophobic residues (32%, with three Tyr, one Trp, and one Phe), a higher percentage of acidic than basic residues (13% vs. 7%), a notable presence of Pro (9%) and Gly (7.5%), and a theoretical pI of 4.91, when calculated using the Expasy server [28]. It lacks Met and Ser.

Furthermore, the presence of six cysteines in the structure of NpCI, likely forming disulphide bonds, agrees with the stability shown by this molecule in the drastic pH conditions used during the purification procedure. The presence of numerous disulphide bonds has been reported in all MCP inhibitors. PCI, TMCPI, and NvCI present three disulphide bonds, while LCI has four, TCI/H1TCI have six, and ACI and SmCI contain seven and nine disulphide bonds, respectively [5,6,8–10,13,14]. The maintenance of the six cysteine residue positions in the two homologous inhibitors indicates that both proteins likely have the same disulphide pattern and the same overall folding, in which a central globular disulphide-stabilized fold of forty-three residues is flanked by the N- and C-terminal tails [11,12]. The homology modelling performed using the *Swiss-Model* server confirmed these similarities, with excellent fitting parameters obtained both globally and along the chains, as shown in Figure S2 in the Supplementary Materials section.

The comparison of the NpCI C-terminal tail with that of other MCP inhibitors, displayed in Figure 5b, showed that such inhibitors predominantly (but not absolutely) have an aliphatic residue at the P1 site. This site can be allocated at positions 3–4 of the tail, i.e., in ACI/TCI, following the last cysteine residue (after the compact central protein core) and preceding the P1' site (the last residue in the longest inhibitors, PCI/LCI), which is known to be cleaved after binding to the carboxypeptidase [37]. No such cleavage occurs for the shortest NpCI or NvCI, or for ACI. Regarding the P2 site, it is possibly allocated at positions 1–2 after the last cysteine; it should be noted that the aromatic residues frequently present in NvCI, LCI, TCI, and other MCP inhibitors are replaced by His in NpCI. Interestingly, the 1–2 positions are among the main points for the interaction and inhibitory action of the inhibitor on putative M14 carboxypeptidase targets [11] and constitute part of the primary binding site (Figure 5b,c). Thus, the Tyr/His substitution at the P2 site of NpCI could account for the strong decrease in its capability to bind and inhibit the enzyme in comparison with other MPC inhibitors, i.e., when compared to NvCI, from 1.0 $\times 10^{-12}$ to 5.5×10^{-9} mol/L for the bCPA enzyme [11]. The expected potential loss of the two hydrogen bonds established between the tyrosinate group of Tyr52 and the Arg71 and Arg127 residues of bCPA (essential for the activity of this enzyme) could be partially responsible for the change in K_i [7,9,11]. Although the C-tail of NvCI is only two residues long, it is nevertheless involved in the primary binding site for the target enzymes [11,29], whilst the secondary binding site extends along the compact central region, as depicted in Figure 5a,b. Presumably, this is also the case for NpCI.

The functional characterization of NpCI also showed that this molecule is a slow inhibitor of bCPA and pCPB, which was determined by taking into account the time necessary for the inhibitory enzyme equilibrium to be established. This is a common behaviour for the majority of characterized MCP inhibitors [5,6,8–14] and is likely determined by the conformation that must be adopted by the inhibitor to introduce the carboxyl tail in the active site of the cognate enzyme [30]. In addition, the K_i values obtained allow us to classify NpCI as a tight-binding inhibitor against both of the M14 MCPs assayed. Furthermore, the shape of the dose–response curves obtained suggests the reversibility of the protease–inhibitor interaction analysed in our work. These features are common for all proteinaceous MCP inhibitors described thus far and could constitute an advantage for biomedical and biotechnological applications.

On the other hand, the decrease in bCPA inhibitory activity produced by the increase in substrate concentration suggests that the substrate used here induced protease–inhibitor complex dissociation. This behaviour is characteristic for competitive inhibitors [38]. However, this behaviour did not seem to apply to pCPB inhibition, suggesting that in this case, the inhibitor and the substrate did not share the same binding site as CPA, a characteristic of non-competitive inhibitors. Nevertheless, for inhibitors that bind to the enzyme in a substrate-like way, as has been described for MCP inhibitors, it can be assumed that the dissociation promoted by the substrate at the assayed concentration is not detectable during the assay time [31].

It should be noted that the absence of inhibitory activity against proteases from other mechanistic classes points to a high specificity of NpCI. This result is in accordance with the narrow specificity shown by the other MCP inhibitors, described in [5,6,8–12,14], with the exception of SmCI, which is also able to inhibit serine proteases [13].

The in vitro inhibition of *P. falciparum* growth by NpCI suggests the potential occurrence of a new antiplasmodial target in the parasite and also agrees with the initial results obtained for other MCP inhibitors, such as PCI, LCI, and benzyl succinate [21]. Considering that a single gene coding for a carboxypeptidase-like enzyme (PfNna1, Q8I2A6 in UniProt) has been described in the *P. falciparum* genome [22], it may be hypothesized that the observed inhibition of parasite growth by NpCI was due to the inhibition of such enzyme [21], either direct or indirect.

PlasmoDB, a molecular database for Plasmodium spp., shows that the maximum expression of this enzyme occurs after 42 h in the intraerythrocytic phase of the life cycle of the parasite [39]. This fact places the occurrence of enzyme activity at the later schizont stage, in agreement with the observed cessation of the parasitic life cycle and the increase in pyknotic (nuclei-packed, cell death) forms.

It should be noted that the IC_{50} value determined for NpCI against the *P. falciparum* in culture was in the low micromolar scale (IC_{50} = 5.5 µmol/L), a figure within the accepted ranges for compounds nowadays investigated as novel lead variants of classical antimalarials [40], particularly when they are not cytotoxic. The great similarity of NpCI to its close homologous NvCI, better known functionally and of reported biological endurance and cell penetration capabilities [12,32], add hopes on the feasibility and interest to investigate its mechanism of action regarding Plasmodium. This could shed light on its target for therapeutic purposes, as well as facilitate its redesign into a smaller active mimicking compound, if convenient.

4. Materials and Methods

4.1. Materials

Enzymes: bovine pancreatic metallocarboxypeptidase A (bCPA) (EC 3.4.17.1), porcine pancreatic metallocarboxypeptidase B (pCPB) (EC 3.4.17.2), bovine pancreatic trypsin (EC 3.4.21.4), bovine pancreatic chymotrypsin A (EC 3.4.21.1), porcine pancreatic elastase (EPP) (EC 3.4.21.36), endoproteinase Lys-C from *Lysobacter enzymogenes* (EC 3.4.21.50) were from provided by Sigma-Aldrich Co. (Saint Louis, MO, USA), papain was obtained from *Carica papaya* (EC 3.4.22.2), *Bacillus licheniformis* subtilisin A (SUBTA) (EC 3.4.21.62) were supplied by Calbiochem Novabiochem Corp (La Jolla, CA, USA) and endoproteinase Glu-C (V8 enzyme from *Staphylococcus aureus*) were purchased from Roche Molecular Biochemicals (Basel, Switzerland).

Synthetic substrates: Substrates N-(4-methoxyphenylazoformyl)-L-phenylalanine (AAFP), N-(4-metoxyphenylazoformyl)-L-arginine (AAFR), Benzoyl-L-arginine-p-nitroanilide-HCl (BAPA), 5-N-Succinyl-alanyl-alanyl-prolyl-phenyl-p-nitroanilide and Leu-p-nitroanilide were purchased from BACHEM (Switzerland), while N-succinyl-alanyl-alanyl-alanyl-p-nitroanilide (N-Suc-(Ala)3-pNA) was obtained from Sigma Chemical Company, (Saint Louis, MO, USA).

Columns and matrixes: HPLC column C8 (3.9 × 150 mm) was purchased from *Waters*, (Milford, MA, USA) and Sepharose CL 6B from Cytiva (Washington, DC, USA).

Plasmodium falciparum strains: Dd2 (clone MRA-150) chloroquine-resistant strain and 3D7 (clone MRA-102) chloroquine-sensitive strain were obtained from MR4 (ATCC, Manassas, VA, USA).

4.2. Methods

4.2.1. Purification of *Nerita peloronta* Carboxypeptidase Inhibitor (NpCI)

Nerita peloronta snails were collected in the tropical sea near Havana (Cuba) and validated by the Cuban Oceanographic Institute. The bodies of the snails were removed from the shell, washed with seawater and homogenized in a home blender. The homogenate was centrifuged for 60 min at 2000× *g*, 4 °C (centrifuge Beckman GS-GKR, Brea, CA, USA) and was filtered through glass wool. The obtained extract was treated with trichloroacetic acid (TCA) (2.5% *v/v*) for 1 h at 4 °C, and then centrifuged at 10 000× *g* for 60 min at 4 °C. The supernatant was adjusted to pH 7.0 with 2 mol/L NaOH and extensively dialyzed against distilled water (v:v 1:200, supernatant/water) using membranes with a molecular weight cut-off of 1000 Da (Amicon, Millipore Corporation, Billerica, MA, USA) and kept at −20 °C. The clarified extract (150.5 mg of total protein) was loaded onto a CPA-ethyloxy-Sepharose CL-6B column (1.0 × 7.0 cm, containing 3.5 mg of CPA/mL gel) previously equilibrated with 5 column volumes (Vc) of Tris-HCl 0.02 mol/L, NaCl 0.5 mol/L, pH 7.5 (equilibration buffer). Non-retained proteins were removed by washing the column with equilibration buffer (5 Vc). The elution was performed with Na_3PO_4 0.05 mol/L, pH 12.0 (5 Vc). The whole process was carried out at room temperature and fractions of 3 mL were collected (2 mL along elution). The linear flow rate was fixed at 17.0 cm/h. The process was monitored by absorbance at 280 nm and bCPA inhibitory activity. The active fraction containing NpCI was then applied to a C8 RP-HPLC column (0.39 × 15.0 cm), equilibrated and washed with 0.1% trifluoroacetic acid (TFA) in water (solution A), and the elution was performed with 0.1% v/v TFA in acetonitrile (solution B) using this gradient: 10% of B during 10 min, followed by a linear gradient from 10 to 40% of B over A along 40 min. The flow rate was 0.75 mL/min (377 cm/h) at room temperature. Protein detection was carried out by absorbance at 214 nm and inhibitory activity against bCPA.

Analysis of Protein concentration: Protein concentration was determined by the bicinchoninic acid (BCA) chemical method [41] and using bovine serum albumin (BSA) as standard, according to manufacturer instructions.

4.2.2. Molecular Characterization of NpCI

Molecular mass determination: Initial LC.ESI-MS mass spectra were obtained using a mass spectrometer with hybrid octagonal configuration (Micromass, Mundelein, IL, USA) with electronebulization Z-spray (nanoESI) as ionization source. The analyser was operated on positive ion mode and calibrated with a reference mix (Reference material: EMsc-02-0910 registered in PPO 4.09.120.98), in a wide mass range (50–2000 Da). ESI–MS spectrum for the intact protein was acquired in a mass range of 400 to 2000 Da.

Determination of total and free cysteines: The number of cysteines present in the NpCI structure was determined by the analysis of MALDI-TOF MS spectra for the native inhibitor and the reduced and carbamidomethylated forms of it. For the free cysteine quantification, the native inhibitor was treated with Ellman's reagent.

NpCI was denatured by treatment with 6 mol/L guanidinium-HCl, in 0.1 mol/L Tris-HCl, pH 8.0, for 5 min at 100 °C. After cooling to room temperature, DTT (10 mmol/L) was added. The reaction was performed in 0.1 mol/L Tris-HCl, pH 8.0, for 30 min, at 56 °C, with burble of N_2. Finally, iodoacetamide, 20 mmol/L, was added and incubated at 37 °C for 30 min. Molecular masses of native and modified NpCI were determined by mass spectrometry, using a MALDI-TOF spectrometer Bruker Ultraflex Extreme. Ionization was achieved with a 337 nm pulsed nitrogen laser, and spectra were acquired in the linear positive ion mode applying a 19 kV acceleration voltage. The 2,5-dihydroxyacetone phosphate (DHAP), prepared at 10 mg/mL in trifluoroacetic acid (TFA) 0.1% / acetonitrile (ACN) 30% was used as matrix for the analysis of protein. The alpha-cyano-4-hydroxycinnamic acid (CHCA), sinapinic acid (SA) and 2,5-dihydroxybenzoic acid (DHB) matrices were also used in some instances. MS spectra were analysed using Bruker Daltonics Flex Analysis Software v.3.4 (https://bruker-daltonics-flexanalysis.updatestar.com/en).

Free cysteines were determined by the incubation of native inhibitor (50 µL) with 10 µL of the Ellman's reagent, 0.2 mol/L, in Na_2HPO_4 0.1 mol/L buffer, pH 8.0 during 5 min. After that, the absorbance at 405 nm was determined in a plate reader (Multiskan EX, Finland). The concentration of thiol groups was calculated using the calibration curve with aqueous solutions of cysteine, with concentrations between 0.05 and 0.6 mg/mL.

Protein sequence determination of NpCI: The freeze-dried NpCI sample, approximately 0.4 mg, after purification by C8 RP-HPLC, was unfolded by treatment with 90 µL of LB buffer (4% SDS or 6 mol/L guanidinium chloride, 1mol/L Tris HCl, pH 7.5) and reduced by adding 10 µL DTT (1 mol/L), with a 30 min incubation at 95 °C. After cooling at 25 °C, the sample was diluted 40 times with Urea buffer (UA; 8 mol/L urea, 0.1 mol/L Tris/HCl pH 8.5), until a volume of 4 mL was reached. Then, it was conditioned and alkylated following the FASP (Filter Aided Sample Preparation) digestion protocol [42], on a 3 KDa Amicon centrifugal filter, at 14000 g, for 10 min, at 10 °C, in each buffer exchange. Briefly, it was washed three times with 500 µL of 8 mol/L urea, 0.1 mol/L Tris-HCl, pH 8.5 buffer, and then treated with 0.05 mol/L iodoacetamide, in 8 mol/L urea, 0.1 mol/L Tris HCl, pH 8.5, in the dark, for 20 min, at 25 °C. Afterwards, the sample was washed three times with 100 µL of UA buffer and three times with 100 µL of 20 mmol/L ammonium bicarbonate buffer, pH 8.5, centrifuged at 14000 g for 15 min, at 10 °C, and freeze-dried in aliquots. Digestion with either trypsin or GluC-endoproteinase was performed at enzyme/protein ratios of 5/100, 1/40 and 1/40 (w/w), at 37 °C, for 18, 1 and 4 h, respectively, in 200 mmol/L triethyl ammonium bicarbonate (TEAB) buffer (pH 8.5), following also the FASP-centrifugal protocol. Samples were either freeze-dried or desalted on C4-ZipTips before MS analyses. An aliquot of the reduced-alkylated protein was subjected to eighteen cycles of automated EDMAN degradation (LF3000 Protein Sequencer, Beckman, Germany). MALDI-TOF.MS analyses were performed in a Bruker Ultraflex Extreme equipment, from Bruker Daltonics, using α-CHCA as a matrix to generate peptide mass fingerprints. The peptide fragments were subsequently subjected to CID fragmentation in the spectrometer, using the LIFT-based approaches [43]. Peptide alignment and protein sequence analyses from the fragmentation spectra were performed using the Bruker Daltonics software and Mascot search engine, with incorporation of the EDMAN degradation data. LC.ESI-MS/MS analysis were performed in an Orbitrap Fusion Lumos Tribid spectrometer (Thermo Fisher Scientific, Waltham, MA, USA), using a μ-precolumn Acclaim C18 PepMap100 and a C18 Acclaim PepMap RSLC (nanoViper, Waltham, MA, USA) analytical column, following the details reported in [44]. Validation of the final derived sequence was achieved by high resolution/high accuracy MALDI.MS analysis on a Bruker timsTOF fleX mass spectrometer.

Sequence analysis: Database searches of NpCI fragments from LC-ESI.MS/MS were performed using the Proteome Discoverer package (Thermo-Instruments, v2.1, Waltham, MA, USA), with a 1% false discovery rate, as well as PSI-Blast [45], versus the protein sequences of Uniprot and nrdb-95% databases. Search parameters were set at 20 ppm fragment tolerance; cleaving enzyme trypsin or Glu-endo; missed cleavages 1; and residue modifications as TMTsixplex (Nterm, K), carbamidomethyl (C); carboxymethyl (C); deamidation (N, Q), oxidation (M, W) and dehydration (N). The sequences of NpCI with significant homologies were analysed for multiple sequence alignments with the program MEGA version 3.1. The PEAKS program (from BSI, 2016 vs.) was also used for data analysis, classification and presentation. A list of the sets of the generated, productively sequenced and assigned peptides of NpCI is shown in Table S1. The protein sequence data reported in this paper has been deposited and will appear in the UniProt Knowledgebase under the accession number C0HM66 (for Carboxypeptidase inhibitor in *Nerita perolonta*).

NpCI 3D modelling: Conformational modelling of NpCI was performed using the *Swiss-Model* (*Expasy*) server [28] and validated using the same server. The best template detected by the server was 5mrv.1, with code corresponding to a PDB structure of NvCI in complex to CPO enzyme [29], followed by 4a94.1, in complex to CPA4 enzyme [11], showing both high homology and local and global similarity with the templates. Main derived parameters, in the first case, were 0.85 for GMQE and 0.82+/− 0.11 for QMEANDisco Global, further displayed in Figure S2 of Supplementary Information.

4.2.3. Kinetic Characterization of NpCI

Inhibition assays were performed by preincubating the inhibitor with the enzymes for 10 min, at room temperature, before adding the substrate. The inhibitory activities of bCPA (3.14×10^{-8} mol/L in the assay) and pCPB (1.5×10^{-8} mol/L in the assay) were evaluated using the substrates AAFP and AAFR (0.1 mmol/L, ~$1K_M$), respectively [46,47]. Hydrolysis of both substrates was followed at 305 nm at 15 s intervals for 3 min, at 25 °C, in a kinetic spectrophotometer UV-1800 (Shimadzu, Kyoto, Japan). The bCPA activity was evaluated in Tris-HCl 0.02 mol/L, NaCl 0.5 mol/L, pH 7.4, while buffer Tris-HCl 0.05 mol/L, NaCl 0.1 mol/L pH 7.5 was used for pCPB.

The Ki values of NpCI against bCPA and pCPB were determined by measuring the enzymatic residual activity (a = v_i/v_0) at different inhibitor concentrations and using a fixed enzyme (bCPA: 7.24×10^{-8} mol/L and pCPB: 2.6×10^{-8} mol/L) and substrate concentrations as described above, where v_i and v_0 are initial velocities in the presence and absence of inhibitor, respectively. The determination of Ki values was carried out on equilibrium conditions ($[E_0]/K_i \leq 10$), using a previously determined preincubation time of 10 min. Ki values were obtained by fitting the experimental data to the equation for tight-binding inhibitors described by Morrison [30] and implemented in GRAFIT software, version 3.01 (England, UK) [48].

In addition, the effect of the substrate concentration in the inhibitory activity of NpCI against bCPA and pCPB was evaluated. Inhibitory assays were developed following the methodology described above but using different substrate concentration (0.5, 1 and 1.5 K_M).

Normality and variance homogeneity were assessed by Kolmogorov–Smirnoff and Bartlett tests, respectively. Then, one-way analysis of variance (ANOVA) followed by Tukey–Kramer's test was performed for determining statistical differences among substrate concentrations. A $p \leq 0.05$ was considered significant.

Moreover, the inhibitory activity of NpCI was evaluated against bovine pancreatic trypsin, chymotrypsin A, PPE, papain and SUBTA. The assay was monitoring at 405 nm at 15 s intervals for 3 min, at 25 °C in a kinetic spectrophotometer, using buffers and substrates previously described for these enzymes [49–51].

4.2.4. Analysis of NpCI Fractions on *P. falciparum* Growth

Plasmodium falciparum cultures: P. falciparum Dd2 (clone MRA-150) and 3D7 (clone MRA-102) strains were used for this study. Erythrocytes were obtained from type O^+ human healthy local donors and collected in Vacuette®tubes with citrate–phosphate/dextrose anticoagulant (Greiner Bio-One, Frickenhausen, Germany). A detailed description of parasite culture, inhibitory studies (as done by NpCI) and synchronization methods have been reported previously [52,53]. A PicoGreen microfluorimetric DNA-based assay was used to monitor parasite growth inhibition as described [52]. Parasite morphology was evaluated from replicate experiments by microscopic analysis of Wright's-stained thin blood smears. Controls without inhibitors or with chloroquine were performed following the same procedure. Inhibition experiments were performed in triplicate at least twice as a reproducibility proof. Changes in growth were estimated by statistical analysis using the Tukey–Kramer's test to compare significant differences between individual groups. A $p \leq 0.05$ was considered significant.

4.2.5. Cytotoxicity Effect of NpCI Fractions

Cytotoxicity effect of NpCI was tested in a cell culture system using human fibroblast cell line 1BR3G (American Type Culture Collection (ATCC)). The cells were grown in Dulbecco's modified Eagle's medium (DMEM) supplemented with 10% (v/v) heat inactivated fetal bovine serum, 2 mmol/L glutamine (Life Technologies Inc., Carlsbad, CA, USA), in a highly humidified atmosphere of 95% air with 5% CO_2, at 37 °C. Growth inhibitory effect was measured in 96-well microplates (3×10^4 cells per well). After 24 h, different concentrations of inhibitor (0.35, 1.76, 3.52, 17.6 and 35.2 µmol/L) were added and the plates were incubated at 37 °C for 24 h. Aliquots of 20 µL of XTT solution were then added to each well. After 5 h, the colour formed was quantitated in a spectrophotometric plate reader at wavelengths of 490 nm and 610 nm. Cytotoxicity experiments were performed in triplicate at least twice as a reproducibility proof. Cell viability was determined using the following equation:

$$\% \ cellular \ viability = \frac{(Abs490nm - Abs610\,nm)}{(Abs490\,nm(control) - Abs610\,nm(control))} * 100. \tag{1}$$

5. Conclusions

Metalloproteases, including metallocarboxypeptidases (MCPs), are ubiquitous and important enzymes in living organisms, constituting biomedical targets to control diseases and infections. A novel MCP inhibitor, NpCI, was isolated from the marine snail *N. peloronta*, sequenced, and characterized. NpCI folds in three regions: the N-tail, compact central region (stabilised by three disulphides), and C-tail, with 8, 43, and 2 residues, respectively. It behaves as a slow- and tight-binding inhibitor for M14 MCPs. NpCI was shown to arrest the growth of the malaria parasite *P. falciparum* in vitro, which may indicate the existence of a novel antimalarial target related to the functional properties of this MCP inhibitor.

Supplementary Materials: The following supporting information can be downloaded at: https://www.mdpi.com/article/10.3390/md21020094/s1, Figure S1: Representative microscopy images of *P. falciparum* Dd2 cultures, incubated or not with different concentrations of inhibitor: at 0.00, control (A); 0.88 (B); 8.8 (C) and 88 (D) μmol/L of NpCI. Images were obtained from observation of Wright's-stained smears from cultures treated for 48 h with different concentrations of NpCI. Figure S2: Parameters derived from the modelling of NpCI to NvCI crystal structures; Table S1: Sets of NpCI peptides from Trypsin and GluC hydrolysis, selected for sequence building.

Author Contributions: Conceptualization, A.C.-M., G.C.-C., M.L.R., J.M.B., F.X.A. and M.A.-d.-R.; Methodology, A.C.-M., Y.S.-G. and G.C.-C.; Investigation, A.C.-M., Y.S.-G., G.C.-C., Y.G.-G. and J.M.B.; Writing–original draft, A.C.-M., G.C.-C. and F.X.A.; Writing—review & editing, A.C.-M., Y.S.-G., G.C.-C., M.L.R., J.M.B., F.X.A. and M.A.-d.-R.; Supervision, M.L.R., F.X.A. and M.A.-d.-R. All authors have read and agreed to the published version of the manuscript.

Funding: This work was partially supported by the CYTED Network Red 210RT0390 and Fundación Carolina (post-doctoral fellowship for Aymara Cabrera-Muñoz) and by grant BIO2016-78057-R, from Ministerio de Ciencia e Innovación, Spain (for GCC and FXA).

Data Availability Statement: Not applicable.

Acknowledgments: We are deeply thankful to Drs. Arndt Asperger and Detlev Suckau, and Bruker Daltonics-Bremen, for kindly analysing and helping in the completion of the protein sequence analysis of NpCI by MS-TDS. We are also thankful to Montserrat Carrascal and the Servei de Proteòmica CSIC-UAB (Bellaterra) for the analysis and help in the resolution of the NpCI sequence by LC-MS/MS.

Conflicts of Interest: Aymara Cabrera-Muñoz, Yusvel Sierra-Gómez, Giovanni Covaleda-Cortes, Mey Ling-Reytor, Yamile González-Gonzáles, Jose M. Bautista, Francesc Xavier Avilés and Maday Alonso-del-Rivero Antigua declare they have no conflict of interest regarding this work.

Abbreviations

AAFP: N-(4-methoxyphenilazoformyl)-L-phenylalanine; AAFR: N-(4-metoxyphenylazoformyl)-L-arginine; ACI: *Ascaris summ* carboxypeptidase inhibitor; BAPA: Benzoyl-L-arginine-p-nitroanilide-HCl; BCA: bicinchoninic acid; bCPA: bovine carboxypeptidase A; BSA: bovine serum albumin; CHCA: alpha-cyano-4-hydroxy-cinnamic acid; CPA4: carboxypeptidase A4; CPO: carboxypeptidase O; DHAP: 2,5-dihydroxyacetone phosphate; DHB: 2,5-dihydroxybenzoic acid; EPP: porcine pancreatic elastase; HTCI: *Haemaphysalis longicornis* carboxypeptidase inhibitor; IC_{50}: Half-maximal inhibitory concentration; K_i: inhibition constant; K_M: Michaelis-Menten constant; LC.ESI-MS: liquid chromatography electrospray ionization tandem mass spectrometric; LCI: leech carboxypeptidase inhibitor; MALDI-TOF MS: matrix-assisted laser desorption/ionization time-of-flight mass spectrometry; MCP: Metallocarboxypeptidase; NpCI: *Nerita peloronta* carboxypeptidase inhibitor; NvCI: *Nerita versicolor* carboxypeptidase inhibitor; PCI: potato carboxypeptidase inhibitor; pCPB: porcine carboxypeptidase B; SA: sinapinic acid; RP-HPLC: reverse phase high performance *liquid chromatography* SmCI: *Sabellastarte magnifica* carboxypeptidase inhibitor; TCA: trichloroacetic acid; TCI: tick carboxypeptidase inhibitor; TFA: trifluoroacetic acid; TFA: trifluoroacetic acid; TMCI: tomato metallocarboxypeptidase inhibitor; Vc: column volumes; v_0: initial velocity for control assay; v_i: initial velocity in the presence of inhibitor.

References

1. Arolas, J.L.; Vendrell, J.; Aviles, F.X.; Fricker, L.D. Metallocarboxypeptidases: Emerging Drug Targets in Biomedicine. *Curr. Pharm. Des.* **2007**, *13*, 349–366. [CrossRef] [PubMed]
2. Janke, C.; Bulinski, J.C. Post-Translational Regulation of the Microtubule Cytoskeleton: Mechanisms and Functions. *Nat. Rev. Mol. Cell Biol.* **2011**, *12*, 773–786. [CrossRef] [PubMed]
3. Fernandez, D.; Pallares, I.; Covaleda, G.X.; Aviles, F.; Vendrell, J. Metallocarboxypeptidases and Their Inhibitors: Recent Developments in Biomedically Relevant Protein and Organic Ligands. *Curr. Med. Chem.* **2013**, *20*, 1595–1608. [CrossRef]
4. Rawlings, N.D.; Barrett, A.J.; Thomas, P.D.; Huang, X.; Bateman, A.; Finn, R.D. The MEROPS Database of Proteolytic Enzymes, Their Substrates and Inhibitors in 2017 and a Comparison with Peptidases in the PANTHER Database. *Nucleic Acids Res.* **2018**, *46*, 624–632. [CrossRef] [PubMed]

5. Hass, G.M.; Nau, H.; Biemann, K.; Grahn, D.T.; Ericsson, L.H.; Neurath, H. The Amino Acid Sequence of a Carboxypeptidase Inhibitor from Potatoes. *Biochemistry* **1975**, *14*, 1334–1342. [CrossRef] [PubMed]
6. Hass, G.M.; Hermodson, M.A. Amino Acid Sequence of a Carboxypeptidase Inhibitor from Tomato Fruit. *Biochemistry* **1981**, *20*, 2256–2260. [CrossRef] [PubMed]
7. Arolas, J.L.; Lorenzo, J.; Rovira, A.; Castellà, J.; Aviles, F.X.; Sommerhoff, C.P. A Carboxypeptidase Inhibitor from the Tick *Rhipicephalus bursa*. *J. Biol. Chem.* **2005**, *280*, 3441–3448. [CrossRef]
8. Gong, H.; Zhou, J.; Liao, M.; Hatta, T.; Harnnoi, T.; Umemiya, R.; Inoue, N.; Xuan, X.; Fujisaki, K. Characterization of a Carboxypeptidase Inhibitor from the Tick *Haemaphysalis longicornis*. *J. Insect Physiol.* **2007**, *53*, 1079–1087. [CrossRef]
9. Reverter, D.; Vendrell, J.; Canals, F.; Horstmann, J.; Avilés, F.X.; Fritz, H.; Sommerhoff, C.P. A Carboxypeptidase Inhibitor from the Medical Leech *Hirudo medicinalis*. *J. Biol. Chem.* **1998**, *273*, 32927–32933. [CrossRef]
10. Homandberg, G.A.; Litwiller, R.D.; Peanasky, R.J. Carboxypeptidase Inhibitors from *Ascaris suum*: The Primary Structure. *Arch. Biochem. Biophys.* **1989**, *270*, 153–161. [CrossRef] [PubMed]
11. Covaleda, G.; Alonso Del Rivero, M.; Chávez, M.A.; Avilés, F.X.; Reverter, D. Crystal Structure of Novel Metallocarboxypeptidase Inhibitor from Marine Mollusk *Nerita versicolor* in Complex with Human Carboxypeptidase A4. *J. Biol. Chem.* **2012**, *287*, 9250–9258. [CrossRef] [PubMed]
12. Covaleda-Cortés, G.; Hernández, M.; Trejo, S.A.; Mansur, M.; Rodríguez-Calado, S.; García-Pardo, J.; Lorenzo, J.; Vendrell, J.; Chávez, M.Á.; Alonso-Del-Rivero, M.; et al. Characterization, Recombinant Production and Structure-Function Analysis of NvCI, A Picomolar Metallocarboxypeptidase Inhibitor from the Marine Snail *Nerita versicolor*. *Mar. Drugs* **2019**, *17*, 511. [CrossRef]
13. Alonso-del-Rivero, M.; Trejo, S.A.; Reytor, M.L.; Rodriguez-De-La-Vega, M.; Delfin, J.; Diaz, J.; González-González, Y.; Canals, F.; Chavez, M.A.; Aviles, F.X. Tri-Domain Bifunctional Inhibitor of Metallocarboxypeptidases A and Serine Proteases Isolated from Marine Annelid *Sabellastarte magnifica*. *J. Biol. Chem.* **2012**, *287*, 15427–15438. [CrossRef] [PubMed]
14. Uratini, Y.; Takiguchi-Hayashi, K.; Miyasaka, N.; Sato, M.; Jin, M.; Arimatsu, Y. Latexin, a Carboxypeptidase A Inhibitor, Is Expressed in Rat Peritoneal Mast Cells and Is Associated with Granular Structures Distinct from Secretory Granules and Lysosomes. *Biochem. J.* **2000**, *346*, 817–826. [CrossRef]
15. Pallarès, I.; Bonet, R.; García-Castellanos, R.; Ventura, S.; Avilés, F.X.; Vendrell, J.; Gomis-Rüth, F.X. Structure of Human Carboxypeptidase A4 with Its Endogenous Protein Inhibitor, Latexin. *Proc. Natl. Acad. Sci. USA* **2005**, *102*, 3978–3983. [CrossRef] [PubMed]
16. Konecny, F. Evaluation of Two Recombinant Plasminogen Activators in Massive Pulmonary Embolism Model and Potato Carboxypeptidase Inhibitor (PCI) Role in Inhibition of Thrombin Activatable Fibrinolysis Inhibitor TAFIa in Lungs. *Recent Pat. Endocr. Metab. Immune Drug Discov.* **2008**, *2*, 45–56. [CrossRef]
17. Mao, S.S.; Holahan, M.A.; Bailey, C.; Wu, G.; Colussi, D.; Carroll, S.S.; Cook, J.J. Demonstration of Enhanced Endogenous Fibrinolysis in Thrombin Activatable Fibrinolysis Inhibitor-Deficient Mice. *Blood Coagul. Fibrinolysis* **2005**, *16*, 407–415. [CrossRef]
18. Willemse, J.L.; Heylen, E.; Nesheim, M.E.; Hendriks, D.F. Carboxypeptidase U (TAFIa): A New Drug Target for Fibrinolytic Therapy. *J. Thromb. Haemost.* **2009**, *7*, 1962–1971. [CrossRef]
19. Aagaard, A.; Listwan, P.; Cowieson, N.; Huber, T.; Ravasi, T.; Wells, C.A.; Flanagan, J.U.; Kellie, S.; Hume, D.A.; Kobe, B.; et al. An Inflammatory Role for the Mammalian Carboxypeptidase Inhibitor Latexin: Relationship to Cystatins and the Tumor Suppressor TIG1. *Structure* **2005**, *13*, 309–317. [CrossRef]
20. Liu, Y.; Howard, D.; Rector, K.; Swiderski, C.; Brandon, J.; Schook, L.; Mehta, J.; Bryson, J.S.; Bondada, S.; Liang, Y. Latexin Is Down-Regulated in Hematopoietic Malignancies and Restoration of Expression Inhibits Lymphoma Growth. *PLoS ONE* **2012**, *7*, e44979. [CrossRef]
21. Aviles Puigvert, F.X.; Lorenzo Rivera, J.; Rodriguez-Vera, M.; QuerolMurillo, E.; Bautista Marugán, M.; Díez Martín, A.; Bautista Santa Cruz, J.M. Therapeutic Agents for Treatment of Malaria. WO/2008077977 A1 patent, 3 July 2008.
22. Rodriguez De La Vega, M.; Sevilla, R.G.; Hermoso, A.; Lorenzo, J.; Tanco, S.; Diez, A.; Fricker, L.D.; Bautista, J.M.; Avilés, F.X. Nna1-like Proteins Are Active Metallocarboxypeptidases of a New and Diverse M14 Subfamily. *FASEB J.* **2007**, *20*, 851–865. [CrossRef] [PubMed]
23. Rodriguez de La Vega Otazo, M.; Lorenzo, J.; Tort, O.; Avilés, F.X.; Bautista, J.M. Functional Segregation and Emerging Role of Cilia-Related Cytosolic Carboxypeptidases (CCPs). *FASEB J.* **2013**, *27*, 424–431. [CrossRef] [PubMed]
24. Tort, O.; Tanco, S.; Rocha, C.; Bièche, I.; Seixas, C.; Bosc, C.; Andrieux, A.; Moutin, M.J.; Avilés, F.X.; Lorenzo, J.; et al. The Cytosolic Carboxypeptidases CCP2 and CCP3 Catalyze Posttranslational Removal of Acidic Amino Acids. *Mol. Biol. Cell* **2014**, *25*, 3017–3027. [CrossRef] [PubMed]
25. Tanco, S.; Tort, O.; Demol, H.; Aviles, F.X.; Gevaert, K.; Van Damme, P.; Lorenzo, J.C. Terminomics Screen for Natural Substrates of Cytosolic Carboxypeptidase 1 Reveals Processing of Acidic Protein C Termini. *Mol. Cell. Proteomics* **2015**, *14*, 177–190. [CrossRef]
26. Covaleda, G.; Trejo, S.A.; Salas-Sarduy, E.; Alonso, M.; Chavez, M.A.; Francesc, X. Intensity Fading MALDI-TOF Mass Spectrometry and Functional Proteomics Assignments to Identify Protease Inhibitors in Marine Invertebrates. *J. Proteomics* **2017**, *2017 165*, 75–92. [CrossRef]
27. Mendiola, J.; Hernández, H.; Sariego, I.; Rojas, L.; Otero, A.; Ramírez, A.; de los Angeles Chávez, M.; Payrol, J.A.; Hernández, A. Antimalarial Activity from Three Ascidians: An Exploration of Different Marine Invertebrate Phyla. *Trans. R. Soc. Trop. Med. Hyg.* **2006**, *100*, 909–916. [CrossRef]

28. Gasteiger, E.; Hoogland, C.; Gattiker, A.; Duvaud, S.; Wilkins, M.R.; Appel, R.D.; Bairoch, A. Protein Identification and Analysis Tools on the ExPASy Server. In *The Proteomics Protocols Handbook*; Walker, J.M., Ed.; Humana Press: Totowa, NJ, USA, 2005; pp. 571–609.
29. Garcia-Guerrero, M.C.; Garcia-Pardo, J.; Berenguer, E.; Fernandez-Alvarez, R.; Barfi, G.B.; Lyons, P.J.; Aviles, F.X.; Huber, R.; Lorenzo, J.; Reverter, D. Crystal Structure and Mechanism of Human Carboxypeptidase O: Insights into Its Specific Activity for Acidic Residues. *Proc. Natl. Acad. Sci. USA* **2018**, *115*, E3932–E3939. [CrossRef]
30. Morrison, J.F. The Slow-Binding and Slow, Tight-Binding Inhibition of Enzyme-Catalysed Reactions. *Trends Biochem. Sci.* **1982**, *7*, 102–105. [CrossRef]
31. Bieth, J. Theoretical and Practical Aspects of Proteinase Inhibition Kinetics. *Methods Enzymol.* **1995**, *248*, 59–84.
32. Waern, I.; Taha, S.; Lorenzo, J.; Montpeyó, D.; Covaleda-Cortés, G.; Avilés, F.X.; Wernersson, S. Carboxypeptidase Inhibition by NvCI Suppresses Airway Hyperreactivity in a Mouse Asthma Model. *Allergy Eur. J. Allergy Clin. Immunol.* **2021**, *76*, 2234–2237. [CrossRef]
33. Soria-Castro, R.; Meneses-Preza, Y.G.; Rodríguez-López, G.M.; Romero-Ramírez, S.; Sosa-Hernández, V.A.; Cervantes-Díaz, R.; Pérez-Fragoso, A.; Torres-Ruíz, J.; Gómez-Martín, D.; Campillo-Navarro, M.; et al. Severe COVID-19 Is Marked by Dysregulated Serum Levels of Carboxypeptidase A3 and Serotonin. *J. Leukoc. Biol.* **2021**, *110*, 425–431. [CrossRef] [PubMed]
34. Shao, Q.; Zhang, Z.; Cao, R.; Zang, H.; Pei, W.; Sun, T. CPA4 Promotes EMT in Pancreatic Cancer via Stimulating PI3K-AKT-MTOR Signaling. *Onco. Targets Ther.* **2020**, *13*, 8567–8580. [CrossRef] [PubMed]
35. Hai, Y.; Cai, Z.M.; Li, P.J.; Wei, M.Y.; Wang, C.Y.; Gu, Y.C.; Shao, C.L. Trends of Antimalarial Marine Natural Products: Progresses, Challenges and Opportunities. *Nat. Prod. Rep.* **2022**, *39*, 969–990. [CrossRef] [PubMed]
36. Kang, H.K.; Seo, C.H.; Park, Y. Marine Peptides and Their Anti-Infective Activities. *Mar. Drugs* **2015**, *13*, 618–654. [CrossRef] [PubMed]
37. Sanglas, L.; Aviles, F.; Huber, R.; Gomis-Rüth, F.X.; Arolas, J.L. Mammalian Metallopeptidase Inhibition at the Defense Barrier of Ascaris Parasite. *Proc. Natl. Acad. Sci. USA* **2009**, *106*, 1743–1747. [CrossRef]
38. Copeland, R.A. *Evaluation of Enzyme Inhibitors in Drug Discovery: A Guide for Medicinal Chemists and Pharmacologists: Second Edition*; John Wiley & Sons, Inc.: Hoboken, NJ, USA, 2013; pp. 1–538. [CrossRef]
39. PlasmoDB. Available online: https://plasmodb.org/plasmo/app/#genome-browser (accessed on 10 October 2022).
40. Pinheiro, L.C.S.; Feitosa, L.M.; Gandi, M.O.; Silveira, F.F.; Boechat, N. The Development of Novel Compounds Against Malaria: Quinolines, Triazolpyridines, Pyrazolopyridines and Pyrazolopyrimidines. *Molecules.* **2019**, *24*, 4095. [CrossRef]
41. Smith, P.K.; Krohn, R.L.; Hermanson, G.T.; Mallia, A.K.; Gartner, F.H.; Provenzano, M.D.; Fujimoto, E.K.; Goeke, N.M.; Olson, B.J.; Klenk, D.C. Measurement of Protein Using Bicinchoninic Acid. *Anal. Biochem.* **1985**, *7*, 6–85. [CrossRef]
42. Wiśniewski, J.R.; Zougman, A.; Nagaraj, N.; Mann, M. Universal Sample Preparation Method for Proteome Analysis. *Nat. Methods* **2009**, *6*, 359–362. [CrossRef]
43. Schnaible, V.; Wefing, S.; Resemann, A.; Suckau, D.; Bücker, A.; Wolf-Kümmeth, S.; Hoffmann, D. Screening for Disulfide Bonds in Proteins by MALDI In-Source Decay and LIFT-TOF/TOF-MS. *Anal. Chem.* **2002**, *74*, 4980–4988. [CrossRef]
44. Gella, A.; Prada-Dacasa, P.; Carrascal, M.; Urpi, A.; González-Torres, M.; Abian, J.; Sanz, E.; Quintana, A. Mitochondrial Proteome of Affected Glutamatergic Neurons in a Mouse Model of Leigh Syndrome. *Front. Cell Dev. Biol.* **2020**, *8*, 660. [CrossRef]
45. Altschul, S.F.; Madden, T.L.; Schäffer, A.A.; Zhang, J.; Zhang, Z.; Miller, W.; Lipman, D.J. Gapped BLAST and PSI-BLAST: A New Generation of Protein Database Search Programs. *Nucleic Acids Res.* **1997**, *25*, 3389–3402. [CrossRef] [PubMed]
46. Mock, W.; Liu, Y.; Stanford, D. Arazoformyl Peptide Surrogates as Spectrophotometric Kinetic Assay Substrates for Carboxypeptidase. *A. Anal. Biochem.* **1996**, *239*, 218–222. [CrossRef] [PubMed]
47. Mock, W.L.; Xhu, C. Catalytic Activity of Carboxypeptidase B and of Carboxypeptidase Y with Anisylazoformyl Substrates. *Bioorg. Med. Chem. Lett.* **1999**, *9*, 187–192. [CrossRef] [PubMed]
48. Leatherbarrow, R.J. *Grafit 3.0*; Erithacus Software Ltd.: Staines, UK, 1992.
49. Erlanger, B.; Kokowsky, N.; Cohen, W. The Preparation and Properties of Two New Chromogenic Substrates of Trypsin. *Arch. Biochem. Biophys.* **1961**, *95*, 271–278. [CrossRef]
50. Wells, J.A.; Cunningham, B.C.; Graycart, T.P.; Estell, D.A. Recruitment of Substrate-Specificity Properties from One Enzyme into a Related One by Protein Engineering. *Biochemistry* **1987**, *84*, 5167–5171. [CrossRef] [PubMed]
51. Schechter, I.; Berger, A. On the Size of the Active Site in Proteases I. Papain. Biochem. *Biophys. Res. Commun.* **1967**, *27*, 157–161. [CrossRef]
52. Moneriz, C.; Marín-García, P.; García-Granados, A.; Bautista, J.M.; Diez, A.; Puyet, A. Parasitostatic Effect of Maslinic Acid. I. Growth Arrest of *Plasmodium falciparum* Intraerythrocytic Stages. *Malar. J.* **2011**, *10*, 82. [CrossRef] [PubMed]
53. Radfar, A.; Méndez, D.; Moneriz, C.; Linares, M.; Marín-García, P.; Puyet, A.; Diez, A.; Bautista, J.M. Synchronous Culture of *Plasmodium falciparum* at High Parasitemia Levels. *Nat. Protoc.* **2009**, *4*, 1899–1915. [CrossRef] [PubMed]

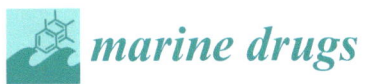

marine drugs

Article

Purification and Molecular Docking Study on the Angiotensin I-Converting Enzyme (ACE)-Inhibitory Peptide Isolated from Hydrolysates of the Deep-Sea Mussel *Gigantidas vrijenhoeki*

Seong-Yeong Heo [1,2], Nalae Kang [1], Eun-A Kim [1], Junseong Kim [1], Seung-Hong Lee [3], Ginnae Ahn [4], Je Hyeok Oh [5], A Young Shin [5], Dongsung Kim [5] and Soo-Jin Heo [1,2,*]

[1] Jeju Bio Research Center, Korea Institute of Ocean Science and Technology (KIOST), Jeju 63349, Republic of Korea; syheo@kiost.ac.kr (S.-Y.H.); nalae1207@kiost.ac.kr (N.K.); euna0718@kiost.ac.kr (E.-A.K.); junseong@kiost.ac.kr (J.K.)
[2] Department of Marine Biotechnology, University of Science and Technology (UST), Daejeon 34113, Republic of Korea
[3] Department of Pharmaceutical Engineering, Soonchunhyang University, Asan 31538, Republic of Korea; shlee80@sch.ac.kr
[4] Department of Food Technology and Nutrition, Chonnam National University, Yeosu 59626, Republic of Korea; gnahn@jnu.ac.kr
[5] Marine Ecosystem and Biological Research Center, Korea Institute of Ocean Science and Technology (KIOST), Busan 49111, Republic of Korea; ohjh@kiost.ac.kr (J.H.O.); shinay@kiost.ac.kr (A.Y.S.); dskim@kiost.ac.kr (D.K.)
* Correspondence: sjheo@kiost.ac.kr; Tel.: +82-64-798-6101

Citation: Heo, S.-Y.; Kang, N.; Kim, E.-A.; Kim, J.; Lee, S.-H.; Ahn, G.; Oh, J.H.; Shin, A.Y.; Kim, D.; Heo, S.-J. Purification and Molecular Docking Study on the Angiotensin I-Converting Enzyme (ACE)-Inhibitory Peptide Isolated from Hydrolysates of the Deep-Sea Mussel *Gigantidas vrijenhoeki*. *Mar. Drugs* **2023**, 21, 458. https://doi.org/10.3390/md21080458

Academic Editors: Francesc Xavier Avilés and Isel Pascual

Received: 27 July 2023
Revised: 15 August 2023
Accepted: 19 August 2023
Published: 21 August 2023

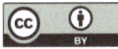
Abstract: The objective of this study was to prepare an angiotensin I-converting enzyme (ACE)-inhibitory peptide from the hydrothermal vent mussel, *Gigantidas vrijenhoeki*. The *G. vrijenhoeki* protein was hydrolyzed by various hydrolytic enzymes. The peptic hydrolysate exhibited the highest ACE-inhibitory activity and was fractionated into four molecular weight ranges by ultrafiltration. The <1 kDa fraction exhibited the highest ACE inhibitory activity and was found to have 11 peptide sequences. Among the analyzed peptides, KLLWNGKM exhibited stronger ACE inhibitory activity and an IC_{50} value of 0.007 µM. To investigate the ACE-inhibitory activity of the analyzed peptides, a molecular docking study was performed. KLLWNGKM exhibited the highest binding energy (−1317.01 kcal/mol), which was mainly attributed to the formation of hydrogen bonds with the ACE active pockets, zinc-binding motif, and zinc ion. These results indicate that *G. vrijenhoeki*-derived peptides can serve as nutritional and pharmacological candidates for controlling blood pressure.

Keywords: hydrothermal vent mussel; *Gigantidas vrijenhoeki*; angiotensin I-converting enzyme; molecular docking; bioactive peptide

1. Introduction

Hypertension is a major healthcare concern that increases the risk of death, stroke, myocardial infarction, arteriosclerosis, cerebral hemorrhage, and other vascular diseases and is affected by various factors, such as salt intake, smoking, stress, and obesity [1,2]. As part of the complex regulatory system of blood pressure, angiotensin I-converting enzyme (ACE) plays a key role in maintaining blood pressure via the renin-angiotensin-aldosterone system [3]. ACE converts the inactive decapeptide, angiotensin I, by cleaving a dipeptide from the C-terminus to produce an active octapeptide, angiotensin II, a potent vasoconstrictor [4,5]. Moreover, it induces the inactivation of bradykinin, an anti-hypertensive vasodilator, and promotes an increase in blood pressure [6,7]. Therefore, ACE inhibition has become a promising approach for maintaining blood pressure within the normal range.

Several synthetic inhibitors, such as captopril, enalapril, lisinopril, and alacepril, have been developed and used extensively for the management of hypertension and cardiovascular disorders [8,9]. However, the use of these synthetic inhibitors are often accompanied by obvious drug-associated adverse effects, including headaches, insomnia, fever, cough, skin rashes, and increased blood potassium levels [8,10]. Therefore, it has become increasingly necessary to develop therapeutic agents that are free from adverse side effects and to develop effective ACE inhibitors derived from natural sources for the treatment and prevention of hypertension.

Several studies have reported that marine organisms are good sources of protein and contain bioactive peptides with potential biological activities, such as osteoblast differentiation [11,12], anti-cancer [13], antioxidative [14], and anti-inflammatory activities [15]. In particular, bioactive peptides with ACE-inhibitory activity isolated from marine organisms, such as *Takifugu bimaculatus* [16], *Ulva intestinalis* [17], *Paralichthys olivaceus* [18], *Mytilus edulis* [19], and *Perna viridis* [20] have been widely reported. Therefore, research on ACE-inhibitory peptides is of considerable interest to the pharmaceutical industry, and marine organisms are regarded as a promising source of ACE-inhibitory peptides [7]. *Gigantidas vrijenhoeki* is a newly discovered hydrothermal vent mussel species, first reported in 2020, and is known to inhabit the Onnuri Vent Fiedl (OVF) Central Indian Ridge [21,22].

The objective of the present study was to prepare protein hydrolysates and ACE-inhibitory peptides from *G. vrijenhoeki*, and to identify any bioactive peptides with ACE-inhibitory activity. In addition, we investigated the interactions between the bioactive compounds and ACE using molecular simulations.

2. Results and Discussion

2.1. Approximate Chemical Composition of G. vrijenhoeki

The approximate chemical composition of *G. vrijenhoeki* is presented in Table 1. The major chemical component of *G. vrijenhoeki* was found to be protein, the content of which accounted for 65.83 ± 4.94% of the total dry weight. The lipid, moisture, ash, and carbohydrate contents of *G. vrijenhoeki* were 16.64 ± 0.89%, 2.28 ± 0.04%, 6.29 ± 1.19% and 8.96 ± 0.57%, respectively. Compared to previous studies, the protein content of *G. vrijenhoeki* was found to be higher or similar to *Chlamys farreri* (66.18%) [23], *Mytilus coruscus* (53.2%) [24], and *Perna canaliculus* (43.0%) [25]. Therefore, *G. vrijenhoeki* can be considered to be richer in protein compared to similar species.

Table 1. Approximate chemical composition of *G. vrijenhoeki*.

Scientific Name	Protein	Lipid	Moisture	Ash	Carbohydrate
G. vrijenhoeki	65.83 ± 4.94	16.64 ± 0.89	2.28 ± 0.04	6.29 ± 1.19	8.96 ± 0.57

2.2. Amino Acid Profile of G. vrijenhoeki

The amino acid composition of *G. vrijenhoeki* muscle is listed in Table 2. Glutamic acid (16.39%), aspartic acid (10.20%), glycine (9.01%), and arginine (8.53%) were dominant in *G. vrijenhoeki* muscle. The major amino acids in fish protein and shellfish hydrolysates are glutamic acid, aspartic acid, and glycine [26]. In particular, in *Mytilidae*, such as *M. edulis*, *M. coruscus*, *P. viridis*, and *P. canaliculus*, glutamic acid, aspartic acid, glycine, and arginine are abundant [20,25,27]. In addition, Ijarotimi et al. (2023) reported that glutamic acid serves as a precursor to arginine, which is a precursor for nitric oxide formation that acts as a vasodilator of the arteries, thus lowering blood pressure [28]. Other studies have also reported the ACE inhibitory activity of protein hydrolysates isolated from blue- and green-lipped mussels [19,29–31]. Therefore, *G. vrijenhoeki* could be a potential source of ACE inhibitory peptides.

Table 2. Total amino acids composition of *G. vrijenhoeki*.

Amino Acid	Content (%)
Aspartic acid	10.20
Glutamic acid	16.39
Serine	5.17
Histidine	2.14
Glycine	9.01
Threonine	5.64
Arginine	8.53
Alanine	4.92
Taurine	0.88
Tyrosine	4.04
Valine	4.61
Methionine	2.73
Phenylalanine	3.65
Isoleucine	4.60
Leucine	6.79
Lysine	6.35
Proline	4.35
Total	100.000

2.3. Preparation of GVHs and Their ACE Inhibitory Activity

G. vrijenhoeki hydrolysates (GVHs) were obtained by enzymatic hydrolysis with nine proteases, including papain, alcalase, flavourzyme, neutrase, bromelain, protamax, pepsin, trypsin, and α-chymotrypsin, under optimal conditions. The nine hydrolysates were evaluated for their ability to inhibit ACE activity. Among all of the enzymatic hydrolysates, the peptic hydrolysate exhibited the highest level of activity relative to the other enzymatic hydrolysates, with an IC_{50} value of 0.266 mg/mL (Table 3). Compared to previous studies, the ACE inhibitory activity of enzymatic hydrolysates from *G. vrijenhoeki* was more effective than those of seahorse (0.81 mg/mL) [8], Yellowbelly (3.98 mg/mL) [9], scallop (10.28 mg/mL) [32], and blue mussel (1.13 mg/mL) [19] hydrolysates. Interestingly, oysters (0.40 mg/mL) [33] exhibit a similar ACE inhibitory activity.

Table 3. ACE inhibitory activity of enzymatic hydrolysates from *G. vrijenhoeki*.

Enzyme	IC_{50} Value (mg/mL)
Papain	0.401 ± 0.001 [f]
Alcalase	0.319 ± 0.003 [d]
Flavourzyme	0.780 ± 0.070 [i]
Neutrase	0.417 ± 0.010 [h]
Bromelain	0.402 ± 0.012 [g]
Protamax	0.281 ± 0.011 [b]
Pepsin	0.266 ± 0.004 [a]
Trypsin	0.334 ± 0.001 [e]
α-chymotrypsin	0.302 ± 0.001 [c]

The concentration of an inhibitor required to inhibit 50% of ACE activity. The values of IC_{50} were determined by triplicate individual experiments. Means with different letters are significantly different ($p < 0.05$).

The peptide hydrolysate from *G. vrijenhoeki* was fractionated by ultrafiltration using membranes of different pore sizes (1 kDa, 5 kDa, and 10 kDa) to obtain fractions of >10 kDa, 5–10 kDa, 1–5 kDa, and <1 kDa. Among all of the fractions, the <1 kDa fraction exhibited the highest ACE inhibitory activity, with an IC_{50} value of 0.025 mg/mL (Table 4). Heo et al. (2017) previously reported that the ACE inhibitory efficiency of a peptide is strongly influenced by the molecular weight thereof. In addition, it has been reported that low-molecular-weight fractions tend to have a more potent ACE inhibitory activity [34,35]. Based on these results, we selected the <1 kDa fraction for further experiments.

Table 4. ACE inhibitory activity of molecular weight fractions of peptic hydrolysate from *G. vrijenhoeki*.

Molecular Weight Fraction	IC_{50} Value (mg/mL)
Pepsin hydrolysates	0.266 ± 0.004 [e]
<1 kDa	0.025 ± 0.022 [a]
1–5 kDa	0.060 ± 0.006 [b]
5–10 kDa	0.067 ± 0.001 [c]
>10 kDa	0.351 ± 0.039 [d]

The concentration of an inhibitor required to inhibit 50% of ACE activity. The values of IC_{50} were determined by triplicate individual experiments. Means with different letters are significantly different ($p < 0.05$).

2.4. Identification of an ACE Inhibitory Peptide

The molecular masses of the ACE-inhibitory peptides were determined. The <1 kDa fraction was subjected to micro Q-TOF mass spectrometry (MS) and tandem MS analysis, and the results revealed that the fraction was composed of 11 peptides (Figure 1). A synthetic peptide with the same sequence was synthesized and evaluated to validate its ACE inhibitory activity. As shown in Table 5, *G. vrijenhoeki* peptide (GVP)-10 ($IC_{50} = 0.007$ μM) exhibited stronger ACE inhibitory activity, followed by GVP-7 ($IC_{50} = 0.024$ μM), GVP-4 ($IC_{50} = 0.067$ μM), GVP-2 ($IC_{50} = 0.162$ μM), GVP-3 ($IC_{50} = 0.292$ μM), GVP-9 ($IC_{50} = 0.435$ μM), GVP-8 ($IC_{50} = 0.513$ μM), GVP-5 ($IC_{50} = 0.582$ μM), GVP-11 ($IC_{50} = 0.795$ μM), GVP-6 ($IC_{50} = 1.390$ μM), and GVP-1 ($IC_{50} = 2.955$ μM). Several reports suggest that the main substrates comprising peptides, such as hydrophobic amino acid residues (aromatic or branched chain) at the C-terminus and positively charged amino acids, are effective for ACE inhibitory activity [1,4,7,30,33,35,36]. This may explain the strong inhibitory activity of GVP-10 (KLLWNGKM) and GVP-7 (ALRPKF), which consist of aromatic amino acids (methionine, M; phenylalanine, F) and positively charged amino acids (lysine, K) at the C-terminus of the analyzed peptide.

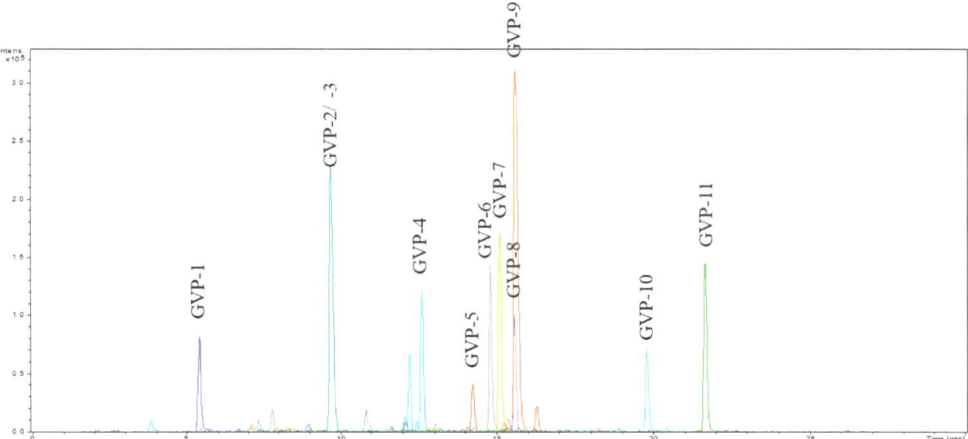

Figure 1. LC-MS chromatogram of <1 kDa fraction from *G. vrijenhoeki* protein.

Table 5. ACE inhibitory activity of peptides from *G. vrijenhoeki* peptic hydrolysate.

Peptide	Peptide Sequence	Molecular Weight (Da)	IC$_{50}$ Value (μM)
GVP-1	KLQE	517.29	2.955 ± 0.165 [k]
GVP-2	KVLH	496.32	0.162 ± 0.002 [d]
GVP-3	KVHL	496.32	0.292 ± 0.013 [e]
GVP-4	LVR	387.27	0.067 ± 0.005 [c]
GVP-5	PSLVG	472.27	0.582 ± 0.008 [h]
GVP-6	LNSL	446.26	1.390 ± 0.011 [j]
GVP-7	ALRPKF	366.23	0.024 ± 0.017 [b]
GVP-8	PGLADMR	380.19	0.513 ± 0.002 [g]
GVP-9	LLR	401.28	0.435 ± 0.007 [f]
GVP-10	KLLWNGKM	495.28	0.007 ± 0.002 [a]
GVP-11	YALPHAL	392.72	0.795 ± 0.015 [i]

The concentration of an inhibitor required to inhibit 50% of ACE activity. The values of IC$_{50}$ were determined by triplicate individual experiments. Means with different letters are significantly different ($p < 0.05$).

2.5. Analysis of Molecular Docking Study

Molecular docking studies are effective analytical tools for investigating ligand-protein interactions to understand structure-activity relationships. Therefore, we investigated whether ACE-inhibitory peptides could interact with ACE proteins and inhibit ACE activity, by performing molecular docking analysis using Discovery Studio (Figure 2). ACE consists of three main active site pockets (S1, S′1 and S′2). These pockets are major active sites in ACE and contain different residues. The S1 pocket includes Ala354, Glu384, and Tyr523 residues, the S1′ pocket includes the Glu162 residue, and the S′2 pocket consists of the Gln281, His353, Lys511, His513, and Tyr520 residues [37]. The HEXXH zinc-binding motif is also a main active site, consisting of the His383, Glu384, and His387 residues, and zinc ions [38]. As shown in Table 6, the relative binding energy between GVP-10 and ACE was the highest, indicating that its binding to ACE was the most stable. The binding energy value of GVP-10 was −1317.01 kcal/mol. It was found to interact with the S1 pocket (Ala354, Glu384, and Tyr523), S′2 pocket (Gln281, His353, Lys511, His513, and Tyr520), and zinc-binding motif (His383, His387, Glu411, and zinc ion). Glycine and aspartic acid of GVP-10 were located in the S1 pocket, forming hydrogen bonds with Ala354, Glu384, and Tyr523. Furthermore, methionine of GVP-10 shared hydrogen bond with Gln281, Lys511, His513, and Tyr520 in the S′2 pocket (Figure 2C). Based on these results, GVP-10 could directly interact with the active sites in the S1 and S′2 pockets, thus contributing to its competitive inhibition modalities [39]. In addition, GVP-10 interacted with a zinc-binding motif. Zinc ions play a key role in maintaining ACE activity, and residues in the zinc-binding motif bind to zinc ions to form tetrahedral coordinates [40]. Previous studies have shown that interactions between ACE-inhibitory peptides and the tetrahedral coordination of zinc ions can inhibit ACE activity [41,42]. Therefore, interactions with zinc ions can inhibit ACE inhibitory activity. Among the components of GVP-10, lysine formed a hydrogen bond with His383, and aspartic acid interacted with His411 and zinc ions through a hydrogen bond, facilitating interaction with the zinc-binding motif. Kaewsahnguan et al. (2021) reported that negatively charged amino acids in the ACE active site can interact with zinc ions to lower the catalytic rate through chelation of the critical zinc atom if enzymatic activity occurs [43].

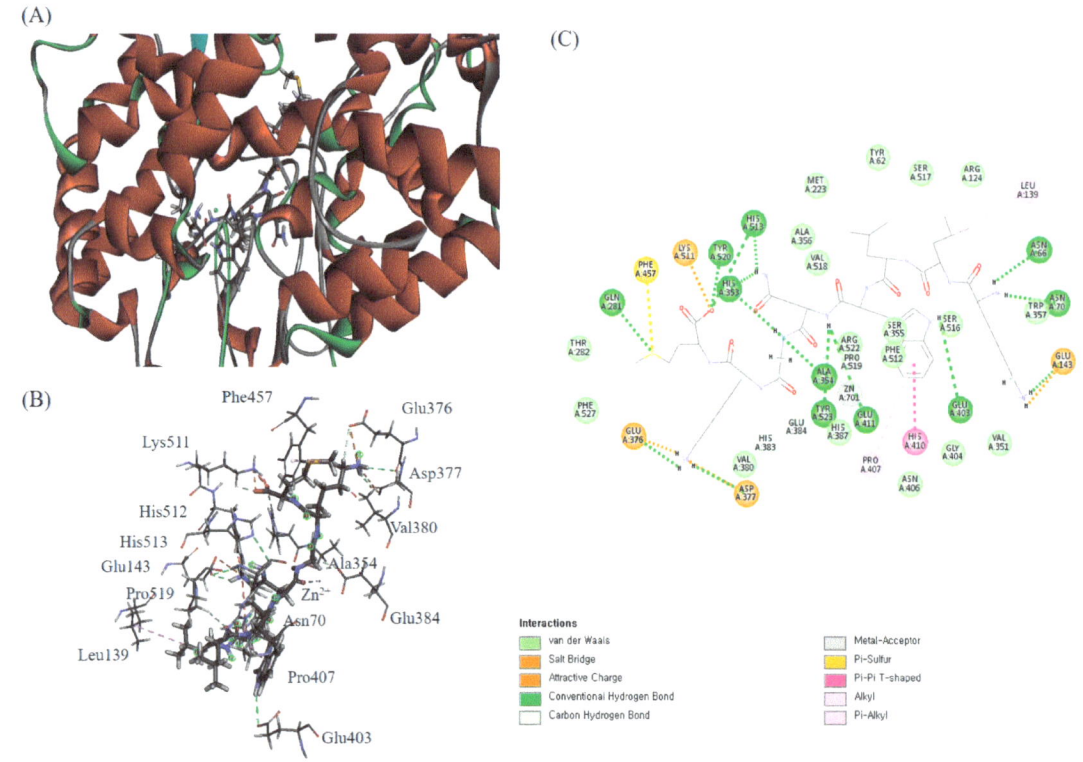

Figure 2. Predicted binding site of GVP-10 with ACE protein (**A**,**B**) and specific points of interaction between GVP-10 and ACE protein (**C**).

Table 6. Interaction between ACE inhibitory peptide and ACE from molecular docking simulation.

Peptide	Peptide Sequence	Binding Energy (kcal/mol)	ACE Residues
GVP-1	KLQE	−449.06	Glu162, Gln281, His353, Ala354, His383, Lys511, Phe512, His513, Tyr520
GVP-2	KVLH	−992.454	Glu162, Gln281, His353, Ala354, Ser355, His383, Glu384, His387, Glu411, Asp415, Asp453, Lys511, His513, Tyr523, Phe527, Zn²⁺
GVP-3	KVHL	−884.496	Glu162, His353, Ala354, Ser355, His383, Glu384, His387, Asp415, Asp453, Lys511, Phe512, His513, Val518, Arg522, Tyr523, Phe523, Phe527, Zn²⁺
GVP-4	LVR	−570.048	Glu162, Gln281, His353, Ala354, His383, Glu384, His387, Glu411, Asp415, Asp453, Lys454, Lys511, Tyr520, Tyr523, Phe527, Zn²⁺
GVP-5	PSLVG	−684.558	His353, Ala354, Ser355, Ala356, His383, Glu384, His387, Phe391, His410, Glu411, Phe512, His513, Val518, Arg522, Tyr523, Phe527, Zn²⁺
GVP-6	LNSL	−607.594	Glu162, His353, Ala354, Ser355, Ala356, His383, Glu384, His387, Phe391, Glu411, Lys511, Phe512, His513, Val518, Arg522, Tyr523, Zn²⁺
GVP-7	ALRPKF	−670.681	Glu162, His353, Ala354, Ser355, Ala356, His383, Glu384, His387, Phe391, His410, Glu411, Asp415, Asp453, Lys511, Phe512, His513, Ser516, Val518, Tyr523, Phe527, Zn²⁺
GVP-8	PGLADMR	−565.024	Gln281, His353, Ala354, Ser355, Ala356, His383, Glu384, His387, Phe391, Pro407, His410, Glu411, Asp415, Asp453, Lys454, Lys511, Phe512, His513, Val518, Tyr523, Phe527, Zn²⁺
GVP-9	LLR	−540.849	Glu162, His353, Ala354, His383, Glu384, His357, Glu411, Asp415, Asp453, Lys454, Tyr523, Phe527, Zn²⁺
GVP-10	KLLWNGKM	−1317.01	Gln281, His353, Ala354, Ser355, Ala356, His383, Glu384, His387, Pro407, His410, Glu411, Lys511, Phe512, His513, Ser516, Ser517, Val518, Pro519, Tyr520, Arg522, Tyr523, Phe527, Zn²⁺
GVP-11	YALPHAL	−782.256	Gln281, His353, Ala354, Ser355, Ala356, His383, Glu384, His387, Phe391, Pro407, His410, Glu411, Asp415, Asp453, Lys454, Lys511, Phe512, His513, Val518, Tyr523, Phe527, Zn²⁺

As shown in Figure 2C, the aspartic acid of GVP-10 interacts with the zinc ion and residue Glu411, leading to the distortion of the tetrahedral geometry of ACE. Moreover, the 11 residues surrounding the ACE active site–Ser355, Ala356, Pro407, His410, Phe512, Ser516, Ser517, Val518, Pro519, Arg522, and Phe527 significantly contributed to the stabilization of the ACE inhibitory peptide-ACE complex.

3. Materials and Methods

3.1. Materials

A deep-sea mussel (*G. vrijenhoeki*) specimen was collected with a video-guided hydraulic grab (Oktopus, Hohenwestedt, Germany) apparatus from the ONNURI vent field in the Indian Ocean (11°14′55.92″ S, 66°15′15.10″ E, at 2014.5 m depth) using the R/V ISABU [21]. The collected sample was immediately rinsed with seawater, directly frozen in a deep freeze, and stored at −80 °C until extraction. Alcalase 2.4 L FG, Neutrase 0.8 L, Flavourzyme 500 MG, and Protamex were purchased from Novo Co. (Novozyme Nordisk, Bagasvaerd, Denmark). Pepsin, trypsin, α-chymotrypsin, bromelain, and papain were purchased from Sigma–Aldrich (St. Louis, MO, USA). All of the other chemicals and reagents used were of analytical grade.

3.2. Chemical Composition of G. vrijenhoeki

The chemical composition of *G. vrijenhoeki* was determined as described by Horwitz et al. [44]. Briefly, the crude protein and lipid contents were determined using the Kjeldahl and Soxhlet methods, respectively. The moisture content was determined by placing the sample in a dry oven, and crude ash was prepared at 550 °C in a dry-type furnace.

3.3. Amino Acid Composition of G. vrijenhoeki

The amino acid composition was analyzed according to a previously developed high-performance liquid chromatography (HPLC) method [14]. The samples were added to 30 mL of 6 N HCl and incubated for 24 h at 130 °C. The mixtures were filtered with a 0.45 μm syringe filter and used for HPLC analysis. The HPLC system used for the analysis consisted of an Ultimated3000 (Thermo Fisher Scientific, Waltham, MA, USA) and a FL detector 1260FLD (Agilent Technologies, Inc., Santa Clara, CA, USA). Analyses were performed in the binary gradient mode. An Inno C18 column (4.6 × 150 mm, 5 μm, YoungJin Biochrom, Gyeonggi, Korea) was used. The chromatogram was obtained using a fluorescence spectrophotometer at 340/450 nm and 266/305 nm and absorbance at 338 nm.

3.4. Preparation of Enzymatic Hydrolysates of G. vrijenhoeki

G. vrijenhoeki enzymatic hydrolysis was performed according to a previous method described by Lee et al. [45]. *G. vrijenhoeki* enzymatic hydrolysates were prepared using alcalase, neutrase, flavourzyme, protamex, pepsin, trypsin,-chymotrypsin, bromelain, and papain under optimal conditions (Table 7). Briefly, 1 g *G. vrijenhoeki* and 10 mg of each enzyme were mixed in 100 mL distilled water. The mixtures were then incubated in a shaking incubator for 24 h. After 24 h, the mixtures were incubated at 100 °C for 10 min to inactivate the enzyme, and the pH was adjusted to 7.0. The mixtures were clarified by centrifugation and filtered through Whatman filter paper. The filtered mixtures were lyophilized and kept at −80 °C for further experiments.

Table 7. Optimal conditions of enzymatic hydrolysis for various enzymes.

Enzyme	Optimal Conditions	
	pH	Temp. (°C)
Alcalase	8.0	50
Flavourzyme	7.0	50
Neutrase	6.0	50
Protamex	6.0	40
Pepsin	2.0	37
Trypsin	8.0	37
α-chymotrypsin	8.0	37
Bromelain	7.0	50
Papain	7.0	60

3.5. Preparation of Molecular Weight Fractionation

GVH was passed through ultrafiltration (UF) membranes (molecular weight cut-offs of 1 kDa, 5 kDa, and 10 kDa) using a laboratory-scale tangential flow filtration (TFF) system (Millipore, Burlington, MA, USA). GVH was subjected to molecular weight fractionation to obtain peptides with molecular weights <1 kDa (1 kDa or smaller), 1–5 kDa (between 1 and 5 kDa), 5–10 kDa (between 5 and 10 kDa), and >10 kDa (10 kDa and larger). All recovered fractions were lyophilized and stored at −80 °C until use.

3.6. Identification of ACE Inhibitory Peptide

The molecular masses and amino acid sequences of the purified peptides were determined using a quadrupole time-of-flight mass spectrometer (Micro Q-TOF III mass spectrometer, Bruker Daltonics, Bremen, Germany) coupled with an electrospray ionization (ESI) source. The fraction was separately infused into the electrospray source after being dissolved in distilled water containing 0.1% formic acid, and the molecular mass was determined from the doubly charged $[M+2H]^2$ states in the mass spectrum. Following molecular mass determination, peptides were automatically selected for fragmentation, and sequence information was obtained by tandem mass spectrometry (MS) analysis.

3.7. Synthesis of the Purified Peptide

The peptide was chemically synthesized at the peptide synthesizer facility of PepTron Inc. (Daejeon, Korea). The peptides were synthesized using the Fmoc solid-phase method with a peptide synthesizer (PeptrEX-R48; Peptron, Inc., Deajeon, Korea). The synthetic peptides were purified using HPCL (Shimadzu, Kyoto, Japan) on a Capcell Pak C18 column (4.6 × 50 mm, 5 μm, Shiseido, Kyoto, Japan). The column was developed at a flow rate of 1.0 mL/min by a linear gradient of acetonitrile containing 0.1% trifluoroacetic acid. The identity of synthetic peptides was confirmed by liquid chromatography-mass spectroscopy (LC-MS) (Shimadzu, Japan), and the purity of the synthetic peptide was confirmed to be over 95%.

3.8. ACE Inhibitory Activity Assay

ACE inhibitory activity was measured using the Dojindo ACE Kit-WET kit (Dojindo Laboratories, Kumamoto, Japan), according to the manufacturer's instructions. The ACE-inhibitory activity was calculated as follows:

$$ACE \ inhibitory \ activity \ (\%) = \frac{A_{control} - A_{sample}}{A_{control} - A_{blank}} \times 100\%$$

where $A_{control}$ is the absorbance of the positive control, A_{blank} is the absorbance of the blank containing distilled water, and A_{sample} is the absorbance of the sample. The IC_{50} value was determined as the concentration of inhibitor required to inhibit 50% of the ACE activity.

3.9. Molecular Docking Analysis

The molecular docking analysis was performed according to the method described by Kang et al. [46] with slight modifications. For molecular docking studies, the crystal structure of ACE (PDB code:1O86) was obtained from the protein data bank (PDB; https://www.rcsb.org/, accessed on 11 October 2022). The structures of the 11 peptides derived from GVH were drawn using the CDOCKER tool. Docking of bioactive peptides to ACE was performed using the Lib Dock tool in Discovery Studio 2022 (Biovia, San Diego, CA, USA).

3.10. Statistical Analysis

All quantitative data are presented as means ± standard deviation and represent at least three individual experiments conducted using fresh reagents. Statistical comparisons of the mean values were performed using analysis of variance (ANOVA) followed by Duncan's multiple range test using SPSS software v29. Differences in mean values were considered statistically significant at * $p < 0.05$, ** $p < 0.01$.

4. Conclusions

In this study, *G. vrijenhoeki* protein was hydrolyzed using alcalase, neutrase, flavourzyme, protamex, pepsin, trypsin, α-chymotrypsin, bromelain, and papain, and their evaluated ACE inhibitory activity. Among enzymatic hydrolysates, peptic hydrolysate showed the highest ACE inhibitory activity compared to other hydrolysates. Subsequently, the peptic hydrolysate was fractionated by ultrafiltration and their fractions significantly improved the ACE inhibitory activity compared to hydrolysate. The low molecular weight fraction (>1 kDa) showed the highest ACE inhibitory activity and identified eleven ACE inhibitory peptides. Among the identified peptides, GVP-10 (KLLWNGKM) exhibited the strongest ACE inhibitory activity with an IC$_{50}$ value of 0.007 μM. Molecular docking studies indicated that GVP-10 was able to bind to residues in the ACE-active pockets (S1 and S'2), interact with zinc-binding motifs, and coordinate with zinc ions. Based on these results, we propose that the ACE-inhibitory peptide isolated from the *G. vrijenhoeki* protein has a beneficial effect in regulating blood pressure.

Author Contributions: Writing an original draft and data curation, S.-Y.H.; Investigation and data acquisition; N.K., E.-A.K. and J.K.; Writing review & editing, S.-H.L. and G.A.; Conceptualization, J.H.O. and A.Y.S.; supervision and project administration, D.K. and S.-J.H. All authors have read and agreed to the published version of the manuscript.

Funding: This research was supported by Korea Institute of Marine Science & Technology (KIMST) funded by the Ministry of Oceans and Fisheries (20170411 and 21210466).

Data Availability Statement: Data is contained within the article.

Conflicts of Interest: The authors declare no conflict of interest.

References

1. Heo, S.-Y.; Ko, S.-C.; Kim, C.S.; Oh, G.-W.; Ryu, B.; Qian, Z.J.; Kim, G.; Park, W.S.; Choi, I.-W.; Phan, T.T.V. A heptameric peptide purified from *Spirulina* sp. gastrointestinal hydrolysate inhibits angiotensin I-converting enzyme-and angiotensin II-induced vascular dysfunction in human endothelial cells. *Int. J. Mol. Med.* **2017**, *39*, 1072–1082. [CrossRef] [PubMed]
2. Ko, S.-C.; Kim, J.-Y.; Lee, J.M.; Yim, M.-J.; Kim, H.-S.; Oh, G.-W.; Kim, C.H.; Kang, N.; Heo, S.-J.; Baek, K. Angiotensin I-Converting Enzyme (ACE) Inhibition and Molecular Docking Study of Meroterpenoids Isolated from Brown Alga, *Sargassum macrocarpum*. *Int. J. Mol. Sci.* **2023**, *24*, 11065. [CrossRef] [PubMed]
3. Xu, Z.; Wu, C.; Sun-Waterhouse, D.; Zhao, T.; Waterhouse, G.I.; Zhao, M.; Su, G. Identification of post-digestion angiotensin-I converting enzyme (ACE) inhibitory peptides from soybean protein Isolate: Their production conditions and in silico molecular docking with ACE. *Food Chem.* **2021**, *345*, 128855. [CrossRef] [PubMed]
4. Bhaskar, B.; Ananthanarayan, L.; Jamdar, S. Purification, identification, and characterization of novel angiotensin I-converting enzyme (ACE) inhibitory peptides from alcalase digested horse gram flour. *LWT* **2019**, *103*, 155–161. [CrossRef]

5. Solanki, D.; Sakure, A.; Prakash, S.; Hati, S. Characterization of Angiotensin I-Converting Enzyme (ACE) inhibitory peptides produced in fermented camel milk (Indian breed) by *Lactobacillus acidophilus* NCDC-15. *J. Food Sci. Technol.* **2022**, *59*, 3567–3577. [CrossRef]

6. Wang, J.; Hu, J.; Cui, J.; Bai, X.; Du, Y.; Miyaguchi, Y.; Lin, B. Purification and identification of a ACE inhibitory peptide from oyster proteins hydrolysate and the antihypertensive effect of hydrolysate in spontaneously hypertensive rats. *Food Chem.* **2008**, *111*, 302–308. [CrossRef]

7. Ishak, N.H.; Shaik, M.I.; Yellapu, N.K.; Howell, N.K.; Sarbon, N.M. Purification, characterization and molecular docking study of angiotensin-I converting enzyme (ACE) inhibitory peptide from shortfin scad (*Decapterus macrosoma*) protein hydrolysate. *J. Food Sci. Technol.* **2021**, *58*, 4567–4577. [CrossRef]

8. Shi, J.; Su, R.-Q.; Zhang, W.-T.; Chen, J. Purification and the secondary structure of a novel angiotensin I-converting enzyme (ACE) inhibitory peptide from the alcalase hydrolysate of seahorse protein. *J. Food Sci. Technol.* **2020**, *57*, 3927–3934. [CrossRef]

9. Su, Y.; Chen, S.; Cai, S.; Liu, S.; Pan, N.; Su, J.; Qiao, K.; Xu, M.; Chen, B.; Yang, S. A novel angiotensin-I-converting enzyme (ACE) inhibitory peptide from *Takifugu flavidus*. *Mar. Drugs* **2021**, *19*, 651. [CrossRef]

10. Ko, S.-C.; Jang, J.; Ye, B.-R.; Kim, M.-S.; Choi, I.-W.; Park, W.-S.; Heo, S.-J.; Jung, W.-K. Purification and molecular docking study of angiotensin I-converting enzyme (ACE) inhibitory peptides from hydrolysates of marine sponge *Stylotella aurantium*. *Process Biochem.* **2017**, *54*, 180–187. [CrossRef]

11. Nguyen, M.H.T.; Qian, Z.-J.; Nguyen, V.-T.; Choi, I.-W.; Heo, S.-J.; Oh, C.H.; Kang, D.-H.; Kim, G.H.; Jung, W.-K. Tetrameric peptide purified from hydrolysates of biodiesel byproducts of *Nannochloropsis oculata* induces osteoblastic differentiation through MAPK and Smad pathway on MG-63 and D1 cells. *Process Biochem.* **2013**, *48*, 1387–1394. [CrossRef]

12. Heo, S.Y.; Ko, S.C.; Nam, S.Y.; Oh, J.; Kim, Y.M.; Kim, J.I.; Kim, N.; Yi, M.; Jung, W.K. Fish bone peptide promotes osteogenic differentiation of MC3T3-E1 pre-osteoblasts through upregulation of MAPKs and Smad pathways activated BMP-2 receptor. *Cell Biochem. Funct.* **2018**, *36*, 137–146. [CrossRef] [PubMed]

13. Ko, S.-C.; Heo, S.-Y.; Choi, S.-W.; Qian, Z.-J.; Heo, S.-J.; Kang, D.-H.; Kim, N.; Jung, W.-K. A heptameric peptide isolated from the marine microalga *Pavlova lutheri* suppresses PMA-induced secretion of matrix metalloproteinase-9 through the inactivation of the JNK, p38, and NF-κB pathways in human fibrosarcoma cells. *J. Appl. Phycol.* **2018**, *30*, 2367–2378. [CrossRef]

14. Kang, N.; Kim, E.-A.; Kim, J.; Lee, S.-H.; Heo, S.-J. Identifying potential antioxidant properties from the viscera of sea snails (*Turbo cornutus*). *Mar. Drugs* **2021**, *19*, 567. [CrossRef] [PubMed]

15. Marasinghe, C.K.; Jung, W.K.; Je, J.Y. Anti-inflammatory action of ark shell (*Scapharca subcrenata*) protein hydrolysate in LPS-stimulated RAW264. 7 murine macrophages. *J. Food Biochem.* **2022**, *46*, e14493. [CrossRef] [PubMed]

16. Cai, S.; Pan, N.; Xu, M.; Su, Y.; Qiao, K.; Chen, B.; Zheng, B.; Xiao, M.; Liu, Z. ACE inhibitory peptide from skin collagen hydrolysate of *Takifugu bimaculatus* as potential for protecting HUVECs injury. *Mar. Drugs* **2021**, *19*, 655. [CrossRef] [PubMed]

17. Sun, S.; Xu, X.; Sun, X.; Zhang, X.; Chen, X.; Xu, N. Preparation and identification of ACE inhibitory peptides from the marine macroalga *Ulva intestinalis*. *Mar. Drugs* **2019**, *17*, 179. [CrossRef]

18. Oh, J.-Y.; Kim, E.-A.; Lee, H.; Kim, H.-S.; Lee, J.-S.; Jeon, Y.-J. Antihypertensive effect of surimi prepared from olive flounder (*Paralichthys olivaceus*) by angiotensin-I converting enzyme (ACE) inhibitory activity and characterization of ACE inhibitory peptides. *Process Biochem.* **2019**, *80*, 164–170. [CrossRef]

19. Neves, A.C.; Harnedy, P.A.; FitzGerald, R.J. Angiotensin converting enzyme and dipeptidyl peptidase-iv inhibitory, and antioxidant activities of a blue mussel (*Mytilus edulis*) meat protein extract and its hydrolysates. *J. Aquat. Food Prod. Technol.* **2016**, *25*, 1221–1233. [CrossRef]

20. Chakraborty, K.; Chakkalakal, S.J.; Joseph, D.; Asokan, P.; Vijayan, K. Nutritional and antioxidative attributes of green mussel (*Perna viridis* L.) from the southwestern coast of India. *J. Aquat. Food Prod. Technol.* **2016**, *25*, 968–985. [CrossRef]

21. Ryu, T.; Kim, J.G.; Lee, J.; Yu, O.H.; Yum, S.; Kim, D.; Woo, S. First transcriptome assembly of a newly discovered vent mussel, *Gigantidas vrijenhoeki*, at Onnuri Vent Field on the northern Central Indian Ridge. *Mar. Genom.* **2021**, *57*, 100819. [CrossRef] [PubMed]

22. Jang, S.-J.; Ho, P.-T.; Jun, S.-Y.; Kim, D.; Won, Y.-J. A newly discovered *Gigantidas bivalve* mussel from the Onnuri Vent Field in the northern Central Indian Ridge. *Deep. Sea Res. Part I Oceanogr. Res. Pap.* **2020**, *161*, 103299. [CrossRef]

23. Wu, Z.X.; Hu, X.P.; Zhou, D.Y.; Tan, Z.F.; Liu, Y.X.; Xie, H.K.; Rakariyatham, K.; Shahidi, F. Seasonal variation of proximate composition and lipid nutritional value of two species of scallops (*Chlamys farreri* and *Patinopecten yessoensis*). *Eur. J. Lipid Sci. Technol.* **2019**, *121*, 1800493. [CrossRef]

24. Li, G.; Li, J.; Li, D. Seasonal variation in nutrient composition of *Mytilus coruscus* from China. *J. Agric. Food Chem.* **2010**, *58*, 7831–7837. [CrossRef]

25. Siriarchavatana, P.; Kruger, M.C.; Miller, M.R.; Tian, H.S.; Wolber, F.M. The preventive effects of greenshell mussel (*Perna canaliculus*) on early-stage metabolic osteoarthritis in rats with diet-induced obesity. *Nutrients* **2019**, *11*, 1601. [CrossRef]

26. Je, J.-Y.; Park, S.Y.; Hwang, J.-Y.; Ahn, C.-B. Amino acid composition and in vitro antioxidant and cytoprotective activity of abalone viscera hydrolysate. *J. Funct. Foods* **2015**, *16*, 94–103. [CrossRef]

27. Jeong, Y.-R.; Park, J.-S.; Nkurunziza, D.; Cho, Y.-J.; Chun, B.-S. Valorization of blue mussel for the recovery of free amino acids rich products by subcritical water hydrolysis. *J. Supercrit. Fluids* **2021**, *169*, 105135. [CrossRef]

28. Ijarotimi, O.S.; Akinola-Ige, A.O.; Oluwajuyitan, T.D. Okra seeds proteins: Amino acid profile, free radical scavenging activities and inhibition of diabetes and hypertensive converting enzymes indices. *Meas. Food* **2023**, *11*, 100101. [CrossRef]

29. Je, J.-Y.; Park, P.-J.; Byun, H.-G.; Jung, W.-K.; Kim, S.-K. Angiotensin I converting enzyme (ACE) inhibitory peptide derived from the sauce of fermented blue mussel, *Mytilus edulis*. *Bioresour. Technol.* **2005**, *96*, 1624–1629. [CrossRef]

30. Jayaprakash, R.; Perera, C.O. Partial purification and characterization of bioactive peptides from cooked New Zealand green-lipped mussel (*Perna canaliculus*) protein hydrolyzates. *Foods* **2020**, *9*, 879. [CrossRef]

31. Suo, S.-K.; Zhao, Y.-Q.; Wang, Y.-M.; Pan, X.-Y.; Chi, C.-F.; Wang, B. Seventeen novel angiotensin converting enzyme (ACE) inhibitory peptides from the protein hydrolysate of *Mytilus edulis*: Isolation, identification, molecular docking study, and protective function on HUVECs. *Food Funct.* **2022**, *13*, 7831–7846. [CrossRef] [PubMed]

32. Zhang, L.; Liu, Y.; Lu, D.; Han, J.; Lu, X.; Tian, Z.; Wang, Z. Angiotensin converting enzyme inhibitory, antioxidant activities, and antihyperlipidaemic activities of protein hydrolysates from scallop mantle (*Chlamys farreri*). *Int. J. Food Prop.* **2015**, *18*, 33–42. [CrossRef]

33. Xie, C.-L.; Kim, J.-S.; Ha, J.-M.; Choung, S.-Y.; Choi, Y.-J. Angiotensin I-converting enzyme inhibitor derived from cross-linked oyster protein. *BioMed Res. Int.* **2014**, *2014*, 379234. [CrossRef] [PubMed]

34. Zhao, Y.; Li, B.; Dong, S.; Liu, Z.; Zhao, X.; Wang, J.; Zeng, M. A novel ACE inhibitory peptide isolated from *Acaudina molpadioidea* hydrolysate. *Peptides* **2009**, *30*, 1028–1033. [CrossRef]

35. Ko, S.-C.; Kang, N.; Kim, E.-A.; Kang, M.C.; Lee, S.-H.; Kang, S.-M.; Lee, J.-B.; Jeon, B.-T.; Kim, S.-K.; Park, S.-J. A novel angiotensin I-converting enzyme (ACE) inhibitory peptide from a marine *Chlorella ellipsoidea* and its antihypertensive effect in spontaneously hypertensive rats. *Process Biochem.* **2012**, *47*, 2005–2011. [CrossRef]

36. Li, Y.; Sadiq, F.A.; Fu, L.; Zhu, H.; Zhong, M.; Sohail, M. Identification of angiotensin I-converting enzyme inhibitory peptides derived from enzymatic hydrolysates of razor clam *Sinonovacula constricta*. *Mar. Drugs* **2016**, *14*, 110. [CrossRef]

37. Li, X.; Feng, C.; Hong, H.; Zhang, Y.; Luo, Z.; Wang, Q.; Luo, Y.; Tan, Y. Novel ACE inhibitory peptides derived from whey protein hydrolysates: Identification and molecular docking analysis. *Food Biosci.* **2022**, *48*, 101737. [CrossRef]

38. Lin, Z.; Lai, J.; He, P.; Pan, L.; Zhang, Y.; Zhang, M.; Wu, H. Screening, ACE-inhibitory mechanism and structure-activity relationship of a novel ACE-inhibitory peptide from *Lepidium meyenii* (Maca) protein hydrolysate. *Food Biosci.* **2023**, *52*, 102374. [CrossRef]

39. Chen, J.; Ryu, B.; Zhang, Y.; Liang, P.; Li, C.; Zhou, C.; Yang, P.; Hong, P.; Qian, Z.J. Comparison of an angiotensin-I-converting enzyme inhibitory peptide from tilapia (*Oreochromis niloticus*) with captopril: Inhibition kinetics, in vivo effect, simulated gastrointestinal digestion and a molecular docking study. *J. Sci. Food Agric.* **2020**, *100*, 315–324. [CrossRef]

40. Soleymanzadeh, N.; Mirdamadi, S.; Mirzaei, M.; Kianirad, M. Novel β-casein derived antioxidant and ACE-inhibitory active peptide from camel milk fermented by *Leuconostoc lactis* PTCC1899: Identification and molecular docking. *Int. Dairy J.* **2019**, *97*, 201–208. [CrossRef]

41. Renjuan, L.; Xiuli, Z.; Liping, S.; Yongliang, Z. Identification, in silico screening, and molecular docking of novel ACE inhibitory peptides isolated from the edible symbiot Boletus griseus-*Hypomyces chrysospermus*. *LWT* **2022**, *169*, 114008. [CrossRef]

42. Pan, D.; Cao, J.; Guo, H.; Zhao, B. Studies on purification and the molecular mechanism of a novel ACE inhibitory peptide from whey protein hydrolysate. *Food Chem.* **2012**, *130*, 121–126. [CrossRef]

43. Kaewsahnguan, T.; Noitang, S.; Sangtanoo, P.; Srimongkol, P.; Saisavoey, T.; Reamtong, O.; Choowongkomon, K.; Karnchanatat, A. A novel angiotensin I-converting enzyme inhibitory peptide derived from the trypsin hydrolysates of salmon bone proteins. *PLoS ONE* **2021**, *16*, e0256595. [CrossRef] [PubMed]

44. Horwitz, W.; Latimer, G.W., Jr. *Official Methods of Analysis*, 15th ed.; Association of Official Analytical Chemists: Gaithersburg, MD, USA, 1990.

45. Lee, H.-G.; Kim, H.-S.; Oh, J.-Y.; Lee, D.-S.; Yang, H.-W.; Kang, M.-C.; Kim, E.-A.; Kang, N.; Kim, J.; Heo, S.-J. Potential antioxidant properties of enzymatic hydrolysates from *Stichopus japonicus* against hydrogen peroxide-induced oxidative stress. *Antioxidants* **2021**, *10*, 110. [CrossRef]

46. Kang, N.; Heo, S.-Y.; Cha, S.-H.; Ahn, G.; Heo, S.-J. In Silico Virtual Screening of Marine Aldehyde Derivatives from Seaweeds against SARS-CoV-2. *Mar. Drugs* **2022**, *20*, 399. [CrossRef]

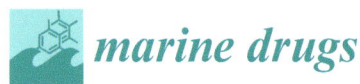

Article

Rapid Mining of Novel *α*-Glucosidase and Lipase Inhibitors from *Streptomyces* sp. HO1518 Using UPLC-QTOF-MS/MS

Jianlin Xu [1,2,3,†], Zhifeng Liu [2,3,†], Zhanguang Feng [2,3], Yuhong Ren [1], Haili Liu [2,*] and Yong Wang [1,2,*]

1   State Key Laboratory of Bioreactor Engineering, East China University of Science and Technology, Shanghai 200237, China; xujianlin@cemps.ac.cn (J.X.); yhren@ecust.edu.cn (Y.R.)
2   CAS-Key Laboratory of Synthetic Biology, CAS Center for Excellence in Molecular Plant Sciences, Institute of Plant Physiology and Ecology, Chinese Academy of Sciences, Shanghai 200032, China; liuzhifeng@cemps.ac.cn (Z.L.); fengzhanguang@cemps.ac.cn (Z.F.)
3   University of Chinese Academy of Sciences, Beijing 100039, China
*   Correspondence: hlliu@cemps.ac.cn (H.L.); yongwang@cemps.ac.cn (Y.W.); Tel.: +86-021-5492-4295 (Y.W.)
†   These authors contributed equally to this work.

Abstract: A rapid and sensitive method using ultra-high performance liquid chromatography/ quadrupole time-of-flight mass spectrometry (UPLC-QTOF-MS/MS) was applied for the analysis of the metabolic profile of acarviostatin-containing aminooligosaccharides derived from *Streptomyces* sp. HO1518. A total of ninety-eight aminooligosaccharides, including eighty potential new compounds, were detected mainly based on the characteristic fragment ions originating from quinovosidic bond cleavages in their molecules. Following an LC-MS-guided separation technique, seven new aminooligosaccharides (**10–16**) along with four known related compounds (**17–20**) were obtained directly from the crude extract of strain HO1518. Compounds **10–13** represent the first examples of aminooligosaccharides with a rare acarviostatin II02-type structure. In addition, all isolates displayed considerable inhibitory effects on three digestive enzymes, which revealed that the number of the pseudo-trisaccharide core(s), the feasible length of the oligosaccharides, and acyl side chain exerted a crucial influence on their bioactivities. These results demonstrated that the UPLC-QTOF-MS/MS-based metabolomics approach could be applied for the rapid identification of aminooligosaccharides and other similar structures in complex samples. Furthermore, this study highlights the potential of acylated aminooligosaccharides with conspicuous *α*-glucosidase and lipase inhibition for the future development of multi-target anti-diabetic drugs.

Keywords: *Streptomyces* sp. HO1518; metabolic profiling; aminooligosaccharides; UPLC-QTOF-MS/MS; diabetes; digestive enzyme inhibitors

Citation: Xu, J.; Liu, Z.; Feng, Z.; Ren, Y.; Liu, H.; Wang, Y. Rapid Mining of Novel *α*-Glucosidase and Lipase Inhibitors from *Streptomyces* sp. HO1518 Using UPLC-QTOF-MS/MS. *Mar. Drugs* **2022**, *20*, 189. https:// doi.org/10.3390/md20030189

Academic Editors: Valentin A. Stonik and Natalia V. Ivanchina

Received: 24 January 2022
Accepted: 23 February 2022
Published: 4 March 2022

Publisher's Note: MDPI stays neutral with regard to jurisdictional claims in published maps and institutional affiliations.

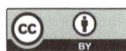
1. Introduction

Type 2 diabetes mellitus (T2DM) is the most prevalent metabolic syndrome characterized by prolonged high levels of blood glucose, reflected by 537 million patients and 6.7 million deaths in 2021. The number of cases of diabetes is estimated to increase further to 783 million by 2045, which placed immense economic and social pressures on patients [1–5]. Currently, *α*-glucosidases (mainly *α*-amylases and disaccharidases), secreted from the intestinal chorionic epithelium capable of converting dietary carbohydrates into glucose, are still recognized as an important pharmacological target for anti-diabetic drug development. Acarbose, a typical anti-diabetes drug functioning as an *α*-glucosidases inhibitor, potently inhibits the *α*-glucosidases in vivo to retard carbohydrate digestion and avoid blood glucose elevation [6,7]. However, the specific kinase Mak1 derived from the human microbiome selectively phosphorylates acarbose at the C6-OH of C_7N cyclohexitol ring in acarbose, leading to its inactivation [8]. Therefore, an urgent demand for the discovery of new *α*-glucosidase inhibitors with high efficacy has declared a public-health imperative for the treatment of T2DM.

Natural products, characteristic of enormous structural diversity and complexity, have been recognized as an attractive source of leading compounds and therapeutic agents attributable to their remarkable pharmacological activities [9]. Traditionally, the bioactivity-based approach remains the most commonly employed screening method to isolate natural products; however, an increasing number of compounds already described are repeatedly isolated during bioassay-guided purification [10,11]. To avoid the rediscovery of known molecules and screen new chemical entities, several dereplication strategies, including ultraviolet-visible spectroscopy (UV-Vis), nuclear magnetic resonance spectroscopy (NMR), or mass spectrometry (MS) have been developed [12,13]. Among them, MS-based dereplication has the advantage of high sensitivity and versatility, enabling users to obtain multiple types of data in a single experiment, which generally serves as the first choice of a structure-based pipeline for the discovery of unknown secondary metabolites [14]. Recently, time-of-flight mass spectrometry (TOF-MS), especially the quadrupole time-of-flight mass spectrometry (QTOF-MS), has become one of the most powerful tools for untargeted analysis of complex mixtures derived from plants and microorganisms and is attributable to their capability of providing accurate mass data and structural information [15]. Because the ultra-high performance liquid chromatography (UPLC) can shorten the analysis time of multi-component extract and increase sensitivity and reproducibility in comparison to conventional HPLC, UPLC coupled to QTOF-MS has become the crucial platform for analyzing the metabolite profiling of certain plants or microbe [16,17].

Marine *Streptomyces*, capable of producing structurally novel and biologically active secondary metabolites, has been recognized as a highly prolific resource of pharmaceutically and industrially meaningful small molecules [18,19]. In our continuing efforts to search for new anti-diabetic lead compounds from the *Streptomyces* species, we have recently discovered a series of rare acylated aminooligosaccharides with intriguing inhibitory activities against α-glucosidases and pancreatic lipase (PL) from the *Streptomyces* sp. HO1518 [20,21]. Structurally, these aminooligosaccharides possess a single or repeated pseudo-trisaccharide unit(s), which are combined with D-glucopyranose groups attached to the reducing and non-reducing terminus through α-(1→4) glycosidic bond. Pseudo-trisaccharide is composed of an acarviosine moiety and a D-glucopyranose group through α-(1→4) quinovosidic bond, and acarviosine is comprised of an unsaturated C_7N cyclohexitol residue and a 4-amino-4,6-dideoxy-D-glucopyranose unit via α-(1→4) pseudo-glycosidic bond. Based on their structure feature, this class of naturally occurring oligosaccharide is referred to as acarviostatins followed by a Roman numeral and two digits, such as acarviostatin I01 (acarbose). The Roman numeral represents the number of the pseudo-trisaccharide cores, the middle digit denotes the number of glucose residues at the non-reducing end, and the last digit corresponds to the number of glucose units at the reducing end [22–24].

Since this family of oligosaccharides displayed conspicuous inhibitory activities against α-glucosidases and PL [20,21], this inspires our great interest to decipher the whole metabolic profiling of aminooligosaccharides in strain HO1518, which may contribute to exploring their structure-activity relationships and screening the optimal antidiabetic candidate molecules. To this end, a rapid and sensitive UPLC-QTOF-MS/MS method was developed to determine aminooligosaccharides secreted by strain HO1518 based on the MS and MS^2 fragmentation patterns of nine reference standards (**1–9**) (Figure 1). This analytical approach resulted in the identification of ninety-eight oligosaccharides, including eighty new ones. Then, guided by the UPLC-QTOF-MS/MS, further study of the fermentation broth of strain HO1518 led to the isolation of seven new aminooligosaccharides (**10–16**) and four known congeners (**17–20**), among which **10–13** represent a new type of pseudo-octasaccharide. Compound **9** was the most potent α-amylase inhibitor with the IC_{50} value of 0.03 μM and was 282-fold more effective than that of acarbose (8.51 μM), while **19** exhibited the strongest activity against lipase with the IC_{50} value of 1.00 μM, and was almost equal to that of the anti-obesity orlistat (0.34 μM).

1 a = 0, b = 3, R = $COCH_3$
2 a = 0, b = 3, R = $COCH_2CH_3$
3 a = 0, b = 3, R = $COCH(CH_3)_2$
4 a = 0, b = 3, R = $COCH_2CH(OH)CH_3$
5 a = 0, b = 3, R = $COCH(CH_3)CH_2CH_3$
6 a = 0, b = 3, R = $COCH_2CH(CH_3)_2$
7 a = 1, b = 3, R = $COCH_3$
8 a = 1, b = 3, R = $COCH(CH_3)_2$
9 a = 1, b = 3, R = H

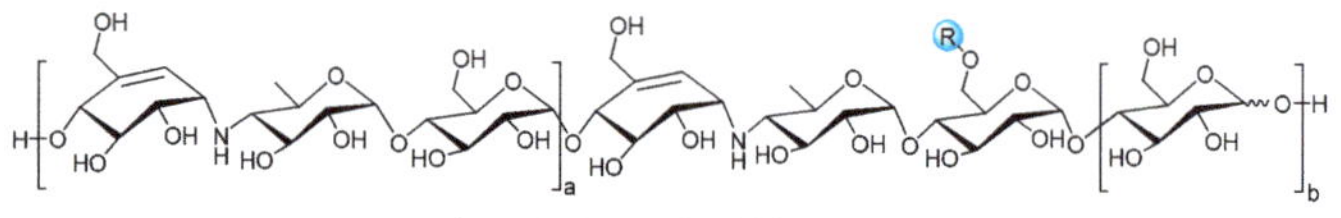

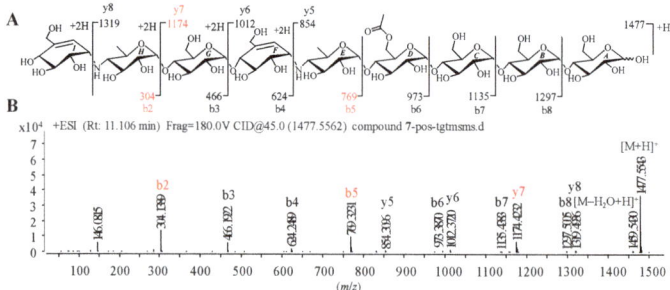

Figure 1. The structures of compounds **1–9**.

2. Results and Discussion

Nine reference compounds D6-*O*-acetyl-acarviostatin I03 (Ac-Aca I03, **1**), D6-*O*-propionyl-acarviostatin I03 (Pr-Aca I03, **2**), D6-*O*-isobutyryl-acarviostatin I03 (isoBu-Aca I03, **3**), D6-*O*-*β*-hydroxybutyryl-acarviostatin I03 (Hbu-Aca I03, **4**), D6-*O*-2-methyl-butyryl-acarviostatin I03 (Mbu-Aca I03, **5**), D6-*O*-isovaleryl-acarviostatin I03 (isoVa-Aca I03, **6**), D6-*O*-acetyl-acarviostatin II03 (Ac-Aca II03, **7**), D6-*O*-isobutyryl-acarviostatin II03 (isoBu-Aca II03, **8**) and acarviostatin II03 (Aca II03, **9**), previously isolated from *Streptomyces* sp. HO1518 by our group, can be grouped into two types, namely acarviostatin I03-type (**1–6**) and acarviostatin II03-type (**7–9**), based on the number of pseudo-trisaccharide units. Since the amine residues of aminooligosaccharides are readily protonated [25], the positive-ion mode HRMS/MS analysis of nine references was performed. Two series of nomenclatures bi and yj, with respect to the fragmentation of glycoconjugates in the FAB-MS/MS spectra, have been adopted in this study [26]. The bi represents fragments containing the sugar moiety counted from the non-reducing end, while the yj refers to ions possessing the aglycone at the reducing end. These fragments can provide multidimensional MS information, including retention times, molecular formulas, base peaks, sugar constituents, as well as the relative abundance of ions.

Given that **1–9** showed similar HRMS/MS fragmentation patterns (Figure S1), the representative D6-*O*-acetyl-acarviostatin II03 (Ac-Aca II03, **7**) harboring two pseudo-trisaccharide cores is taken as an example of how to take advantage of MS/MS data to identify the structure of acarviostatins. In the positive HRESIMS/MS spectrum of **7**, a strong protonated molecular ion at *m*/*z* 1477 was observed (Figure 2B). The high-intensity peaks in **7** were *m*/*z* 304 (b2), 769 (b5) and 1174 (y7), which resulted from the cleavages of two quinovosidic bonds. The peak intensity of some fragments with secondary amine residues, such as 146, was relatively high, which is conducive for the structure identification of aminooligosaccharides. In addition, the crucial ions at *m*/*z* 973 (b6), 1135 (b7), 1298 (b8), 854 (y5), 1012 (y6), 1174 (y7) and 1398 (y8) in **7**, were 42 mass units more than those of its deacyl product **9**, revealing that the location of the acetyl group of **7** was assigned at C-D6. Therefore, the structure of Ac-Aca II03 was established.

Figure 2. Positive HRESIMS/MS fragmentation and spectrum of **7**. (**A**) Positive-ion HRESIMS/MS fragmentation pattern of **7**; (**B**) HRESIMS/MS spectra of **7**.

It is worth noting that these most abundant fragments in **7** were produced by the rupture of the quinovosidic bonds between the quinovopyranose and glucose units. Similarly, the relatively high fragment ions in the other eight standards also originated from the dissociation of the quinovosidic bond, suggesting that the cleavage of this bond was easy to achieve when compared with those of pseudo-glycosidic, glycosidic and acyl bonds (Figure S1). The resultant fragments were thus regarded as characteristic fragment ions, as outlined in Table 1. In brief, the standards **1–6** sharing one pseudo-trisaccharide have the same base peak at m/z 304, whereas the other references **7–9** possessing two pseudo-trisaccharides have the mutual fragment ions at m/z 304 and 769.

Table 1. Information of reference aminooligosaccharides **1–9**.

Compounds	Formula	t_R (min)	$[M + H]^+$	Characteristic Fragment Ions
1	$C_{39}H_{65}NO_{29}$	10.99	1012.3715	304.1395, 1012.3703
2	$C_{40}H_{67}NO_{29}$	13.10	1026.3872	304.1395, 1026.3862
3	$C_{41}H_{69}NO_{29}$	15.43	1040.4028	304.1481, 1040.4034
4	$C_{41}H_{69}NO_{30}$	11.31	1056.3977	304.1386, 1056.3943
5	$C_{42}H_{71}NO_{29}$	17.93	1054.4184	304.1388, 1054.4172
6	$C_{42}H_{71}NO_{29}$	18.04	1054.4184	304.1388, 1054.4200
7	$C_{58}H_{96}N_2O_{41}$	11.11	1477.5561	304.1389, 769.3231, 1174.4232, 1477.5543
8	$C_{60}H_{100}N_2O_{41}$	14.40	1505.5874	304.1391, 769.3228, 1202.4547, 1505.5877
9	$C_{56}H_{94}N_2O_{40}$	9.27	1435.5456	304.1386, 769.3219, 1132.4094, 1435.5427

On the basis of the features of mass spectrometry data of reference, aminooligosaccharides, potential fragmentation rules of oligosaccharides were summarized. First, the glycosidic, pseudo-glycosidic and quinovosidic bonds in acarviostatins could be dissociated to some extent, and the quinovosidic bond was more fragile than two other ordinary bonds. Therefore, the most abundant signals in the positive HRMS/MS spectra were produced by the quinovosidic bond cleavages, which played pivotal roles in the structural determination of undescribed acarviostatins. Second, the fragments harboring a single or repeated amine-containing moiety (moieties) tended to display higher intensity, largely attributable to the considerably strong basicity of secondary amine residues that readily formed protonated molecules, which offered important information for the structure identification of new oligosaccharides. Third, some diagnostic product ions bi and yj in the acylated aminooligosaccharides could be applied for the assignment of the location of the acyloxy side chain.

After the establishment of the fragmentation rules of aminooligosaccharides, the UPLC-QTOF-MS/MS data of the crude extract of *Streptomyces* sp. HO1518 was analyzed. The result showed that, except for those of nine reference acarviostatins, a considerable number of newly appeared protonated molecular ions at m/z 812, 1115, 1132, 1273, 1597, 1759, etc., were detected. Further analysis of the quasi-molecular signals implied that the predicted aminooligosaccharides in strain HO1518 possess 0–3 repeating pseudo-trisaccharide moieties accompanied with a 0–1 glucose unit attached to the non-reducing end and 0–5 glucose residues on the reducing termini. In most cases, the hydroxy group at C6 of the glucose unit in pseudo-trisaccharide moiety at the proximal of the reducing terminus was acylated by an acyl group with 2–6 carbon chain. The assembly of the repeating pseudo-trisaccharide units with different numbers of glucose residues at the reducing and/or non-reducing end, together with the diversity of acyl side chain led to the identification of ninety-eight aminooligosaccharides in strain HO1518 (Figures S6–S8), among which eighty are new compounds, including seventy-three acylated aminooligosaccharides and seven precursors. The structure of each oligosaccharide in the extract was determined on the basis of the molecular ion peak, characteristic fragments mainly corresponded to quinovosidic bond cleavages, as well as the qualitative retention time (Tables S10–S12).

According to the abundant fragment ion peaks (m/z 304, 466, 146) arising from the cleavage of the first quinovosidic bond numbered at the non-reducing terminus, all the aminooligosaccharides are directly divided into three groups, namely acarviostatins with glucose(s) at the reducing end (Aca-glu), acarviostatins with glucose(s) at both ends (glu-Aca-glu), and acarviostatins with an incomplete pseudo-trisaccharide at the non-reducing end (incAca-glu) (Figure 3). The structures of sixty-three oligosaccharides can be categorized as group Aca-glu, which accounts for a major portion (more than 64%) of the metabolic profiling of strain HO1518. Amongst them, acarviostatin II05 (Aca II05) contains up to five glucose units at the reducing end, while D6-*O*-propionyl-acarviostatin III03 (Pr-Aca III03) possesses three pseudo-trisaccharides. The abundant MS^2 fragment ion at m/z 304, produced by the loss of the acarviosine moiety at the non-reducing end, is the basic and characteristic peak for group Aca-glu. The structures of fifteen aminooligosaccharides are assigned as group glu-Aca-glu. Due to the presence of an additional glucose unit appended to the non-reducing terminus in group glu-Aca-glu compared with those in group Aca-glu, the typical peak ion of aminooligosaccharides is m/z 466. Group incAca-glu contains twenty aminooligosaccharides. The rare absence of an unsaturated cyclohexitol unit in the partial pseudo-trisaccharide core at the non-reducing termini results in a high-intensity characteristic MS/MS fragment at m/z 146, corresponding to the loss of the 4-amino-4,6-dideoxy-D-glucopyranose unit in the non-reducing end. Moreover, when discriminating aminooligosaccharides harbor more than one pseudo-trisaccharide core, the above-mentioned characteristic peak in each group combined with the second typical fragment ion peaks at m/z 769 for Aca-glu, 931 for glu-Aca-glu, and 611 for incAca-glu and would be greatly helpful for the judgment of their structures.

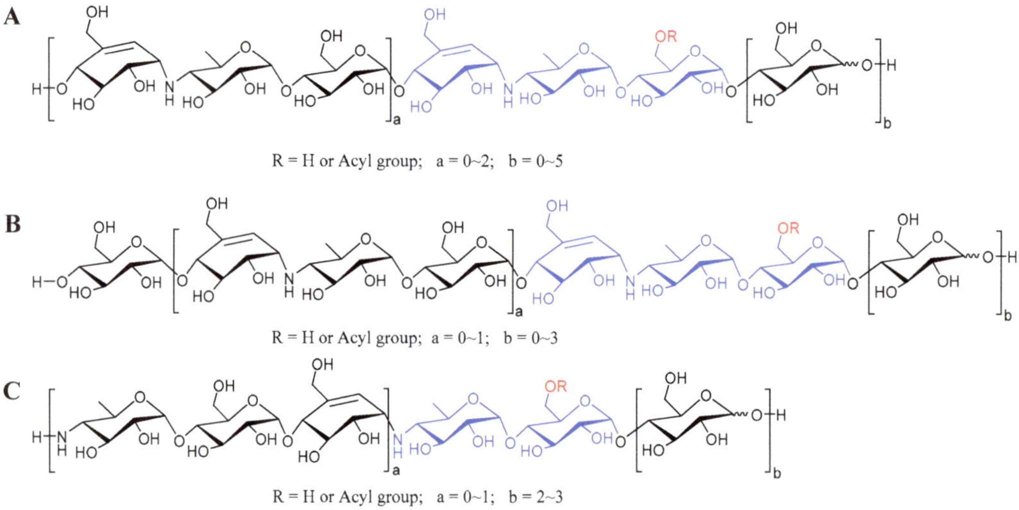

Figure 3. The general structures of aminooligosaccharides from *Streptomyces* sp. HO1518. (**A**) The general structures of acarviostatins with glucoses at the reducing terminus; (**B**) The general structures of acarviostatins with glucoses at the reducing and non-reducing terminus; (**C**) The general structures of acarviostatins with an incomplete pseudo-trisaccharide at the non-reducing terminus.

Some aminooligosaccharides, in particular the acylated acarviostatins, share identical m/z values and molecular formulas, suggesting that these compounds should be structural isomers. The reasons for this were attributed to the different assembly sequences of the same number of monosaccharides or the isomerism of the acyl side chains. For example, the protonated molecular ion at m/z 1012 in the extracted ion chromatograms (EIC) shows two peaks (Figure S9A). The minor peak with a retention time of 10.19 min was assigned as D6-*O*-acetyl-acarviostatin I12 (Ac-Aca I12) attributable to the most abundant fragment at m/z 466 (Figure S9B), while the major peak appearing at a retention time of 11.19 min was inferred as D6-*O*-acetyl-acarviostatin I03 (Ac-Aca I03) due to the most abundant ion at *m/z* 304 (Figure S9C). Therefore, these abundant signals produced by the cleavage of quinovosidic bonds could confirm the number of the D-glucopyranose attached to the reducing and/or non-reducing terminus. In addition, it is worth mentioning that twenty aminooligosaccharides belonging to group incAca-glu represent a new type of oligosaccharides. To the best of our knowledge, this is the first report of acylated aminooligosaccharides directly ending with 4-amino-4-deoxy-D-quinovopyranose unit at the non-reducing end.

Motivated by the metabolic profile of aminooligosaccharides, the LC-MS guided fractionation procedure was performed to acquire new oligosaccharides. The extract of the strain HO1518 was prepared and subjected to C_{18} column chromatography to yield six fractions. After careful analysis of these fractions using LC-HRMS/MS, the molecular weights related to various aminooligosaccharides were found to enrich the fractions F1 and F2. Then, several new ion peaks at *m/z* 1273, 1329, 1343, 1491, and 1519 in group Aca-glu were selected as target compounds (Figure S5). In addition, many newly appeared quasi-molecular ion peaks of acarviostatins, especially those in group incAca-glu, also inspired our great interest to further perform the chemical search of strain HO1518 for the discovery of new anti-diabetic agents. Nevertheless, to our regret, we failed to acquire these novel compounds due to the trace amount of these two groups of oligomers.

Under the guidance of the aforementioned quasi-molecular peaks, seven new aminooligosaccharide congeners (**10–16**) and four known related compounds (**17–20**) were isolated (Figure 4). Compound **10**, white amorphous powder, was assigned a HRESIMS ion peak at *m/z* 1273.4938 ([M + H]$^+$, calcd for 1273.4927), which matched a molecular formula of $C_{50}H_{84}N_2O_{35}$ with 10 degrees of hydrogen deficiency (Figure S27). The 1D and 2D NMR spectra, especially the 1D-selective TOCSY, 2D-TOCSY, HSQC, HMBC, and HSQC-TOCSY, allowed the construction of the gross structure of **10** (Figure 5). This deduction was further supported by several crucial fragments at *m/z* 304 (b2), 769 (b5), and 970 (y6) observed in the HRESIMS/MS spectrum of **10**, corresponding to the fission of the quinovosidic bond (Figure 6). The molecular formula of **11** was determined as $C_{53}H_{88}N_2O_{36}$ (*m/z* 1329.5234 ([M + H]$^+$, calcd for 1329.5190) by HRESIMS, suggesting that **11** was an acetylated derivative of **10**. A careful analysis of ^{1}H and ^{13}C NMR spectra between **10** and **11** revealed that the hydroxyl group at C-D6 was acetylated in **11**, which was further verified by the ^{1}H-^{1}H COSY cross peak of H-2′/H-3′ and the HMBC correlations from H-2′ (δ_H 2.48) and H-3′ (δ_H 1.13) to C-1′ (δ_C 180.8) as well as H-3′ to C-2′ (δ_C 30.6) (Figure 5). Similarly, the carbon signals (δ_C 180.1, 33.9, 18.3 and 18.2 for **12**, and δ_C 176.2, 42.9, 25.5, 21.7 and 21.7 for **13**) indicated **12** and **13** to be isobutyryl and isovaleryl substituted analogs of **10**, respectively.

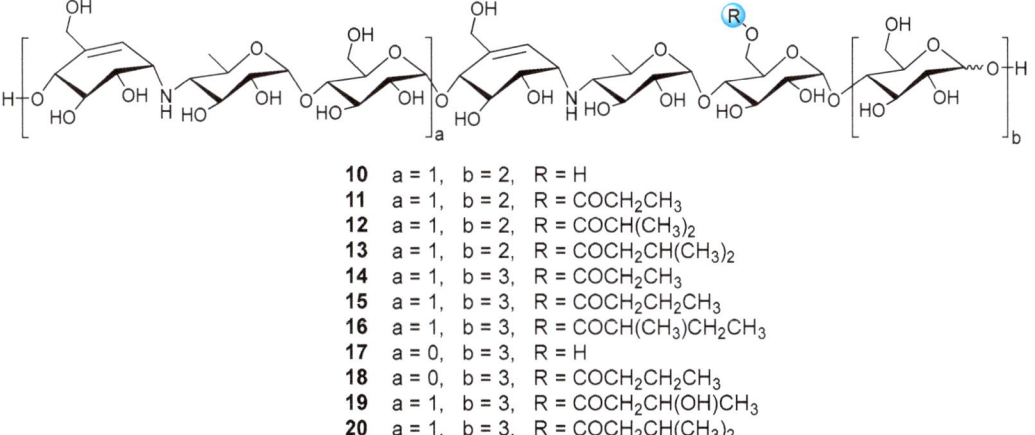

10	a = 1,	b = 2,	R = H
11	a = 1,	b = 2,	R = COCH$_2$CH$_3$
12	a = 1,	b = 2,	R = COCH(CH$_3$)$_2$
13	a = 1,	b = 2,	R = COCH$_2$CH(CH$_3$)$_2$
14	a = 1,	b = 3,	R = COCH$_2$CH$_3$
15	a = 1,	b = 3,	R = COCH$_2$CH$_2$CH$_3$
16	a = 1,	b = 3,	R = COCH(CH$_3$)CH$_2$CH$_3$
17	a = 0,	b = 3,	R = H
18	a = 0,	b = 3,	R = COCH$_2$CH$_2$CH$_3$
19	a = 1,	b = 3,	R = COCH$_2$CH(OH)CH$_3$
20	a = 1,	b = 3,	R = COCH$_2$CH(CH$_3$)$_2$

Figure 4. The structures of compounds **10–20**.

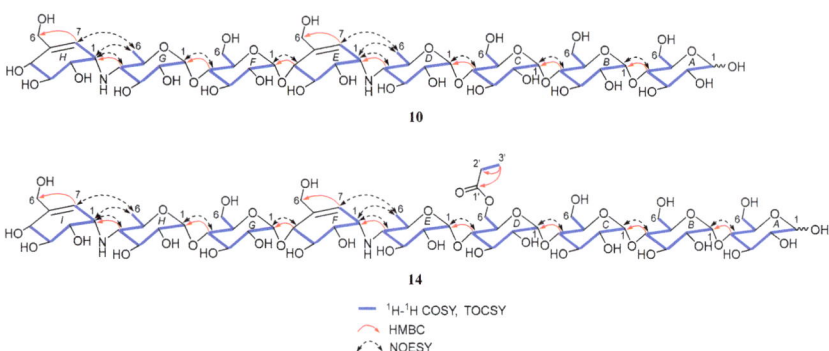

Figure 5. Key 2D NMR correlations of compounds **10** and **14**.

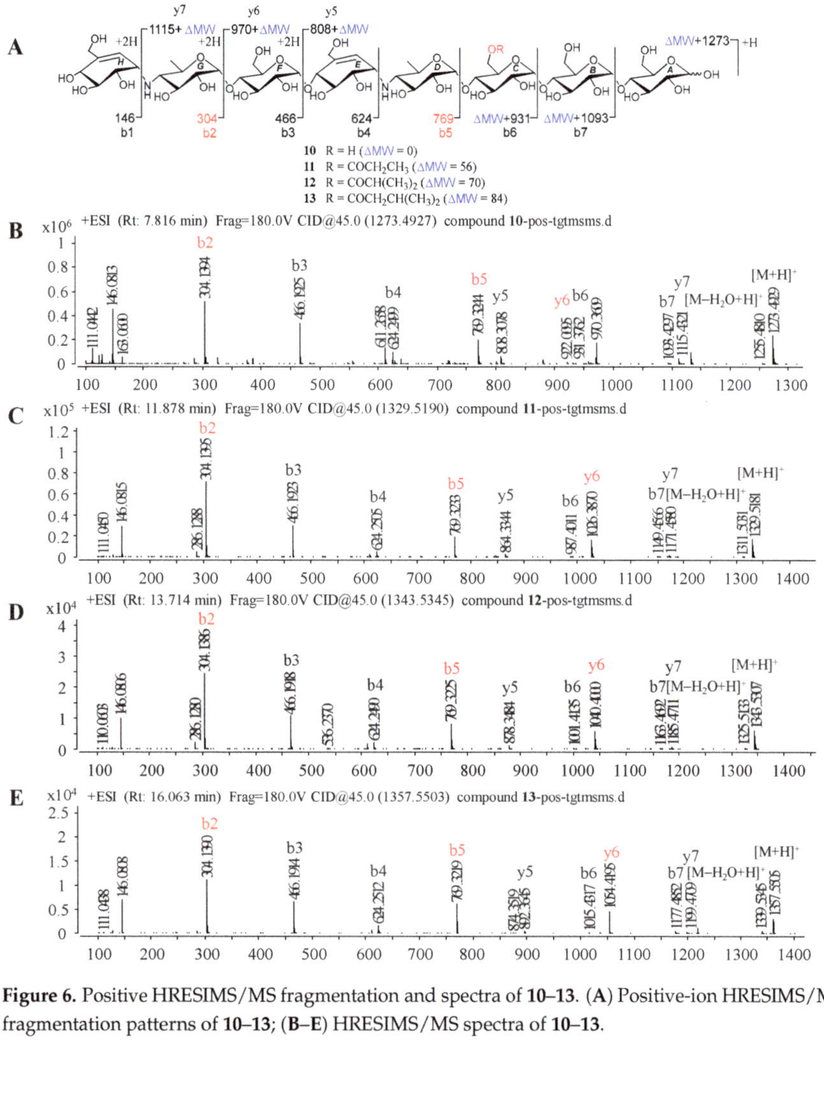

Figure 6. Positive HRESIMS/MS fragmentation and spectra of **10–13**. (**A**) Positive-ion HRESIMS/MS fragmentation patterns of **10–13**; (**B–E**) HRESIMS/MS spectra of **10–13**.

The molecular formula of **14** was assigned as $C_{59}H_{98}N_2O_{41}$ by HRESIMS ion peak at m/z 1491.5715 ([M + H]$^+$, calcd for 1491.5718), which was 162 mass units more than that of **11**. Detailed inspection of the NMR spectroscopic data of **11** and **14** suggested that they should feature an analogous planar structure (Figure 4), with the major difference being the presence of an additional glucose unit at the reducing end in **14** (δ_C 102.3, 79.9, 76.1, 74.3, 74.1 and 63.5). After a careful comparison of ^1H and ^{13}C NMR data of **15** and **16** (Table S2) with those of **14**, three compounds were found to share the identical acarviostatin II03-type core skeleton, but the side chain differentiated. The propionyl functionality in **14** was replaced by the butyryl group in **15** (δ_H 2.45, 1.65, 1.18 and 0.94) or the 2-methyl-butyryl group in **16** (δ_H 2.52, 1.63, 1.51, 1.13 and 0.88), which could be supported by the ^1H-^1H COSY cross-peaks (H-2′/H-3′/H-4′ in **15**, and H-5′/H-2′/H-3′/H-4′ in **16**) and the HRMS/MS spectra (Figure 5 and Figure S2).

T2DM is one of the most serious chronic diseases worldwide, which is closely linked to disturbances of glucose and lipid metabolism. Inhibiting α-glucosidase and lipase involved in the breakdown of carbohydrates and fats can reduce glucose and free fatty acid absorption in the gastrointestinal tract, which contributes to avoiding postprandial hyperglycemia and restoring normal levels of insulin secretion of pancreatic β-cells in diabetic patients [27–29]. Thus, compounds **9–20** were evaluated for their inhibitory activities against PPA, sucrase and PL, as presented in Table 2.

Table 2. The inhibitory activities of **9–20** against PPA, sucrase and PL.

Compounds	IC$_{50}$ Values (µM) [a]		
	Against PPA	**Against Sucrase**	**Against PL**
9	0.030 ± 0.001	17.24 ± 0.76	7.64 ± 0.13
10	0.084 ± 0.001	13.05 ± 0.55	12.66 ± 0.76
11	0.079 ± 0.001	4.34 ± 0.24	7.22 ± 0.10
12	0.085 ± 0.006	6.79 ± 0.06	5.48 ± 0.18
13	0.092 ± 0.001	7.06 ± 0.09	1.56 ± 0.04
14	0.035 ± 0.001	2.56 ± 0.12	4.21 ± 0.03
15	0.059 ± 0.007	10.67 ± 2.60	4.46 ± 0.14
16	0.052 ± 0.003	7.28 ± 0.10	1.34 ± 0.03
17	0.296 ± 0.007	11.12 ± 0.24	31.56 ± 4.13
18	0.402 ± 0.008	3.80 ± 0.78	11.68 ± 2.52
19	0.061 ± 0.005	9.67 ± 0.10	1.00 ± 0.12
20	0.080 ± 0.003	9.93 ± 0.50	1.43 ± 0.08
acarbose	8.513 ± 0.240	2.34 ± 0.23	191.00 ± 15.17
orlistat	-	-	0.34 ± 0.06

[a] Values are expressed as the mean $\pm$ SD.

All the compounds showed inhibition of three metabolic enzymes under the assay conditions. Twelve isolates (**9–20**) showed remarkable inhibition of PPA, with the IC$_{50}$ values ranging from 0.03 to 0.40 µM (Figure S3). Compounds **9–16**, **19** and **20** possessing the repeated pseudo-trisaccharide moieties exhibited more potential α-amylase inhibitory effects than those with a single pseudo-trisaccharide (**17** and **18**), among which **9** (IC$_{50}$ = 0.03 µM) was 282-fold more effective than that of acarbose (IC$_{50}$ = 8.51 µM). Nevertheless, the more pseudo-trisaccharide cores might pose an unfavorable effect for sucrase inhibition by comparison with the suppressing activities of **9**, **10**, and **17**. When the hydroxyl group occurred at C-6 in **10** (IC$_{50}$ = 13.05 µM) was acylated, **11–13** presented stronger inhibitory activity against sucrase with IC$_{50}$ values of 4.34, 6.79 and 7.06 µM, respectively, which implied that the acyl group shows a positive contribution to their inhibitory potency toward sucrase. Furthermore, twelve compounds displayed considerable inhibitory ability against PL with IC$_{50}$ values in a range of 1.00–31.56 µM, while acarbose was inactive with an IC$_{50}$ value of 191.00 µM. Of these compounds, **13**, **16**, **19** and **20**, sharing an acarviostatin II03-type structure, showed potent inhibitory effects against lipase with IC$_{50}$ values of 1.56, 1.34, 1.00 and 1.43 µM, respectively, which was nearly equal to the positive control orlistat

(IC_{50} = 0.34 μM). It is noteworthy, that increasing the acyl chain length in aminooligosaccharides contributes to enhancing their lipase inhibitory activities, as referred to **9–20**. These biological results highlight the potential of acylated aminooligosaccharides with prominent α-glucosidase and lipase inhibition for the future development of multi-target anti-diabetic drugs.

The significant PL inhibitory activity for aminooligosaccharides prompted us to further investigate the potential molecular recognition mechanism between this class of compounds and PL, thus the molecular docking simulations were implemented using a previously reported crystal structure of human PL (PDB ID: 1LPB) [30,31]. To better understand the binding mode of different aminooligosaccharides, the anti-obesity drug orlistat was firstly docked into the same domain for comparative purposes. As shown in Figure 7A, orlistat abrogated the activity of human PL by occupying the substrate binding canyon of PL and stabilized itself via strong interactions with a series of key residues (G76, F77, D79, S152 and R256) in the catalytic active site. Based on this, three characteristic aminooligosaccharides **9** (IC_{50} = 7.64 μM), **10** (IC_{50} = 12.66 μM), **17** (IC_{50} = 31.56 μM) as well as acarbose (negative control) belonging to acarviostatins II03, II02, I03 and I01 type, respectively, were selected as ligands for further detailed study.

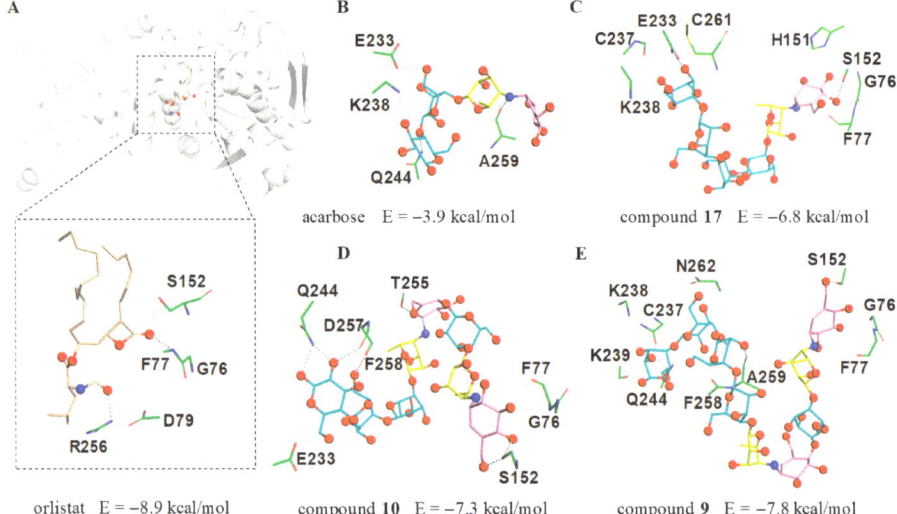

Figure 7. The docking results of human PL (PDB ID: 1LPB) with inhibitors. (**A**) The possible interactions between 1LPB and orlistat; (**B**) acarbose; (**C**) acarviostatin I03; (**D**) acarviostatin II02; (**E**) acarviostatin II03. Wheat: orlistat; pink: C_7N cyclohexitol; yellow: 4-amino-4,6-dideoxy-D-glucopyranose; cyan: D-glucopyranose.

As we anticipated, the cyclohexitol ring of the pseudo-trisaccharide unit for **9**, **10** and **17** could be perfectly docked into the catalytic cavity of PL by forming three hydrogen bonds with G76, F77 and S152, whereas the pseudo-tetrasaccharide acarbose, only located outside the catalytic pocket with no bonding site observed in the catalytic active center, indicates that the chain length and the pseudo-trisaccharide core(s) of aminooligosaccharides were crucial in hinting PL activity (Figure 7B–E). Besides the common residues mentioned above, **17** also interacted with four residues E233, C237, K238, and C261, while **10** showed interactions with the five residues E233, Q244, T255, D257, and F258. Notably, compound **9** (calculated binding energy = −7.8 kcal/mol), possessing an extra seven polar contacts with PL, exhibits a higher potency toward lipase than **10** and **17** (calculated binding energy = −7.3 and −6.8 kcal/mol), suggesting that the total strength of individual contact between ligand and PL is a definitive factor to forming a stable substrate-enzyme complex.

These results were consistent with the aforementioned biological results and demonstrated the pseudo-trisaccharide unit(s) along with the glucose residues of aminooligosaccharides played a crucial role in their lipase inhibitory activity.

3. Materials and Methods

3.1. General Experimental Procedures

The optical rotations were performed on an Anton Paar MCP-500 spectropolarimeter (Anton Paar, Graz, Austria) at 20 °C. UV spectra were recorded on a JASCO V-550 UV/VIS spectrophotometer (Jasco Corporation, Tokyo, Japan). IR data were measured using a FT-IR Vertex 70 v spectrometer (Bruker, Fällanden, Switzerland). The 1D and 2D NMR spectra were acquired using a Bruker Avance 500 MHz spectrometer with TMS as an internal standard (Bruker, Fällanden, Switzerland). HRESIMS data were collected on a Thermo Q Exactive high-resolution mass spectrometer (Thermo Fisher Scientific, Waltham, MA, USA). HRMS/MS data were recorded on an Agilent Q-TOF 6545 mass spectrometer (Agilent Technologies, Santa Clara, CA, USA) equipped with an electrospray ionization source (ESI). MCI gel CHP20/P120 (Mitsubishi Chemical Corporation, Tokyo, Japan) and SiliaSphere C_{18} (50 μm, Silicycle, QuébecK, QC, Canada) were used for column chromatography. UPLC analysis was performed using an Agilent 1200Series LC system (Agilent Technologies, Santa Clara, CA, USA) equipped with a binary pump, an online degasser, an autoplate-sampler, and a thermostatically controlled column compartment. The Thermo ultimate 3000 (Thermo Fisher Scientific, Waltham, MA, USA), equipped with an Alltech 3300 ELSD detector and VWD detector was used for HPLC. Preparative HPLC was performed using a SilGreen C_{18} column (250 × 20 mm, 5 μm, 12 nm, Greenherbs CO., Ltd., Beijing, China), while semi-preparative HPLC was performed utilizing a TSK-gel 100 V C_{18} column (250 × 10 mm, 5 μm, 12 nm, Tosoh Corporation, Tokyo, Japan).

3.2. Reagents

The HPLC-grade methanol and acetonitrile were purchased from CINC High Purity Solvents (Shanghai) Co., Ltd. (Shanghai, China). The other solvents were of analytical grade (Sinopharm Chemical Reagent Co., Ltd., Beijing, China). Porcine pancreatic α-amylase (PPA) and PL were purchased from Sigma Aldrich Co. (St Louis, MO, USA). Sucrase and acarbose were obtained from Shanghai yuanye Bio-Technology Co., Ltd. (Shanghai, China). Orlistat was bought from Shanghai xushuo Bio-Technology Co., Ltd. (Shanghai, China). Standards **1–9** were previously isolated from *Streptomyces* sp. HO1518 by our group.

3.3. Bacterial Material

The *Streptomyces* sp. HO1518 was isolated from a sediment sample collected from the Rizhao coastal area, Shandong Province of China, in summer 2010. This strain (Voucher Specimen No. M2018176) is preserved at the China Center for Type Culture Collection (CCTCC), Wuhan University.

3.4. UPLC Analysis

The ethanol extract of strain HO1518 was separated using an XBridge C_{18} column (4.6 × 150 mm, 3.5 μm; Waters, Milford, MA, USA). The mobile phase was composed of A (0.01% aqueous ammonia) and B (acetonitrile) with a flow rate of 0.3 mL/min. The column temperature was maintained at 40 °C, and the injection volume was 1 μL. The elution program was as follows: 0–1 min, 5% B; 1–21 min, 5–35% B; 21–26 min, 35–65% B; 26–27 min, 65–100% B; 27–28.5 min, 100% B; 28.5–29 min, 100–5% B; 29–30 min, 5% B.

3.5. QTOF-MS/MS Analysis

HRMS/MS spectra were performed on an Agilent Q-TOF 6545 mass spectrometer equipped with an electrospray ionization source (ESI). The operating parameters were set as follows: drying gas (nitrogen, N_2) flow rate, 6.0 L/min; drying gas temperature, 320 °C; nebulizer, 45 psig; sheath gas temperature, 350 °C; sheath gas flow, 12 L/min; capillary,

3500 V; skimmer, 65 V; OCT RF V, 750 V; and fragmentor voltage, 180 V. For MS/MS experiments, the collision energy was adjusted from 10V to 45V to optimize signals and obtain maximal structural information from the ions of interest. The system was operated under the Masshunter workstation software, version B.02.00 (Agilent Technologies, Santa Clara, CA, USA). Each sample was analyzed in positive-ion mode to provide sufficient information for structural identification. The mass range was set at m/z 50–2000.

3.6. Fermentation, Extraction and Isolation

The 70 L fermented broth of strain HO1518 was filtered to remove mycelia and the supernatant was subjected to XAD-16 resin by column chromatography, eluting with anhydrous ethanol to obtain the crude extract. The ethanol extract (9.2 g) was separated into 6 fractions (Frs. 1–6) on a C_{18} reverse-phase (RP) silica gel column by step gradient elution with MeOH/H_2O (5–100%, v/v). Since the majority of aminooligosaccharide derivatives were present in Frs. 1 and 2, the MS-guided fractionation was carried out.

Fr. 1 (4.2 g) was subjected to reversed-phase C_{18} silica gel using the gradient elution with MeOH/H_2O (5–100%, v/v) to obtain six subfractions (Frs. 1-1–1-6). Fr. 1-1 (0.2 g) was chromatographed over the MCI column and further purified by a preparative RP HPLC system equipped with a preparative SilGreen C_{18} column (MeCN/H_2O, 8 mL/min, 6:94) to produce **10** (1.6 mg, t_R 9.6 min). Fr. 1-3 (0.3 g) was fractionated by HPLC using an isocratic mobile phase of 10% MeCN/H_2O to obtain **19** (4.5 mg, t_R 15.1 min), whereas Fr. 1-4 (0.4 g) was successively separated by MCI and HPLC with an isocratic mobile phase of 10% MeCN/H_2O to acquire **14** (13.2 mg, t_R 40.5 min). Fr. 1-5 (0.8 g) was repeatedly purified by HPLC (MeCN/H_2O, 8 mL/min, 16:84) to yield **18** (10.2 mg, t_R 14.3 min). Fr. 1-6 (0.8 g) was fractionated by the MCI column, which was purified by HPLC on a preparative SilGreen C_{18} column (MeCN/H_2O, 8 mL/min, 18:82) to yield **16** (4.2 mg, t_R 12.2 min) and **20** (6.2 mg, t_R 12.8 min). Fr. 2 (3.9 g) was subjected to the MCI column, eluting with MeOH/H_2O (5–100%, v/v) to afford four subfractions (Frs. 2-1–2-4). Fr. 2-1 (0.2 g) was purified by HPLC with an isocratic phase of 18% MeOH/H_2O to yield **17**. Fr. 2-2 (0.5 g) was separated by the reversed-phase C_{18} silica gel column, and then purified by HPLC (MeCN/H_2O, 8 mL/min, 16:84) to obtain **12** (1.9 mg, t_R 10.4 min) and **15** (5.9 mg, t_R 11.9 min). Fr. 2-3 (0.3 g) was purified by HPLC using 10% MeCN/H_2O to produce **11** (2.2 mg, t_R 17.0 min), while Fr. 2-4 (0.2 g) was separated by the RP HPLC system (MeCN/H_2O, 8 mL/min, 6:94) to afford **13** (2.0 mg, t_R 44.3 min).

Acarviostatin II02 (Aca II02, **10**): White amorphous powder, $[\alpha]_D^{25}$ +127.2 (*c* 1.05, H_2O). UV (H_2O) end absorption; IR ν_{max} 3319, 1663, 1396, 1149, 1031 cm^{-1}. ^{1}H (500 MHz) and ^{13}C (125 MHz) NMR spectroscopic data, see Table S1; positive ESIMS: m/z 1273 [M + H]$^+$; HRESIMS: m/z 1273.4938 [M + H]$^+$ (calcd for $C_{50}H_{84}N_2O_{35}$, 1273.4927).

D6-*O*-Propionyl-acarviostatin II02 (Pr-Aca II02, **11**): White amorphous powder, $[\alpha]_D^{25}$ +142.4 (*c* 1.01, H_2O). UV (H_2O) end absorption; IR ν_{max} 3337, 1726, 1407, 1149, 1026 cm^{-1}. ^{1}H (500 MHz) and ^{13}C (125 MHz) NMR spectroscopic data, see Table S1; positive ESIMS: m/z 1329 [M + H]$^+$; HRESIMS: m/z 1329.5234 [M + H]$^+$ (calcd for $C_{53}H_{88}N_2O_{36}$, 1329.5190).

D6-*O*-Isobutyryl-acarviostatin II02 (isoBu-Aca II02, **12**): White amorphous powder, $[\alpha]_D^{25}$ +136.1 (*c* 1.02, H_2O). UV (H_2O) end absorption; IR ν_{max} 3329, 1721, 1365, 1147, 1014 cm^{-1}. ^{1}H (500 MHz) and ^{13}C (125 MHz) NMR spectroscopic data, see Table S1; positive ESIMS: m/z 1343 [M + H]$^+$; HRESIMS: m/z 1343.5365 [M + H]$^+$ (calcd for $C_{54}H_{90}N_2O_{36}$, 1343.5346).

D6-*O*-Isovaleryl-acarviostatin II02 (isoVa-Aca II02, **13**): White amorphous powder, $[\alpha]_D^{25}$ +143.0 (*c* 0.99, H_2O). UV (H_2O) end absorption; IR ν_{max} 3305, 1647, 1407, 1150, 1013 cm^{-1}. ^{1}H (500 MHz) and ^{13}C (125 MHz) NMR spectroscopic data, see Table S1; positive ESIMS: m/z 1357 [M + H]$^+$; HRESIMS: m/z 1357.5520 [M + H]$^+$ (calcd for $C_{55}H_{92}N_2O_{36}$, 1357.5503).

D6-*O*-Propionyl-acarviostatin II03 (Pr-Aca II03, **14**): White amorphous powder, $[\alpha]_D^{25}$ +136.3 (*c* 0.90, H_2O). UV (H_2O) end absorption; IR ν_{max} 3304, 1734, 1402, 1148, 1023 cm^{-1}. ^{1}H (500 MHz) and ^{13}C (125 MHz) NMR spectroscopic data, see Table S2; positive ESIMS: m/z 1491 [M + H]$^+$; HRESIMS: m/z 1491.5727 [M + H]$^+$ (calcd for $C_{59}H_{98}N_2O_{41}$, 1491.5718).

D6-*O*-Butyryl-acarviostatin II03 (Bu-Aca II03, **15**): White amorphous powder, $[\alpha]_D^{25}$ +150.3 (*c* 0.53, H$_2$O). UV (H$_2$O) end absorption; IR ν_{max} 3324, 1729, 1568, 1149, 1024 cm^{-1}. ^{1}H (500 MHz) and ^{13}C (125 MHz) NMR spectroscopic data, see Table S2; positive ESIMS: *m/z* 1505 [M + H]$^+$; HRESIMS: *m/z* 1505.5872 [M + H]$^+$ (calcd for C$_{59}$H$_{98}$N$_2$O$_{41}$, 1505.5874).

D6-*O*-2-Methyl-butyryl-acarviostatin II03 (Mbu-Aca II03, **16**): White amorphous powder, $[\alpha]_D^{25}$ +130.1 (*c* 1.03, H$_2$O). UV (H$_2$O) end absorption; IR ν_{max} 3303, 1645, 1406, 1149, 1014 cm^{-1}. ^{1}H (500 MHz) and ^{13}C (125 MHz) NMR spectroscopic data, see Table S2; positive ESIMS: *m/z* 1519 [M + H]$^+$; HRESIMS: *m/z* 1519.6039 [M + H]$^+$ (calcd for C$_{61}$H$_{102}$N$_2$O$_{41}$, 1519.6031).

3.7. PPA Inhibition Assay

The PPA inhibitory activities of compounds **9–20** were conducted based on a previously reported method. Commercial α-amylase inhibitor acarbose was used as the positive control [20].

3.8. Sucrase Inhibition Assay

The sucrase inhibition assay of compounds **9–20** was evaluated according to the previously reported method. Acarbose was also used as the positive control [21].

3.9. PL Inhibition Assay

The lipase inhibition assay of compounds **9–20** was performed according to the method outlined by McDougall et al. with slight modification [32]. Orlistat was measured as a positive control.

3.10. Molecular Docking

The molecular docking simulations were performed by AutoDock Vina software, version 1.5.7 [33]. The crystal structure of human PL was downloaded from the RSCB Protein Data Bank (PDB ID: 1LPB). The binding site parameters (*x*: 4.342 Å; *y*: 24.299 Å; *z*: 47.471 Å) and the grid box dimensions (30 × 30 × 30 Å) were set. The results of molecular docking were evaluated on the basis of the binding energy, criteria of binding structure, and possible interactions between ligand and the critical catalytic triad of protein 1LPB.

4. Conclusions

In summary, the hyphenated system UPLC-QTOF-MS/MS that could provide qualitative retention time and reliable mass spectrometry information was utilized to reveal the metabolic profiling of aminooligosaccharides secreted by *Streptomyces* sp. HO1518. A total of ninety-eight aminooligosaccharides, including eighty new compounds, were detected and characterized from the extract of stain HO1518. Among them, twenty structural intriguing oligomers that ended with the 4-amino-4-deoxy-D-quinovopyranose unit at the non-reducing terminus were reported for the first time. The subsequent MS-guided fractionation method resulted in the isolation of seven new oligosaccharides (**10–16**) and four known analogs (**17–20**). Notably, compounds **10–13** are the first reported examples of oligosaccharides with a rarely occurring acarviostatin II02-type structure. All the compounds exhibited significant inhibitory activities against three digestive enzymes, among which compounds **9–16**, **19** and **20** sharing two pseudo-trisaccharides were the most effective inhibitors of α-amylase and lipase. Furthermore, primary structure-activity relationships of **9–20** revealed that the number of the pseudo-trisaccharide core and acyl side chain play pivotal roles in their biological activity, which was evidenced by molecular docking analysis. These results of this study highlighted the advantages of UPLC-QTOF-MS/MS for the rapid structural identification of oligosaccharides, and this strategy could be extended to other investigations for high-throughput analysis of natural products with similar structures. More importantly, this study not only provided new lead compounds for further scientific research towards anti-diabetic drug discovery, but also shed light on the structural optimization of aminooligosaccharides analogs for medicinal scientists.

Supplementary Materials: The following supporting information can be downloaded at: https://www.mdpi.com/article/10.3390/md20030189/s1, Figures S1–S9: HRMS data for an extract of strain HO1518, Figures S10–S154: HRESIMS, IR, UV, and 1D and 2D NMR spectra of compounds **10–16**, Tables S1–S9: NMR data of **10–16**, Tables S10–S12: information of 98 acarviostatins [20,21,34–41].

Author Contributions: Y.W. designed and coordinated this study and reviewed the manuscript; H.L. and Y.R. reviewed and edited the manuscript; J.X., Z.L. and Z.F. performed MS data analysis, fermentation, isolation and biological evaluations experiments; Z.L. performed the docking analysis; J.X., H.L. and Z.L. elucidated structures and wrote the paper. All authors have read and agreed to the published version of the manuscript.

Funding: This work was supported by the National Key R&D Program of China (No. 2018YFA0900600), the National Natural Science Foundation of China (Nos. 41876084, 31670099), the Strategic Priority Research Program "Molecular mechanism of Plant Growth and Development" of the Chinese Academy of Sciences (Nos. XDB27020202, XDB27020103), the Construction of the Registry and Database of Bioparts for Synthetic Biology of the Chinese Academy of Sciences (No. ZSYS-016), the Program of Shanghai Academic Research Leader (No. 20XD1404400), the International Partnership Program of the Chinese Academy of Sciences (No. 153D31KYSB20170121), the Tianjin Synthetic Biotechnology Innovation Capacity Improvement Project (No. TSBICIP-KJGG-002-15), and the National Key Laboratory of Plant Molecular Genetics, SIPPE, CAS.

Institutional Review Board Statement: Not applicable.

Informed Consent Statement: Not applicable.

Data Availability Statement: Not applicable.

Acknowledgments: We are grateful to Shizheng Bu and Yining Liu for NMR, HRESIMS and ESIMS/MS data acquisitions (the Core Facility Center of the Institute of the CAS Centre for Excellence in Molecular Plant Science, Chinese Academy of Sciences).

Conflicts of Interest: The authors declare no conflict of interest.

References

1. Xie, K.B.; Zhang, X.L.; Sui, S.Y.; Ye, F.; Dai, J.G. Exploring and applying the substrate promiscuity of a C-glycosyltransferase in the chemo-enzymatic synthesis of bioactive C-glycosides. *Nat. Commun.* **2020**, *11*, 5162. [CrossRef] [PubMed]
2. Targher, G.; Corey, K.E.; Byrne, C.D.; Roden, M. The complex link between NAFLD and type 2 diabetes mellitus-mechanisms and treatments. *Nat. Rev. Gastroenterol. Hepatol.* **2021**, *18*, 599–612. [CrossRef] [PubMed]
3. Wagner, R.; Heni, M.; Tabák, A.G.; Machann, J.; Schick, F.; Randrianarisoa, E.; de Angelis, M.H.; Birkenfeld, A.L.; Stefan, N.; Peter, A.; et al. Pathophysiology-based subphenotyping of individuals at elevated risk for type 2 diabetes. *Nat. Med.* **2021**, *27*, 49–57. [CrossRef] [PubMed]
4. Magkos, F.; Hjorth, M.F.; Astrup, A. Diet and exercise in the prevention and treatment of type 2 diabetes mellitus. *Nat. Rev. Endocrinol.* **2020**, *16*, 545–555. [CrossRef] [PubMed]
5. Roden, M.; Shulman, G.I. The integrative biology of type 2 diabetes. *Nature* **2019**, *576*, 51–60. [CrossRef] [PubMed]
6. Liu, D.; Gao, H.; Tang, W.; Nie, S.P. Plant non-starch polysaccharides that inhibit key enzymes linked to type 2 diabetes mellitus. *Ann. N. Y. Acad. Sci.* **2017**, *1401*, 28–36. [CrossRef]
7. Bailey, C.J.; Day, C. The future of new drugs for diabetes management. *Diabetes Res. Clin. Pract.* **2019**, *155*, 107785. [CrossRef]
8. Balaich, J.; Estrella, M.; Wu, G.J.; Jeffrey, P.D.; Biswas, A.; Zhao, L.P.; Korennykh, A.; Donia, M.S. The human microbiome encodes resistance to the antidiabetic drug acarbose. *Nature* **2021**, *600*, 110–115. [CrossRef]
9. Newman, D.J.; Cragg, G.M. Natural products as sources of new drugs over the nearly four decades from 01/1981 to 09/2019. *J. Nat. Prod.* **2020**, *83*, 770–803. [CrossRef]
10. Wolfender, J.L.; Litaudon, M.; Touboul, D.; Queiroz, E.F. Innovative omics-based approaches for prioritisation and targeted isolation of natural products—New strategies for drug discovery. *Nat. Prod. Rep.* **2019**, *36*, 855–868. [CrossRef]
11. Xu, J.L.; Chen, Y.C.; Liu, Z.M.; Li, S.N.; Wang, Y.; Ren, Y.H.; Liu, H.X.; Zhang, W.M. Lithocarpins E−G, potent anti-tumor tenellone-macrolides from the deep-sea fungus *Phomopsis lithocarpus* FS508. *Chin. J. Chem.* **2021**, *39*, 1104–1112. [CrossRef]
12. Covington, B.C.; McLean, J.A.; Bachmann, B.O. Comparative mass spectrometry-based metabolomics strategies for the investigation of microbial secondary metabolites. *Nat. Prod. Rep.* **2017**, *34*, 6–24. [CrossRef] [PubMed]
13. Nothias, L.F.; Nothias-Esposito, M.; da Silva, R.; Wang, M.X.; Protsyuk, I.; Zhang, Z.; Sarvepalli, A.; Leyssen, P.; Touboul, D.; Costa, J.; et al. Bioactivity-based molecular networking for the discovery of drug leads in natural product bioassay-guided fractionation. *J. Nat. Prod.* **2018**, *81*, 758–767. [CrossRef]
14. Henke, M.T.; Kelleher, N.L. Modern mass spectrometry for synthetic biology and structure-based discovery of natural products. *Nat. Prod. Rep.* **2016**, *33*, 942–950. [CrossRef]

15. Alvarez-Rivera, G.; Ballesteros-Vivas, D.; Parada-Alfonso, F.; Ibañez, E.; Cifuentes, A. Recent applications of high resolution mass spectrometry for the characterization of plant natural products. *Trends Anal. Chem.* **2019**, *112*, 87–101. [CrossRef]
16. Bozicevic, A.; Dobrzynski, M.; De Bie, H.; Gafner, F.; Garo, E.; Hamburger, M. Automated comparative metabolite profiling of large LC-ESIMS data sets in an ACD/MS workbook suite add-in, and data clustering on a new open-source web platform FreeClust. *Anal. Chem.* **2017**, *89*, 12682–12689. [CrossRef]
17. Panusa, A.; Petrucci, R.; Marrosu, G.; Multari, G.; Gallo, F.R. UHPLC-PDA-ESI-TOF/MS metabolic profiling of *Arctostaphylos pungens* and *Arctostaphylos uva-ursi*. A comparative study of phenolic compounds from leaf methanolic extracts. *Phytochemistry* **2015**, *115*, 79–88. [CrossRef] [PubMed]
18. Robertsen, H.L.; Musiol-Kroll, E.M. Actinomycete-derived polyketides as a source of antibiotics and lead structures for the development of new antimicrobial drugs. *Antibiotics* **2019**, *8*, 157. [CrossRef]
19. Niu, G.Q. Genomics-driven natural product discovery in actinomycetes. *Trends Biotechnol.* **2018**, *36*, 238–241. [CrossRef]
20. Liu, H.-L.; E, H.-C.; Xie, D.-A.; Cheng, W.-B.; Tao, W.-Q.; Wang, Y. Acylated aminooligosaccharides with inhibitory effects against α-amylase from *Streptomyces* sp. HO1518. *Mar. Drugs* **2018**, *16*, 403. [CrossRef]
21. Xu, J.L.; Liu, H.L.; Liu, Z.F.; Ren, Y.H.; Wang, Y. Acylated aminooligosaccharides from the yellow sea *Streptomyces* sp. HO1518 as both α-glucosidase and lipase inhibitors. *Mar. Drugs* **2020**, *18*, 576. [CrossRef] [PubMed]
22. McCranie, E.K.; Bachmann, B.O. Bioactive oligosaccharide natural products. *Nat. Prod. Rep.* **2014**, *31*, 1026–1042. [CrossRef] [PubMed]
23. Xu, J.L.; Liu, Z.F.; Zhang, X.W.; Liu, H.L.; Wang, Y. Microbial oligosaccharides with biomedical applications. *Mar. Drugs* **2021**, *19*, 350. [CrossRef] [PubMed]
24. Truscheit, E.; Frommer, W.; Junge, B.; Müller, L.; Schmidt, D.D.; Wingender, W. Chemistry and biochemistry of microbial α-glucosidase inhibitors. *Angew. Chem. Int. Ed.* **1981**, *20*, 744–761. [CrossRef]
25. Lang, Y.Z.; Zhao, X.; Liu, L.L.; Yu, G.L. Applications of mass spectrometry to structural analysis of marine oligosaccharides. *Mar. Drugs* **2014**, *12*, 4005–4030. [CrossRef]
26. Domon, B.; Costello, C.E. A systematic nomenclature for carbohydrate fragmentations in FAB-MS/MS spectra of glycoconjugates. *Glycoconj. J.* **1988**, *5*, 397–409. [CrossRef]
27. Padhi, S.; Nayak, A.K.; Behera, A. Type II diabetes mellitus: A review on recent drug based therapeutics. *Biomed. Pharmacother.* **2020**, *131*, 110708. [CrossRef]
28. Al-Mrabeh, A.; Zhyzhneuskaya, S.V.; Peters, C.; Barnes, A.C.; Melhem, S.; Jesuthasan, A.; Aribisala, B.; Hollingsworth, K.G.; Lietz, G.; Mathers, J.C.; et al. Hepatic lipoprotein export and remission of human type 2 diabetes after weight loss. *Cell Metab.* **2020**, *31*, 233–249. [CrossRef]
29. Bray, G.A.; Heisel, W.E.; Afshin, A.; Jensen, M.D.; Dietz, W.H.; Long, M.; Kushner, R.F.; Daniels, S.R.; Wadden, T.A.; Tsai, A.G.; et al. The science of obesity management: An endocrine society scientific statement. *Endocr. Rev.* **2018**, *39*, 79–132. [CrossRef]
30. Egloff, M.P.; Marguet, F.; Buono, G.; Verger, R.; Cambillau, C.; van Tilbeurgh, H. The 2.46 Å resolution structure of the pancreatic lipase-colipase complex inhibited by a C11 alkyl phosphonate. *Biochemistry* **1995**, *34*, 2751–2762. [CrossRef]
31. Van Tilbeurgh, H.; Egloff, M.P.; Martinez, C.; Rugani, N.; Verger, R.; Cambillau, C. Interfacial activation of the lipase-procolipase complex by mixed micelles revealed by X-ray crystallography. *Nature* **1993**, *362*, 814–820. [CrossRef] [PubMed]
32. McDougall, G.J.; Kulkarni, N.N.; Stewart, D. Berry polyphenols inhibit pancreatic lipase activity in vitro. *Food Chem.* **2009**, *115*, 193–199. [CrossRef]
33. Trott, O.; Olson, A.J. AutoDock Vina: Improving the speed and accuracy of docking with a new scoring function, efficient optimization, and multithreading. *J. Comput. Chem.* **2010**, *31*, 455–461. [CrossRef] [PubMed]
34. Schmidt, D.D.; Frommer, W.; Junge, B.; Müller, L.; Wingender, W.; Truscheit, E.; Schäfer, D. α-Glucosidase inhibitors. New complex oligosaccharides of microbial origin. *Naturwissenschaften* **1977**, *64*, 535–536. [CrossRef] [PubMed]
35. Fukuhara, K.; Murai, H.; Murao, S. Isolation and structure-activity relationship of some amylostatins (F-lb Fraction) produced by *Streptomyces diastaticus* subsp *amylostaticus* No. 9410. *Agric. Biol. Chem.* **1982**, *46*, 1941–1945.
36. Geng, P.; Qiu, F.; Zhu, Y.Y.; Bai, G. Four acarviosin-containing oligosaccharides identified from *Streptomyces coelicoflavus* ZG0656 are potent inhibitors of α-amylase. *Carbohydr. Res.* **2008**, *343*, 882–892. [CrossRef]
37. Qian, M.X.; Nahoum, V.; Bonicel, J.; Bischoff, H.; Henrissat, B.; Payan, F. Enzyme-catalyzed condensation reaction in a mammalian α-amylase. High resolution structural analysis of an enzymeinhibitor complex. *Biochemistry* **2001**, *40*, 7700–7709. [CrossRef]
38. Weiss, S.C.; Skerra, A.; Schiefner, A. Structural basis for the interconversion of maltodextrins by MalQ, the amylomaltase of *Escherichia coli*. *J. Biol. Chem.* **2015**, *290*, 21352–21364. [CrossRef]
39. Si, D.Y.; Zhong, D.F.; Xu, Q.M. Two butylated aminooligosaccharides isolated from the culture filtrate of *Streptomyces luteogriseus*. *Carbohydr. Res.* **2001**, *335*, 127–132. [CrossRef]
40. Zhong, D.F.; Si, D.Y.; He, W.Y.; Zhao, L.M.; Xu, Q.M. Structural revision of isovalertatins M03, M13, and M23 isolated from the culture of *Streptomyces luteogriseus*. *Carbohydr. Res.* **2001**, *331*, 69–75. [CrossRef]
41. Si, D.Y.; Zhong, D.F.; He, W.Y.; Zhao, L.M. Structural revision of isovalertatins D03 and D23 isolated from the culture filtrate of *Streptomyces luteogriseus*. *Chin. Chem. Lett.* **2001**, *12*, 327–330.

MDPI AG
Grosspeteranlage 5
4052 Basel
Switzerland
Tel.: +41 61 683 77 34

Marine Drugs Editorial Office
E-mail: marinedrugs@mdpi.com
www.mdpi.com/journal/marinedrugs

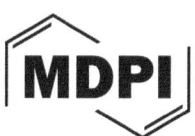

www.ingramcontent.com/pod-product-compliance
Lightning Source LLC
LaVergne TN
LVHW072338090526
838202LV00019B/2439